Articulation
and
Phonological Disorders

Fourth Edition

Articulation and Phonological Disorders

John E. Bernthal
University of Nebraska–Lincoln

Nicholas W. Bankson
James Madison University

Allyn and Bacon
Boston • London • Toronto • Sydney • Tokyo • Singapore

Executive editor: Stephen D. Dragin
Editorial assistant: Liz McGuire
Editorial-production administrator: Susan Brown
Editorial-production service: Matrix Productions
Cover administrator: Linda Knowles
Cover designer: Susan Paradise
Prepress buyer: Linda Cox
Manufacturing buyer: David Suspanic

Internet: www.abacon.com
America Online: keyword: College Online

Library of Congress Cataloging-in-Publication Data

Articulation and phonological disorders / [edited by] John E. Bernthal, Nicholas W. Bankson.— 4th ed.
     p. cm.
     Rev. ed. of: Articulation and phonological disorders / John E. Bernthal, Nicholas W. Bankson. 3rd ed. c1993.
     Includes bibliographical references and indexes.
     ISBN 0–205–19693–4
     1. Articulation disorders.   I. Bernthal, John E.   II. Bankson, Nicholas W.
     [DNLM: 1. Articulation Disorders.   2. Voice Disorders.
3. Phonetics   WM 475 A792 1997]
     RC424.7.B47   1997
     616.85′8—dc21
     DNLM/DLC
     for Library of Congress
                                                 97–13185
                                                CIP

This book is dedicated in loving memory
to our friend and wife

Lou Ann Bankson
1938–1996

Her zest for living
Her love of children
Her willingness to help those in need
Remain with us

JEB
NWB

Contents

Preface

This book has the same goals as the three previous editions, which is to present a comprehensive review of information important to the study of clinical phonology. It includes an introduction to the normal aspects of speech sound articulation, normal phonological development, possible factors related to the presence of phonological disorders, the assessment and remediation of phonological disorders, instrumentation available for acoustical analyses relevant to clinical phonology, and phonology as it relates to language and dialectal variations.

As in past editions, this text is primarily concerned with those phonological disorders not etiologically associated with known or obvious sensory, structural, or neuromotor deficits. Such disorders traditionally have been labeled *functional* articulation disorders, a category that has come to be viewed clinically as a catch-all, frequently including all individuals with phonological errors of unknown cause. It is recognized, however, that a phonological disorder of unknown etiology may be caused by one or more subtle organic, learning, or environmental factors.

Those readers acquainted with previous editions of this text will notice some changes in organizational structure, as well as updated information concerning topics covered in previous editions, plus new areas of coverage related to dialects, instrumentation, dyspraxia, and phonological awareness. Once again, we have attempted to synthesize the literature and present it in a manner meaningful to a student studying clinical phonology.

This book has been divided into nine chapters (one less than the previous edition—our attempt at downsizing!). Chapter 1 reviews normal aspects of articulation and provides an introduction to the phonological system of American English. This information is typically covered in courses other than clinical phonology; for those lacking such course work or in need of review, however, this content is presented.

Chapters 2 and 3 focus on normal phonological acquisition in children and review the process through which children develop production and perceptual skills at both the prelinguistic and linguistic levels. Since speech-language pathologists must distinguish delayed or deviant phonological development from normal development, they must recognize and understand normal phonological development. This chapter reflects primarily an update of the literature.

Chapter 4 was added in our last edition in response to our increasing awareness of the multicultural nature of our society and the fact that the linguistic systems of our clients are often influenced by languages and dialects other than Standard American English. Two major dialectal variations found in our society were reviewed in the previous edition, Black English Vernacular and Spanish-influenced English. This edition has been expanded to include dialectal variations influenced by Asian and Native American languages.

Chapter 5 reviews factors related to the development of normal and disordered phonology. Since this text is primarily focused on disorders of unknown or functional etiology, review of cognitive-linguistic as well as psychosocial factors as they relate to phonological disorders is presented. In addition, potential etiological variables associated with impairments of the speech and hearing mechanism are reviewed. This chapter reflects an update of the literature in these areas.

Chapter 6 is concerned with procedures for obtaining speech samples from which to assess phonological behavior. Included in this discussion are the assessment battery, screening measures, and speech discrimination (perception measures).

Chapter 7 deals with determining the need for intervention by examining such factors as intelligibility, severity, stimulability, error patterns, and developmental considerations. When intervention is indicated, identification of treatment targets and factors to consider in the target selection are discussed.

A major addition to the third edition was the review of computer software designed for phonological analysis of children's speech samples. Since the publication of the last edition, such computer software has become commonplace and thus the reader will note that this edition contains no reviews of commercially available software but only an overview of such instruments. However, because of the increased use of acoustic analysis techniques as a tool to supplement more traditional methods of phonological analysis, we asked the authors of this chapter to include a discussion of such analysis procedures. Although these techniques are not used routinely outside research labs, but because the cost of analysis instrumentation continues to become less expensive as well as more portable, this technology may soon become a part of the clinical battery of the practicing speech-language pathologist.

Chapter 8 is a large and comprehensive chapter dealing with the remediation of phonological disorders. This chapter begins with a description of basic treatment consideration (e.g., sequencing of instrumental components, intervention style), followed by presentation of motor-based approaches to intervention and linguistic-based approaches. Included is a review of pertinent literature and a discussion of remediation issues, as well as selected treatment programs and approaches that represent a number of different clinical and theoretical points of view. In addition, the chapter contains a section dealing with children with developmental verbal dyspraxia and a presentation of information concerning phonological awareness.

As stated, this text is designed to introduce the student to the clinical management of individuals with phonological disorders. Although the reader does not need an extensive background in speech-language pathology to understand this presentation, knowledge of phonetic transcription, basic anatomy and physiology of the speech mechanism, and language acquisition is advantageous.

The following people reviewed the manuscript for this revision and offered suggestions for changes: Judith Brasseur, California State University, Chico; Angela Massenberg, Eastern Michigan University; Toni B. Morehouse, University of Nebraska-Lincoln; Karen E. Pollock, University of Memphis; Dennis M. Ruscello, West Virginia University; Ann Bosma Smit, Kansas State University; and Tina T. Smith, University of South Carolina.

Chapter *1*

Normal Aspects of Articulation

RAY KENT
University of Wisconsin–Madison

Introduction

Speech has been defined as *a system that relates meaning with sound*. Meaning itself arises in **language**. A *language* is *an arbitrary system of signs or symbols used according to pre-scribed rules to convey meaning within a linguistic community*. Of course, once an arbitrary association of symbol with meaning has been made, the users of that language must be con-sistent in this association if they want to communicate with one another. The word *dog* has a meaning in the English language, but this word can be communicated to other users of English by speaking, by writing, or by signing it with the manual symbols used by the deaf. Speech is but one modality for the expression of language; however, speech has special importance because it is the primary, first-learned modality for hearing language users. Speech is a system in the sense that it consistently and usefully relates the meanings of a language with the sounds by which the language is communicated.

Not all sound variations in speech are related to meaning. When a person suffers from a cold, he or she has a different way of talking, but so long as the cold is not so severe as to make speech unintelligible, the relation of sound to meaning is basically the same as when the person is healthy. The acoustic signal of speech—that is, the vibrations of air molecules in response to the energy source of human speech—carries more information than just the expression of meaning. As we listen to a speaker, we often make judgments not only about the intended meaning but also about the speaker's age and sex (if the speaker isn't visible), the speaker's mood, the speaker's state of health, and perhaps even the speaker's dialectal background. Thus, on hearing a simple question—"Could you tell me the time, please?"—

1

we might deduce that the speaker is a young southern woman in a hurry, an elderly British gentleman in a cheerful mood, or a young boy quite out of breath.

Structure of Language

To derive a speaker's meaning, the listener is basically concerned with the **phonemes** in the speech message. From a linguistic perspective, phonemes are sound units related to decisions about meaning. In the list, *cat hat mat bat sat fat that chat*, each word rhymes with every other word because all end with the same sound. However, the words differ in their initial sounds, and these differences can change the meaning of the syllables. In fact, the linguist identifies the phonemes in a given language by assembling lists of words and then determining the sound differences that form units of meaning. The layman usually thinks of words as the units of meaning, but the linguist recognizes a smaller form called the **morpheme**. For example, the linguist describes the words *walked* and *books* as having two morphemes: *walk + past tense* for *walked*, and *book + plural* for *books*. If two sounds can be interchanged without changing word meaning, or if they never occur in exactly the same combination with other sounds, then they are not different phonemes. Hence, phonemes are the minimal sound elements that represent and distinguish language units (words or morphemes).

A **phonemic transcription** (which is always enclosed in virgules /   /) is less detailed than a **phonetic transcription** (which is enclosed in brackets [   ]). A phonetic transcription is sensitive to sound variations within a phoneme class. An individual variant of this kind is called an *allophone*. Thus, a phoneme is a family of allophones. Phonemes are the minimal set of sound classes needed to specify the meaningful units (words or morphemes) of the language. Allophones are a more numerous set of distinct sounds, some of which may belong to the same phoneme family. As a very simple example, the word *pop* begins and ends with the same phoneme but often begins and ends with a different allophone. If the final /p/ is produced by holding the lips together after they close, then this sound is the unreleased allophone of the /p/ phoneme. However, the initial /p/ must be released before the vowel is formed, so this sound is the released allophone of the /p/ phoneme. The /p/ phoneme also includes a number of other allophones, though perhaps not as obvious as these two.

To understand more clearly the difference between phonemes and allophones, say the following word-pairs to yourself as you try to detect a difference in the production of the italicized sounds.

> *k*eep - *c*oop   (phoneme /k/)
>
> m*a*n - b*a*t   (phoneme /æ/)
>
> te*n* - te*n*th   (phoneme /n/)

In the first pair of words, the phoneme /k/ is articulated toward the front of the mouth in the first word and toward the back of the mouth in the second. Despite the differences in the place of tongue contact, the two sounds are heard by speakers of English to be the same phoneme. Speakers of other languages, such as Arabic, may hear the two sounds as different phonemes. The tongue-front and tongue-back versions are allophones of the /k/ phoneme.

In the next pair of words, *man* and *bat*, the pertinent difference might be more easily heard than felt through articulation. In the word *man*, the vowel is nasalized (produced with sound transmission through the nose) owing to the influence of the surrounding nasal consonants. But in the word *bat*, the vowel /æ/ is not normally nasalized. The phonetic environment of the vowel—that is, its surrounding sounds—determines whether or not the vowel is nasalized. The nasal and nonnasal versions of the vowel are allophones of the /æ/ phoneme.

Finally, in comparing /n/ in the words *ten* and *tenth*, you might notice that your tongue is more toward the front (just behind the upper front teeth) in the word *tenth*. The final *th* sound exerts an articulatory influence on the preceding /n/, causing it to be dentalized or produced at the teeth. Again, the two types of /n/ are simply allophones of the /n/ phoneme.

Allophonic variation is of two types: *complementary distribution* and *free variation*. In complementary distribution, two (or more) allophones never occur in exactly the same phonetic environment, so that the occurrence of one is complementary (nonoverlapping) to the occurrence of the other. For example, the front and back /k/ discussed above are in complementary distribution. The front /k/ occurs in the environment of vowels made in the front of the mouth and the back /k/ occurs in the environment of vowels made in the back of the mouth. Similarly, the nasal and nonnasal allophones of /æ/ are in complementary distribution, determined by the presence or absence of nasals in the phonetic environment. The nasalized /æ/ occurs only when this vowel is preceded or followed by nasal sounds. Allophones are said to be in free variation when they can occur in the same phonetic context. For example, the released /p/ and the unreleased /p/ are in free variation in word-final position in words like *pop* or *map*. As indicated above, the final /p/ can be released audibly with a small burst as the lips open or it can be unreleased if the lip closure is maintained.

The discipline of linguistics is concerned primarily with the structure of language. The disciplines of psychology and speech pathology are concerned primarily with the processing of language—with its formulation and its reception. The linguistic study of language structure has influenced the study of language processing, and, to some degree, the reverse is true as well. Descriptions of language processing often use terms, such as syntax, semantics, phonology, and phonetics, that denote traditional areas of linguistic study. These terms have come to have a duel usage, one referring to structure and another to processing.

Figure 1.1 is a diagram of an information processing model of verbal formulation and utterance production. The diagram attempts to show how different types of information are processed in the act of speaking. The cognitive level is where a thought is initiated. This is a prelinguistic, propositional level that involves decisions such as the identification of participants and actions. For example, the cognitive processing that preceded formulation of the sentence, *the dog chased the cat*, involved the identification of a dog and a cat as participants and chasing or pursuit as an action. However, the words *dog*, *cat*, and *chased* were not actually selected. Rather, propositions or relations associated with these words were established.

Information from the cognitive level is used to make decisions at the syntactic and semantic levels. Syntax involves the ordering of words in a sentence and semantics involves the selection of words. Research on verbal formulation indicates that syntactic and semantic processing are interactive (hence, the arrows between them in the diagram). Deciding upon a particular syntactic structure for a sentence can influence word selection, and sel-

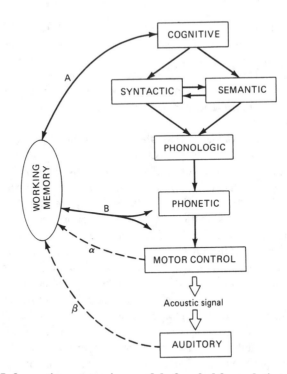

FIGURE 1.1   **Information processing model of verbal formulation and utterance production.**

Adapted from J. K. Bock, "Toward a cognitive psychology of syntax: Information processing contributions to sentence formulation." *Psychological Review*, 89 (1982): 1–47.

ection of particular words can limit or direct syntactic decisions. The semantic level is sometimes called lexicalization, or the choice of lexical units. Lexicalization appears to be a two-stage process. The first stage is selection of a lexical concept, not a phonologically complete word. Phonologic specification, that is, specification of the word's sound pattern, is accomplished in the second stage of the process. The phonologic level in Figure 1.1 is the level at which the evolving sentence comes to have phonologic structure. Various decisions are made at this level to insure that a sound pattern accurately represents the syntactic and semantic decisions made earlier. The phonologic information then directs decisions at the phonetic level, where the details of the sound pattern are worked out. We might think of the phonetic level as producing a detailed phonetic representation of the utterance.

The output of the phonetic level is sufficient to specify the phonetic goals to be satisfied in speech production. Actual motor instructions are determined by a motor control level. This level selects the muscles to be activated and controls the timing and strength of the muscle contractions. This is no small task. Speech requires rapid changes in the activation of about 100 muscles. Once the muscles have done their work, the acoustic speech signal is produced. This signal is then processed by the speaker and the listener(s) as auditory information. For the speaker, the auditory processing completes a feedback loop.

One component that remains to be explained in Figure 1.1 is working memory and its connections to other parts of the diagram. Working memory is a speaker's operational memory, the memory that is used to keep track of the information involved in sentence production. But this memory is limited, so it is in the interest of efficient processing to minimize demands on it. Therefore, the theory goes, two kinds of processing are involved in utterance production. One is **controlled processing**; this kind makes demands on working memory. The other is **automatic processing**, which does not require allocation of working memory. Verbal formulation is performed with both controlled processing and automatic processing. Controlled processing can be identified in Figure 1.1 by the arrows labeled A and B. Note that syntactic, semantic, and phonologic processing are automatic; that is, the speaker does not have direct access to these operations. It is for this reason that slips of the tongue are not detected until they are actually spoken.

Feedback is provided by two channels, labeled α and β in Figure 1.1. Channel α represents information from touch and movement. Channel β represents auditory feedback.

Researchers have concluded that when we ordinarily produce a sentence, we don't make all of the syntactic, semantic, and phonologic decisions before beginning to speak. Rather, it is likely that we will utter a few words and then formulate the remainder of the utterance.

According to this view of verbal formulation, producing a sentence involves highly interactive levels of processing and a complex time pattern for this processing. It would not be surprising, then, to discover that articulation is affected by syntactic, semantic and phonologic variables.

The following discussion of articulatory phonetics presents basic information on speech sound production. For the student who has had a course in phonetics, this chapter should be a summary review. The student without such background should be able to acquire at least the basics of articulatory phonetics. The topics to be discussed are these:

The Speech Mechanism
Vowels
    Monophthongs (single vowels)
    Diphthongs
Consonants
    Stops
    Nasals
    Fricatives
    Affricates
    Liquids
    Glides
Suprasegmentals
Coarticulation
Aerodynamics
Acoustics
Afference
Sensory Information
Phonology

Fundamentals of Articulatory Phonetics

The Speech Mechanism

The anatomy of the speech production system is not within the scope of this chapter, but some general anatomical descriptions are needed to discuss the fundamentals of articulatory phonetics. The basic aspects of speech production can be understood by an examination of six principal organs or subsystems, illustrated in Figure 1.2. The *respiratory system*, consisting of the lungs, airway, rib cage, diaphragm, and associated structures, provides the basic air supply for generating sound. The *larynx*, composed of various cartilages and muscles, generates the voiced sounds of speech by vibration of the vocal folds, or it allows air to pass from lungs to the vocal tract (the oral and nasal cavities) for voiceless sounds. The *velopharynx*—the soft palate (or velum) and associated structures of the velopharyngeal port—joins or separates the oral and nasal cavities so that air passes through the oral cavity, the nasal cavity, or both. The *tongue*, primarily a complex of muscles, is the principal articulator of the oral cavity; it is capable of assuming a variety of shapes and positions in vowel and consonant articulation. For articulatory purposes, the tongue is divided into five major parts: the tip or apex, the blade, the back or dorsum, the root, and the body. These divisions are illustrated in Figure 1.3. The *lips*, along with the jaw, are the most visible of the articulators; they are involved in the production of vowels and consonants. The *jaw*, the

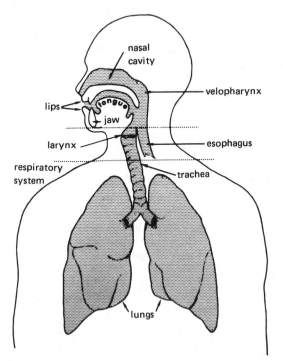

FIGURE 1.2   Organs of speech production.

massive bony structure and its associated muscles, supports the soft tissues of both tongue and lower lip. It participates in speech production by aiding tongue and lip movements and by providing skeletal support for these organs.

Other anatomical features shown in Figure 1.2 provide general orientation or are relevant in a significant way to the processes of speech and hearing.

The respiratory system and larynx work together to provide the upper airway with two major types of air flow: a series of pulses of air created by the action of the vibrating vocal folds (for voiced sounds like the sounds in the word *buzz*), and a continuous flow of air that can be used to generate noise energy in the vocal tract (for voiceless sounds like the *s* in *see*). The basic function of the respiratory system in speech is to push air into the airway composed of the larynx and the oral and nasal cavities. The basic function of the larynx is to regulate the air flow from the lungs to create both voiced and voiceless segments. The upper airway, often called the vocal tract, runs from the larynx to the mouth or nose and is the site of what is commonly called speech articulation. For the most part, this process is accomplished by movements of the *articulators*: tongue, lips, jaw, and velopharynx. The vocal tract may be viewed as a flexible tube that can be lengthened or shortened (by moving the larynx up and down in the neck or by protruding and retracting the lips) and constricted at many points along its length by actions of tongue, velopharynx, and lips. Speech articulation is thus a matter of lengthening, shortening, and constricting the tube known as the vocal tract.

This entire process is controlled by the nervous system, which must translate the message to be communicated into a pattern of signals that run to the various muscles of the speech mechanism. As these muscles contract, a variety of things can happen: Air may be pushed out of the lungs, the vocal folds may start to vibrate, the velopharynx may close, the jaw may lower, or the lips may protrude. The brain has the task of coordinating all the different muscles so that they contract in the proper sequence to produce the required phonetic

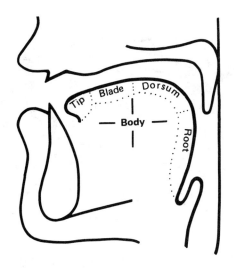

FIGURE 1.3   Divisions of tongue into five functional parts for speech articulation.

result. The margin for error is small; sometimes an error of just a few milliseconds in the timing of a muscle contraction can result in a misarticulation.

It is appealing to suppose that speech production is controlled at some relatively high level of the brain by discrete units, such as phonemes. However, a major problem in the description of speech articulation is to relate the discrete linguistic units that operate at a high level of the brain to the muscle contractions that result in articulatory movements. For example, to say the word *stop*, a speaker's brain must send nerve instructions, in the proper sequence, to the muscles of the respiratory system, larynx, tongue, lips, and velopharynx. The full understanding of speech production therefore involves a knowledge of **phonology** (the study of how sounds are put together to form words and other linguistic units), **articulatory phonetics** (the study of how the articulators make individual sounds), **acoustic phonetics** (the study of the relationship between articulation and the acoustic signal of speech), and **speech perception** (the study of how phonetic decisions are made from the acoustic signal).

Vowel Articulation: Traditional Phonetic Description

A vowel sound is usually formed as sound energy from the vibrating vocal folds escapes through a relatively open vocal tract of a particular shape. Because a syllable must contain a vowel or vowel-like sound, vowels sometimes are called *syllable nuclei*. Each vowel has a characteristic vocal tract shape that is determined by the position of the tongue, jaw, and lips. Although other parts of the vocal tract, like the velum, pharyngeal walls, and cheeks, may vary somewhat with different vowels, the positions of the tongue, jaw, and lips are of primary consequence. Therefore, individual vowels can be described by specifying the articulatory positions of tongue, jaw, and lips. Furthermore, because the jaw and tongue usually work together to increase or reduce the mouth opening (Figure 1.4), for general

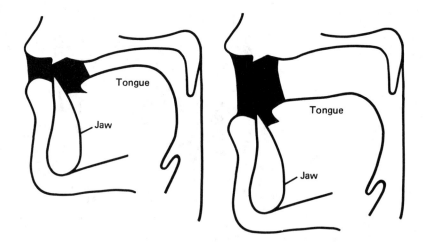

FIGURE 1.4   Variations in mouth opening (darkened area) related to lowering of jaw and tongue.

phonetic purposes vowel production can be described by specifying the positions of just two articulators, tongue and lips. Usually, the vocal folds vibrate to produce voicing for vowels, but exceptions, such as whispered speech, do occur.

The two basic lip articulations can be demonstrated with the vowels in the words *he* and *who*. Press your finger against your lips as you say first *he* and then *who*. You should feel the lips push against your finger as you say *who*. The vowel in this word is a rounded vowel, meaning that the lips assume a rounded, protruded posture. Vowels in English are described as being either rounded, like the vowel in *who*, or unrounded, like the vowel in *he*. Figure 1.5 illustrates the lip configuration for these two vowels.

The tongue moves in essentially two dimensions within the oral cavity, as shown in Figure 1.6. One dimension, front-back, is represented by the motion the tongue makes as you alternately say *he, who* or *map, mop*. The other dimension, high-low, is represented by the motion the tongue makes as you say *heave-have* or *who-ha*. With these two dimensions of tongue movement, we can define four extreme positions of the tongue within the oral cavity, as shown in Figure 1.7. The phonetic symbols for these four vowels also are shown in the illustration. With the tongue high and forward in the mouth, the high-front vowel /i/ as in *he* is produced. When the tongue is low and forward in the mouth, the low-front vowel /æ/ as in *have* is produced. A tongue position that is high and back in the mouth yields the high-back vowel /u/. Finally, when the tongue is low and back in the mouth, the vowel is the low-back /ɑ/. The four vowels, /i/, /æ/, /u/, and /ɑ/, define four points which establish the *vowel quadrilateral*, a four-sided figure against which tongue position for vowels can be described. In Figure 1.8, the vowels of English have been plotted by phonetic symbol and key word within the quadrilateral. As an example, notice the vowel /ɪ/ as in *bit* has a tongue position that is forward in the mouth and not quite as high as that for /i/. The tongue position for any one vowel can be specified with terms such as low-high, front for /ɪ/ as in *bit*, low-mid, front for /ɛ/ as in *bet*, mid-central for /ɝ/ as in *Bert*, and low-mid, back for /ɔ/ as in *bought*.

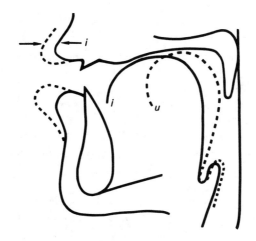

FIGURE 1.5   Vocal tract configurations for /i/ and /u/. Note lip rounding for /u/.

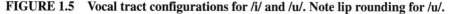

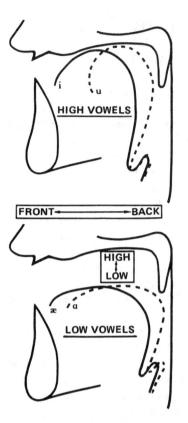

FIGURE 1.6   The two major dimensions of tongue position, front-back and high-low.

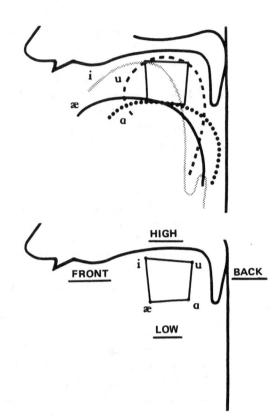

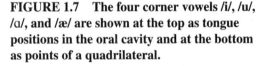

FIGURE 1.7   The four corner vowels /i/, /u/, /ɑ/, and /æ/ are shown at the top as tongue positions in the oral cavity and at the bottom as points of a quadrilateral.

The vowels of English can be categorized as follows with respect to tongue position:

Front vowels: /i/   /ɪ/   /e/   /ɛ/   /æ/
Central vowels: /ɝ/   /ʌ/   /ɚ/   /ə/
Back vowels: /u/   /ʊ/   /o/   /ɔ/   /ɑ/
High vowels: /i/   /ɪ/   /u/   /ʊ/
Mid vowels: /e/   /ɛ/   /ɝ/   /ʌ/   /ɚ/   /ə/   /o/   /ɔ/
Low vowels: /æ/   /ɑ/

The vowels can also be categorized with respect to lip rounding, with the following being rounded: /u/, /ʊ/, /o/, /ɔ/, and /ɝ/. All other vowels are unrounded. Notice that, in English, the rounded vowels are either back or central vowels; front rounded vowels do not occur.

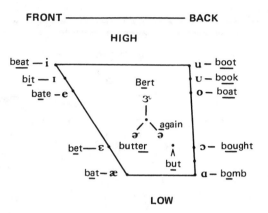

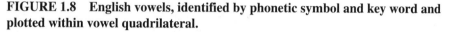

FIGURE 1.8   English vowels, identified by phonetic symbol and key word and plotted within vowel quadrilateral.

Vowel production is also commonly described as *tense (long)* or *lax (short)*. Tense vowels are longer in duration and supposedly involve a greater degree of muscular tension. Lax vowels are relatively short and involve less muscular effort. One way of demonstrating the distinction between tense and lax is to feel the fleshy undersurface of your jaw as you say /i/ as in *he* and /ɪ/ as in *him*. Most people can feel a greater tension for /i/ (a tense vowel) than for /ɪ/ (a lax vowel). The tense vowels are /i/, /e/, /ɝ/, /u/, /o/, /ɔ/, and /ɑ/. The remaining vowels are considered lax, but opinion is divided for the vowel /æ/ as in *bat*.

In standard production, all English vowels are voiced (associated with vibrating vocal folds) and nonnasal (having no escape of sound energy through the nose). Therefore, the descriptors *voiced* and *nonnasal* usually are omitted. However, it should be remembered that vowels are sometimes devoiced, as in whispering, and nasalized, as when they precede or follow nasal consonants. For phonetic purposes it is usually sufficient to describe a vowel in terms of the three major characteristics of tenseness—laxness, lip configuration, and tongue position. Examples of vowel description are given as follows:

/i/	tense, unrounded, high-front
/o/	tense, rounded, high-mid, back
/ɝ/	tense, rounded, mid-central
/ʊ/	lax, rounded, low-high, back

Closely related to the vowels are the *diphthongs*, which, like vowels, are produced with an open vocal tract and serve as the nuclei for syllables. But unlike vowels, diphthongs are formed with an articulation that gradually changes during production of the sound. Diphthongs are dynamic sounds, because they involve a progressive change in vocal tract shape. An example of the articulation of /aɪ/ is shown in Figure 1.9. Many phoneticians regard diphthongs as combinations of two vowels, one called the *onglide* portion and the other called the *offglide* portion. This vowel + vowel description underlies the phonetic symbols

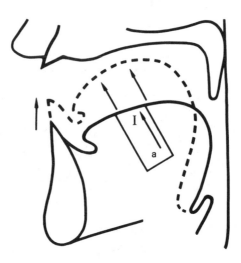

FIGURE 1.9   Articulation of diphthong /aɪ/ (as in *eye*), represented as onglide (/a/) and offglide (/ɪ/) configurations.

for the diphthongs, which have the *digraph* (two-element) symbols /aɪ/, /aʊ/, /ɔɪ/, /eɪ/, and /oʊ/. Key words for these sounds are as follows:

/aɪ/	*I, buy, why, ice, night*
/aʊ/	*ow, bough, trout, down, owl*
/ɔɪ/	*boy, oil, loin, hoist*
/eɪ/	*bay, daze, rain, stay*
/oʊ/	*bow, no, load, bone*

Whereas the diphthongs /aɪ/, /aʊ/, and /ɔɪ/ are truly phonemic diphthongs, /eɪ/ and /oʊ/ are not; they are variants of the vowels /e/ and /o/, respectively. The diphthongal forms /eɪ/ and /oʊ/ occur in strongly stressed syllables, whereas the monophthongal (single-vowel) forms /e/ and /o/ tend to occur in weakly stressed syllables. For example, in the word *vacation*, the first syllable (weakly stressed) is produced with /e/ and the second syllable (strongly stressed) is produced with /eɪ/. Stressed syllables tend to be long in duration and therefore allow time for the articulatory movement of the diphthong. The diphthongs /aɪ/, /aʊ/, and /ɔɪ/ do not alternate with monophthongal forms. To produce a recognizable /aɪ/, /aʊ/, or /ɔɪ/, a speaker must use a diphthongal movement.

As shown in Figure 1.10, the onglide and offglide segments of the diphthongs are roughly located by the positions of the digraph symbols on the vowel quadrilateral. For example, in diphthong /aɪ/, the tongue moves from a low-back to nearly a high-front position. However, it should be noted that these onglide and offglide positions are only approximate and that substantial variation occurs across speakers and speaking conditions.

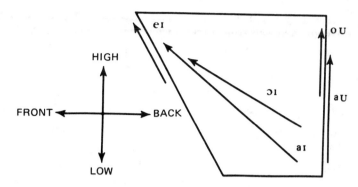

FIGURE 1.10   Diphthong articulation shown as onglide to offglide arrows in the vowel quadrilateral.

Vowel Articulation: Description by Distinctive Features

The phonetic descriptions considered to this point are one method of classifying vowel sounds. An alternative is a method relying on *distinctive features*, as defined by the linguists Noam Chomsky and Morris Halle (1968). The distinctive features are a set of binary (two-valued) features designed to describe the phonemes in all languages of the world. A convenient example of a binary feature is nasality. In general terms, a given speech sound is either nasal or nonnasal, meaning that sound energy is transmitted through the nose (nasal) or is not (nonnasal). If nasality is described as a binary feature, then sounds can be classified as +nasal (indicating the nasal transmission of sound) or –nasal (indicating the absence of nasal transmission). Hence, a positive value (+nasal) means that the property is present or is relevant to description of the sound. In some ways, distinctive feature analysis is similar to the guessing game of Twenty Questions in which the participants have to identify an object by asking questions that can be answered with only yes or no. Chomsky and Halle proposed a set of 13 binary features, which, given the appropriate yes (+) or no (–) answers, can describe all phonemes used in the languages of the world.

In the Chomsky-Halle system, the voiced vowels are specified primarily with the features shown in Table 1.1. First, notice the three major class features of *sonorant, vocalic,* and *consonantal.* A sonorant sound is produced with a vocal cavity configuration in which spontaneous voicing is possible. Essentially, the vocal tract above the larynx is sufficiently open so that no special laryngeal adjustments are needed to initiate voicing. For nonsonorants, or *obstruents,* the cavity configuration does not allow spontaneous voicing. Special mechanisms must be used to produce voicing during the nonsonorant sounds. Vocalic sounds are produced with an oral cavity shape in which the greatest constriction does not exceed that associated with the high vowels /i/ and /u/ and with vocal folds that are adjusted so as to allow spontaneous voicing. This feature, then, describes the degree of opening of the oral cavity together with the vocal fold adjustment. Finally, consonantal sounds have a definite constriction in the *midsagittal,* or midline, region of the vocal tract; nonconsonantal sounds do not. Vowels are described as +sonorant, +vocalic, and –consonantal. Taken

TABLE 1.1   Distinctive Features for Selected Vowel Sounds. The Class Features Distinguish Vowels from Various Consonants; Therefore, All Vowels Have the Same Values for These Features.

	i	ɪ	ɛ	æ	ʌ	ɝ	u	ʊ	ɔ	ɑ
CLASS FEATURES										
Sonorant	+	+	+	+	+	+	+	+	+	+
Vocalic	+	+	+	+	+	+	+	+	+	+
Consonantal	–	–	–	–	–	–	–	–	–	–
CAVITY FEATURES										
High	+	+	–	–	–	–	+	+	–	–
Low	–	–	–	+	–	–	–	–	+	+
Back	–	–	–	–	–	–	+	+	+	+
Rounded	–	–	–	–	–	+	+	+	+	–
Nasal	–	–	–	–	–	–	–	–	–	–
MANNER OF ARTICULATION FEATURE										
Tense	+	–	–	+	–	+	+	–	+	+

together, these three features indicate that vowels are produced with a relatively open oral cavity, with no severe constriction in the midsagittal plane, and with a vocal fold adjustment that allows for spontaneous vocal fold vibration.

Vowels are also described with respect to cavity features and manner of articulation features, some of which are shown in Table 1.1 (the others will be discussed with respect to consonants later in this chapter). The cavity features of primary concern in vowel description are:

> Tongue Body Features: High–Nonhigh; Low–Nonlow; Back–Nonback (see Figure 1.11a, b, c)
>
> High sounds are produced by raising the body of the tongue above the level that it occupies in the neutral (or resting) position, as shown in Figure 1.11a.
>
> Low sounds are produced by lowering the body of the tongue below the level that it occupies in the neutral position; see Figure 1.11b.
>
> Back sounds are produced by retracting the body of the tongue from the neutral position, as shown in Figure 1.11c.
>
> Rounded–Nonrounded
>
> Rounded sounds have a narrowing or protrusion of the lips.
>
> Nasal–Nonnasal
>
> Nasal sounds are produced with a lowered *velum*, so that sound energy escapes through the nose.

Table 1.1 shows that most vowels can be distinguished using the cavity features. For example, /i/ and /u/ differ in the back and rounded features, and /æ/ and /i/ differ in the high and low features. Most other distinctions can be made by referring to a manner of articulation

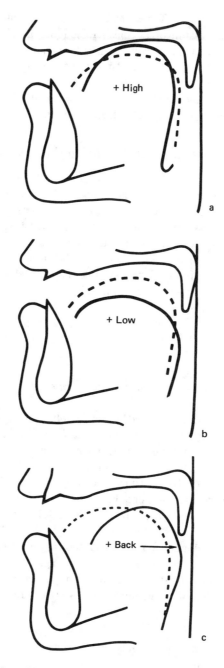

FIGURE 1.11 a, b, and c Vocal tract drawings illustrating the tongue body features high, low, and back relative to the neutral tongue position (broken line).

called tense–nontense. Tense sounds are produced with a deliberate, accurate, maximally distinct gesture that involves considerable muscular effort. The tense-nontense distinction is best illustrated with the vowel pairs /i/–/ɪ/ and /u/–/ʊ/. Vowels /i/ and /u/ are tense vowels because they are lengthened and are produced with marked muscular effort. As mentioned earlier, the difference in muscular effort can be felt by placing your fingers in the fleshy area just under the chin, saying alternately /i/–/ɪ/. A greater tension occurs during production of the tense vowel /i/ than during the nontense vowel /ɪ/.

Consonant Articulation: Traditional Phonetic Description

The consonants generally differ from the vowels in terms of the relative openness of the vocal tract and the function within the syllable. Vowels are produced with an open vocal tract; most consonants are made with a complete or partially constricted vocal tract. Within a syllable, vowels serve as a nucleus, meaning that a syllable must contain one and only one vowel (the only exceptions to this rule are the diphthongs, which are like vowels plus vowel glides, and certain syllabic consonants to be discussed later). Consonants are added to the vowel nucleus to form different syllable shapes, such as the following, where V represents a vowel and C represents a consonant.

VC shape:	*on, add, in*
CV shape:	*do, be, too*
CVC shape:	*dog, cat, man*
CCVC shape:	*truck, skin, clap*
CCVCC shape:	*screams, squint, scratched*

Consonants are described by degree or type of closure and by the location at which the complete or partial closure occurs. The *manner* of consonant articulation refers to the degree or type of closure, and the *place* of consonant articulation refers to the location of the constriction. In addition, consonants are described as *voiced* when the vocal folds are vibrating and *voiceless* when the vocal folds are not vibrating. Thus, an individual consonant can be specified by using three terms: one to describe *voicing*, one to describe *place*, and one to describe *manner*. Tables 1.2 and 1.3 show combinations of these terms used to specify the consonants of English.

Table 1.2 contains four columns, showing place of articulation, phonetic symbol and key word, manner of articulation, and voicing. The terms for place of articulation usually signify two opposing structures that accomplish a localized constriction of the vocal tract. Notice in the following definitions the two structures involved for the place terms.

Bilabial: two lips (*bi = two* and *labia = lip*)

Labial/velar: lips, and also a constriction between the *dorsum* or back of the tongue and the velum

Labiodental: lower lip and upper teeth

Linguadental or interdental: tip of tongue and upper teeth (*lingua = tongue*)

Lingua-alveolar: tip of tongue and the *alveolar ridge*

TABLE 1.2   Classification of Consonants by Manner and Voicing within Place

Place of Articulation	Phonetic Symbol and Key Word	Manner of Articulation	Voicing
Bilabial	/p/ (pay)	Stop	–
	/b/ (bay)	Stop	+
	/m/ (may)	Nasal	+
Labial/velar	/ʌ/ (which)	Glide (semivowel)	–
	/w/ (witch)	Glide (semivowel)	+
Labiodental	/f/ (fan)	Fricative	–
	/v/ (van)	Fricative	+
Linguadental (interdental)	/θ/ (thin)	Fricative	–
	/ð/ (this)	Fricative	+
Lingua-alveolar	/t/ (two)	Stop	–
	/d/ (do)	Stop	+
	/s/ (sue)	Fricative	–
	/z/ (zoo)	Fricative	+
	/n/ (new)	Nasal	+
	/l/ (Lou)	Lateral	+
	/ɾ/ (butter)	Flap	+
Linguapalatal	/ʃ/ (shoe)	Fricative	–
	/ʒ/ (rouge)	Fricative	+
	/tʃ/ (chin)	Affricative	–
	/dʒ/ (gin)	Affricative	+
	/j/ (you)	Glide (semivowel)	+
	/r/ (rue)	Rhotic	+
Linguavelar	/k/ (back)	Stop	–
	/g/ (bag)	Stop	+
	/ŋ/ (bang)	Nasal	+
Glottal (laryngeal)	/h/ (who)	Fricative	–
	/ʔ/ —	Stop	+(–)

> Linguapalatal: blade of tongue and palatal area behind the alveolar ridge
>
> Linguavelar: dorsum or back of tongue and roof of mouth in the velar area
>
> Glottal: the two vocal folds

Each of these places of articulation is discussed more fully below. To get a feeling for these different places of consonant articulation, concentrate on the first sounds in each word as you say the sequence: *pie, why, vie, thigh, tie, shy, guy, hi.* Notice from Figure 1.12 that the initial sounds constitute a progression from front to back in place of articulation.

Table 1.3 provides a breakdown of English consonants by place and voicing within manner classes. The manner of production associated with complete closure is the *stop*, which is formed when two structures completely block the passage of air from the vocal tract, building up air pressure behind the closure. Usually, when the closure is released, the air pressure built up behind the constriction causes a burst of escaping air. The burst is audible in words like *pie* and *two*.

TABLE 1.3   Classification of Consonants by Place and Voicing within Manner

Manner	Place	Voiced	Voiceless
Stop	Bilabial	b	p
	Alveolar	d	t
	Velar	g	k
	Glottal	------ ʔ -----------------	
Fricative	Labiodental	v	f
	Linguadental	ð	θ
	Alveolar	z	s
	Palatal	ʒ	ʃ
	Glottal		h
Affricative	Palatal	dʒ	tʃ
Nasal	Bilabial	m	
	Alveolar	n	
	Velar	ŋ	
Lateral	Alveolar	l	
Rhotic	Palatal	r	
Glide	Palatal	j	
	Labial/Velar	w	ʍ

Fricatives, like the initial sounds in *sue* and *zoo*, are made with a narrow constriction so that the air creates a noisy sound as it rushes through the narrowed passage.

Affricates, as in *church* and *judge*, are combinations of stop and fricative segments; that is, a period of complete closure is followed by a brief fricative segment. The stop + fricative nature of the affricates explain why these sounds are represented by the digraph symbols /tʃ/ and /dʒ/.

Nasals, as in the word *meaning* /minɪŋ/, are like stops in having a complete oral closure (bilabial, lingua-alveolar, or linguavelar) but are unlike stops in having an open velopharyngeal port so that sound energy passes through the nose rather than the mouth.

The *lateral* /l/ as in *lay* is formed by making a lingua-alveolar closure in the midline but with no closure at the sides of the tongue. Therefore, the sound energy from the vibrating folds escapes laterally, or through the sides of the mouth cavity.

The *rhotic* (or *rhotacized*) /r/ as in *ray* is a complex phoneme sometimes called *retroflex* in the phonetic literature. Retroflex literally means *turning* or *turned back* and refers to the appearance of the tongue tip, as viewed in X-ray films, for some /r/ productions. But in other productions of /r/, the tongue has a bunched appearance in the center or near the front of the mouth cavity. Because /r/ is produced in at least these two basic ways, the general term *rhotic* (Ladefoged, 1975) is preferable to the narrower term *retroflex*. This issue is discussed in more detail below.

The /ʍ/, /w/, and /j/ sounds are said to have a *glide* (semivowel) manner of production. These sounds are characterized by a gliding, or gradually changing, articulatory shape. For example, in /ʍ/ and its voiced counterpart /w/, the lips gradually move from a rounded and

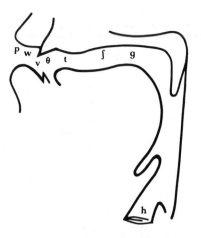

FIGURE 1.12   Places of articulation are marked by location of the phonetic symbols for the initial sounds in *pie, why, vie, thigh, tie, shy, guy, hi*.

narrowed configuration to the lip shape required by the following vowel simultaneously with a change in tongue position from high-back (like that for /u/) to the position for the following vowel. The glides always are followed by vowels.

In the following summary, manner of articulation is discussed for different places of articulation, proceeding from front to back.

Bilabial Sounds

In American English, the only consonant phonemes produced with a complete or partial closure (bilabial production) are the voiceless and voiced stops /p/ as in *pay* and /b/ as in *bay*, the nasal /m/ as in *may*, and the voiced and voiceless glides /w/ as in *witch* and /ʍ/ as in *which*. The vocal tract configurations for /p/, /b/, and /m/ are shown in Figure 1.13. These three sounds share a bilabial closure but differ in voicing and nasality. The stops /p/ and /b/ are called voiced and voiceless *cognates*, which means that they differ only in voicing. The production of these bilabial sounds is usually marked by a closed jaw position because the jaw closes somewhat to assist the constriction at the lips. The tongue is virtually unconstrained for /p/, /b/, and /m/, so that these bilabial sounds often are made simultaneously with the tongue position for preceding or following vowels. In other words, when we say words like *bee*, *pa*, and *moo*, the tongue is free to assume the required shape for the vowel during the closure for the bilabial, as illustrated in Figure 1.14.

The glides /w/ and /ʍ/ have a specified tongue position, roughly like that for the high-back vowel /u/, so these sounds cannot interact as freely with preceding or following sounds. Students (and even some practicing clinicians) sometimes fail to appreciate the importance of tongue articulation for /w/ and /ʍ/; for these sounds, both the tongue and lips execute gliding movements, as shown for the word *we* in Figure 1.15.

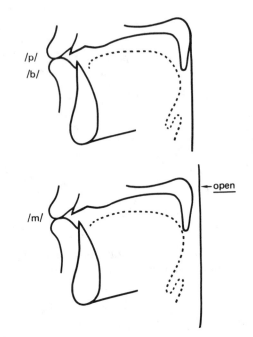

FIGURE 1.13   Vocal tract configurations for /p/, /b/, and /m/. Note labial closure for all three sounds and the open velopharynx for /m/.

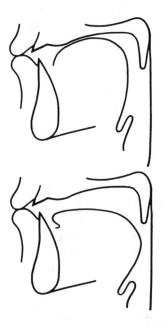

FIGURE 1.14   Variation in tongue position during a bilabial closure. Top: tongue position during *pea*; bottom: tongue position for *pa*.

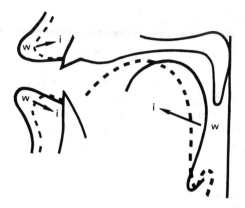

FIGURE 1.15   Illustration of gliding motion of tongue and lips for the word *we* (/wi/).

Labiodental Sounds

The voiceless and voiced *fricatives* /f/ as in *fan* and /v/ as in *van* are the only labiodental sounds in American English. The articulation is illustrated in Figure 1.16. Frication noise is generated by forcing air through the constriction formed by the lower lip and the upper teeth, principally the incisors. The noise is quite weak, very nearly the weakest of the fricatives. Like the labial sounds /p/, /b/, and /m/, the labiodentals allow the tongue to assume its position for preceding or following sounds. The jaw tends to close to aid the lower lip in its constricting gesture.

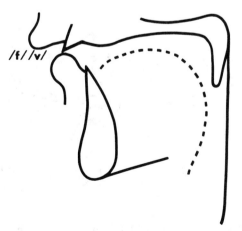

FIGURE 1.16   Vocal tract configuration for /f/ and /v/. Note labiodental constriction.

Interdental Sounds

There are only two interdentals, both fricatives: the voiceless /θ/ (e.g., *thaw*) and voiced /ð/ (e.g., *the*). They are illustrated in Figure 1.17. The frication noise is generated as air flows through the narrow constriction created by the tongue tip and the edge of the incisors. The weak frication noise is not much different from that for /f/ or /v/. The weak intensity of these sounds should be remembered in articulation testing, and the clinician should include both visual and auditory information in evaluating this pair of sounds. Jaw position for /θ/ and /ð/ usually is closed to aid the tongue in making its constriction. These sounds may be produced with either an interdental projection of the tongue or tongue contact behind the teeth.

Alveolar Sounds

The alveolar place of production is used for two stops: the voiceless /t/ (e.g., *too*) and the voiced /d/ (e.g., *do*); a nasal: /n/ (e.g., *new*); a lateral: /l/ (e.g., *Lou*); and two fricatives: the voiceless /s/ (e.g., *sue*) and the voiced /z/ (e.g., *zoo*). Not surprisingly, given the frequent and diverse movements of the tongue tip in the alveolar region, motions of the tongue tip are among the fastest articulatory movements. For example, the major closing and release movement for the stops /t/ and /d/ is made within about 50 milliseconds, or a twentieth of a second. For /t/ and /d/, an airtight chamber is created as the tongue tip closes firmly against the alveolar ridge and the sides of the tongue seal against the lateral oral regions. The site of tongue tip closure actually varies to a limited degree with phonetic context. When /t/ or /d/ are produced before the dental fricatives /θ/ and /ð/, the stop closure is made in the dental region. This context-dependent modification of alveolar consonant production is termed *dentalization* and is illustrated for /t/ in Figure 1.18.

The nasal /n/ is similar in basic tongue shape and movement to the stops /t/ and /d/. But /n/ differs from both /t/ and /d/ in having an open velopharyngeal port, making /n/ nasalized.

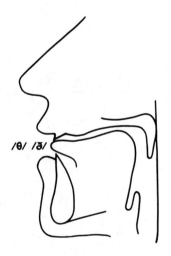

FIGURE 1.17   Vocal tract configuration for /θ/ and /ð/. Note linguadental constriction.

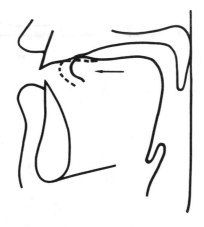

FIGURE 1.18   Dentalization of /t/. The normal alveolar closure is shown by the solid line and the dental closure is shown by the broken line.

But /n/ further differs from /t/ in that /n/ is voiced; /t/ is not. Because /n/ and /d/ are very similar in lingual articulation and voicing, failure to close the velopharyngeal port for /d/, as might happen with some speech disorders, results in /n/. Like /t/ and /d/, /n/ is dentalized when produced in the same syllable and adjacent to a dental sound like /θ/; compare, for example, the /n/ in *nine* /naɪn/ with the /n/ in *ninth* /naɪnθ/.

The lateral /l/ is a *liquid* formed with midline closure and a lateral opening, usually at both sides of the mouth (see Figure 1.19). Because of the midline closure made by the tongue tip against the alveolar ridge, sound energy escapes through the sides of the oral cavity. Although /l/ is the only lateral sound in English, there are at least two major allophones. Historically, these allophones are termed *light* and *dark*, but phoneticians disagree as to exactly how these allophones are formed. Wise (1957a, 1957b) explained that the light /l/ is made with linguadental contact whereas the dark /l/ is made with a lingua-alveolar contact. However, Kantner and West (1960) contend that the light /l/ has a greater lip spread and a lower and flatter tongue position than the dark /l/. An important feature of /l/, presumably, is a raising of the tongue toward the velum or palate. Giles (1971) concluded from X-ray pictures of speech that for allophonic variations of /l/, the position of the tongue dorsum falls into three general groups regardless of phonetic context: prevocalic, postvocalic, and syllabic (with syllabic being similar to postvocalic /l/). The postvocalic allophones had a more posterior dorsal position than the prevocalic allophones. Tongue tip contact occasionally was not achieved for the postvocalic allophones in words like *Paul*. Otherwise, the only variation in tongue tip articulation was dentalization influenced by a following dental sound. Apparently, then, /l/ can be produced with either a relatively front (light /l/) or back (dark /l/) dorsal position, but the light and dark variants are perhaps just as well termed prevocalic and postvocalic. Lingua-alveolar contact is not essential at least for /l/ in postvocalic position, which explains why postvocalic /l/ in words like *seal* may sound like /o/ or /ʊ/. The fricatives /s/ and /z/ are made with a narrow constriction between the tongue tip and the alveolar ridge (Figure 1.20).

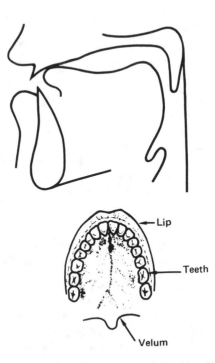

FIGURE 1.19   Articulation of /l/, shown in side view of a midline section (top) and as regions of tongue closure (shaded areas) against roof of mouth.

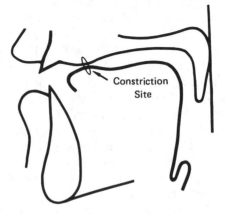

FIGURE 1.20   Vocal tract configuration for /s/ and /z/. Note lingua-alveolar constriction.

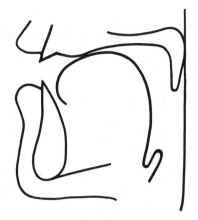

FIGURE 1.21   Vocal tract configuration for /ʃ/ and /ʒ/. Note linguapalatal constriction.

Palatal Sounds

The palatal sounds include the voiceless and voiced fricatives /ʃ/ (e.g., *shoe*) and /ʒ/ (e.g., *rouge*), the voiceless and voiced affricates /tʃ/ (e.g., *chin*) and /dʒ/ (e.g., *gin*), the glide /j/ (e.g., *you*), and the rhotic or retroflex /r/ (e.g., *rue*). For these sounds, the blade or tip of the tongue makes a constriction in the palatal region, the area just behind the alveolar ridge (see Figure 1.21).

The fricatives /ʃ/ and /ʒ/, like /s/ and /z/, are sibilants associated with intense noisy energy. For /ʃ/ and /ʒ/, this noise is generated as air moves rapidly through a constriction formed between the blade of the tongue and the front palate. Similarly, the affricates /tʃ/ and /dʒ/ are made in the palatal area as stop + fricative combinations. The airstream is first interrupted during the stop phase and then released during the fricative phase that immediately follows. In English, the only affricates are the palatal /tʃ/ and /dʒ/.

The glide /j/ is similar to the high-front vowel /i/ (as in *he*). The tongue is initially far forward and high in the mouth and subsequently moves toward the position for the following vowel. The similarity between /j/ and /i/ can be demonstrated by saying the biblical pronoun *ye* while noting the tongue position. Because the glide /j/ must be followed by a vowel, its articulation involves a gliding motion from the high-front position to some other vowel shape. The gliding motion can be felt during articulation of the words *you, yea, ya.*

As mentioned briefly above, the articulation of /r/ is highly variable. It sometimes is produced as a retroflexed consonant, in which case the tongue tip points upward and slightly backward in the oral cavity. But /r/ also can be produced with a bunching of the tongue, either in the middle of the mouth or near the front of the mouth. These basic articulations are illustrated in Figure 1.22. Some speakers also round their lips for /r/, and some constrict the lower pharynx by pulling the root of the tongue backward. Because /r/ is variably produced, it seems advisable to use *rhotic* or *rhotacized* (Ladefoged, 1975) rather than *retroflex* as a general articulatory descriptor. Given the complicated articulation of /r/, it is not surprising that it should present a major problem to children learning to talk. The

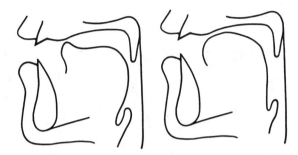

FIGURE 1.22 **The two major articulations of /r/:** *left,* **the retroflexed articulation;** *right,* **the bunched articulation.**

variation in tongue shape and position also complicates a speech clinician's attempts to teach /r/ articulations to a child who misarticulates the sound.

Velar Sounds

A velar constriction, formed by elevation of the tongue dorsum toward the roof of the mouth, occurs for the voiceless and voiced stops /k/ and /g/ and for the nasal /ŋ/. This artic-ulation is illustrated in Figure 1.23, which shows that the constriction can be made with the tongue relatively toward the front or relatively toward the back. The tongue placement is generally determined by the vowel context, with a front placement for velars adjacent to

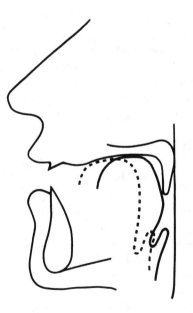

FIGURE 1.23 **Vocal tract configurations for velar consonants. Note variation in site of closure.**

front vowels (e.g., /g/ in *geese*) and a back placement for velars adjacent to back vowels (e.g., /g/ in *goose*). The nasal /ŋ/ has a tongue constriction similar to that for /k/ and /g/ but has an open velopharyngeal port for nasalization. The velar and bilabial places of articulation are similar in that both are used in English only for stops and nasals.

Glottal Sounds

The glottis, or chink between the vocal folds, is primarily involved only with two sounds, the voiceless fricative /h/ and the stop / ʔ / (a stoppage of air at the vocal folds). The fricative is produced with an opening of the vocal folds so that a fricative noise is generated as air moves at high speed through the glottis. A similar vocal fold adjustment is used in whisper.

It can be seen from Tables 1.2 and 1.3 that more types of sounds are made at some places of articulation than at others. Moreover, some sounds occur more frequently in the English language than others, contributing to a further imbalance in the use of places of articulation. Actual data on the frequency of occurrence of English consonants, grouped by place of articulation, are shown in Figure 1.24. In this circle graph, based on data from Dewey (1923), the relative frequencies of occurrence of different places of articulation are shown by the relative sizes of the pieces of the graph. Notice that alveolar sounds account for almost 50 percent of the sounds in English. The rank order of frequency of occurrence for place of articulation, from most to least frequent, is: alveolar, palatal, bilabial, velar, labiodental, interdental, and glottal. Within each place-of-articulation segment in Figure 1.24, the individual consonants are listed in rank order of frequency of occurrence. For

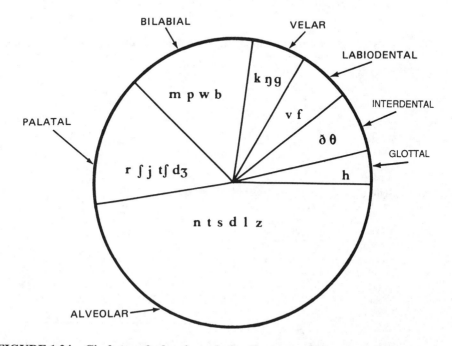

FIGURE 1.24   Circle graph showing relative frequency of occurrence of consonants made at different places of articulation. Based on data from Dewey (1923).

example, /n/ is the most frequently occurring alveolar consonant (in fact, it is the most frequently occurring of all consonants). Because of the differences in frequency of occurrence of consonants, a misarticulation affecting one place of articulation can be far more conspicuous than a misarticulation affecting another place. Therefore, statistical properties of the language are one consideration in the assessment and management of articulation disorders.

Consonant Articulation: Description by Distinctive Features

Distinctive features, discussed earlier with respect to vowels, can be used as an alternative to the place-manner chart to describe consonants. One simple example is the feature of voiced: All voiced consonants can be assigned the feature value of +voiced, and all voiceless consonants can be assigned the value of −voiced. Some important features for consonants are defined briefly below and are used for consonant classification in Table 1.4. These definitions are based on Chomsky and Halle (1968).

Consonantal sounds have a radical or marked constriction in the midsagittal region of the vocal tract. This feature distinguishes the "true" consonants from vowels and glides.

Vocalic sounds do not have a radical or marked constriction of the vocal tract and are associated with spontaneous voicing. The voiced vowels and liquids are vocalic; the voiceless vowels and liquids, glides, nasal consonants, and obstruents (stops, fricatives, and affricates) are *nonvocalic* (that is, −vocalic).

TABLE 1.4   Distinctive Feature Classifications for Selected Consonants

Consonants

Feature	p	b	m	t	d	n	s	l	θ	k
Consonantal	+	+	+	+	+	+	+	+	+	+
Vocalic	−	−	−	−	−	−	−	−	−	−
Sonorant	−	−	+	−	−	+	−	+	−	−
Interrupted	+	+	−	+	+	−	−	−	−	+
Strident	−	−	−	−	−	−	+	−	−	−
High	(−)	(−)	(−)*	−	−	−	−	−	−	+
Low	(−)	(−)	(−)	−	−	−	−	−	−	−
Back	(−)	(−)	(−)	−	−	−	−	−	−	+
Anterior	+	+	+	+	+	+	+	+	+	−
Coronal	−	−	−	+	+	+	+	+	+	−
Rounded	−	−	−	−	−	−	−	−	−	−
Distributed	+	+	+	−	−	−	−	−	+	−
Lateral	−	−	−	−	−	−	−	+	−	−
Nasal	−	−	+	−	−	+	−	−	−	−
Voiced	−	+	+	−	+	+	−	+	−	−

*Feature values enclosed in parentheses indicate that the feature in question may not be specified for this sound. For example, tongue position for /p/, /b/, and /m/ is not really specified, as it is free to assume the position required for the following vowel.

Sonorant sounds have a vocal configuration that permits spontaneous voicing, which means that the airstream can pass virtually unimpeded through the oral or nasal cavity. This feature distinguishes the vowels, glides, nasal consonants, and lateral and rhotacized consonants from the stops, fricatives and affricates (the class of obstruents).

Interrupted sounds have a complete blockage of the airstream during a part of their articulation. Stops and affricates are +interrupted, which distinguishes them from fricatives, nasals, liquids, and glides. Sometimes the feature *continuant* is used rather than interrupted, with opposite values assigned, that is, +continuant sounds are –interrupted and vice versa.

Strident sounds are those fricatives and affricates produced with intense noise: /s/, /z/, /ʃ/, /ʒ/, /tʃ/, /dʒ/. The amount of noise produced depends on characteristics of the constriction, including roughness of the articulatory surface, rate of air flow over it, and angle of incidence between the articulatory surfaces.

High sounds are made with the tongue elevated above its neutral (resting) position (see Figure 1.11a).

Low sounds are made with the tongue lowered below its neutral position (see Figure 1.11b).

Back sounds are made with the tongue retracted from its neutral position (see Figure 1.11c).

Anterior sounds have an obstruction that is farther forward than that for the palatal /ʃ/. Anterior sounds include the bilabials, labiodentals, linguadentals, and lingua-alveolars.

Coronal sounds have a tongue blade position above the neutral state. In general, consonants made with an elevated tongue tip or blade are +coronal.

Rounded sounds have narrowed or protruded lip configuration.

Distributed sounds have a constriction extending over a relatively long portion of the vocal tract (from back to front). For English, this feature is particularly important to distinguish the dental fricatives /θ/ and /ð/ from the alveolars /s/ and /z/.

Lateral sounds are coronal consonants made with midline closure and lateral opening.

Nasal sounds have an open velopharynx allowing air to pass through the nose.

Voiced sounds are produced with vibrating vocal folds.

The feature assignments in Table 1.4 are for general illustration of the use of features. The features should be viewed with some skepticism, as several different feature systems have been proposed, and any one system is subject to modification. It should be understood that distinctive features are one type of classification system. It should also be realized that distinctive features have an intended linguistic function that may not always be compatible with their application to the study of articulation disorders. The issue is beyond the scope of this chapter, but the interested reader is referred to Walsh (1974) and Parker (1976).

The relationship between the traditional place terms of phonetic description and the distinctive features is summarized below. For each traditional place term, the associated features are listed. As an example, a bilabial stop is +anterior, –coronal, and +distributed. (The placement of both features within brackets indicates that they are considered together in sound description.)

Bilabial
$$\begin{bmatrix} +\text{anterior} \\ -\text{coronal} \\ +\text{distributed} \end{bmatrix}$$

Labiodental
$$\begin{bmatrix} +\text{anterior} \\ -\text{coronal} \\ -\text{distributed} \end{bmatrix}$$

Interdental
$$\begin{bmatrix} +\text{anterior} \\ +\text{coronal} \\ +\alpha\text{distributed}^* \end{bmatrix}$$

Alveolar
$$\begin{bmatrix} +\text{anterior} \\ +\text{coronal} \\ -\alpha\text{distributed}^* \end{bmatrix}$$

Palatal
$$\begin{bmatrix} -\text{anterior} \\ +\text{high} \\ -\text{back} \end{bmatrix}$$

Velar
$$\begin{bmatrix} -\text{coronal} \\ +\text{high} \\ +\text{back} \end{bmatrix}$$

Suprasegmentals

The phonetic characteristics discussed to this point are *segmental*, which means that the units involved in the description are the size of phonemes or phonetic segments. *Suprasegmentals* are characteristics of speech that involve larger units, such as syllables, words, phrases, or sentences. Among the suprasegmentals are stress, intonation, loudness, pitch level, juncture, and speaking rate. Briefly defined, the suprasegmentals, also called *prosodies*, or *prosodic features*, are properties of speech that have a domain larger than a single segment. This definition does not mean that a single segment cannot, at times, carry the bulk of information for a given suprasegmental; on occasion, a segment, like a vowel, can convey most of the relevant information. Most suprasegmental information in speech can be described by the basic physical quantities of amplitude (or intensity), duration, and fundamental frequency (f_0) of the voice. Stated briefly, amplitude refers to the perceptual attribute of loudness; duration, to the perceptual attribute of length; and fundamental frequency, to the perceptual attribute of vocal pitch.

---

*The symbol α is a "dummy variable" and is used here to indicate that the Chomsky-Halle features can distinguish the interdental and alveolar consonants only if they differ with respect to the feature *distributed*. Thus, if interdentals are regarded as −distributed, then alveolars must be +distributed. (See Ladefoged, 1971 for development of this issue.)

Stress

Stress refers to the degree of effort, prominence, or importance given to some part of an utterance. For example, if a speaker wishes to emphasize that someone should take the red car (as opposed to a blue or green one), the speaker might say "Be sure to take the *red* car," stressing *red* to signify the emphasis. There are several varieties of stress, but all generally involve something akin to the graphic underline used to denote emphasis in writing. Although underlining is seldom used in writing, stress is almost continually used in speech. In fact, any utterance of two or more syllables may be described in terms of its stress pattern. Because stress has influences that extend beyond the segment, stress usually is discussed with respect to syllables. The pronouncing guide of a dictionary places special marks after individual syllables to indicate stress. For example, the word *ionosphere* is rendered as (i-*an*ʹ ə-sferʹ), with the marks ʹ and ʹ signifying the primary and secondary stress for the syllables.

The International Phonetic Alphabet (IPA) uses a different stress notation from that commonly found in dictionaries. In IPA the stress mark precedes the syllable to which it refers, and the degree of stress is indicated by whether *any* stress mark is used and by the *location* of the stress mark in the *vertical* dimension. The strongest degree of stress is indicated by a mark above the symbol line: ʹan (rather like a superscript); the second degree of stress is indicated by a mark below the symbol line: ˌaɪ (like a subscript); and the third degree of stress is simply unmarked: ə. The word *ionosphere* is rendered as /ˌaɪʹɑn ə ˌsfir/, with three degrees of stress marked.

Acoustically, stress is carried primarily by the vowel segment within a syllable. The acoustic correlates, roughly in order of importance, are fundamental frequency (especially with a rise in fundamental frequency on or near the stressed syllable), vowel duration (greater duration with increased stress), relative intensity (greater intensity with increased stress), sound quality (reduction of a vowel to a weaker, unstressed form, like /ɑ/ to /ə/, vowel substitution, and consonant changes), and disjuncture (pauses or intervals of silence) (Rabiner, Levitt, and Rosenberg, 1969).

Another form of unstressed (or weakly stressed) syllable is the syllabic consonant. This type of consonant, usually an /l/, /m/, or /n/ (but infrequently /r/), acts like a vowel in forming a syllable nucleus. Examples of syllabic consonants are the final sounds in the words *battle* /bætl̩/, *something* /sʌm ʔ m̩/, and *button* /bʌtn̩/. The syllabic function of a consonant is designated by a small vertical mark placed under the phonetic symbol. Syllabic consonants are most likely to occur when the consonant is *homorganic* (shares place of articulation) with a preceding consonant because it is economical or efficient simply to maintain the articulatory contact for both sounds. Additional information on stress will be provided following some basic definitions of related terms.

Intonation

Intonation is the vocal pitch contour of an utterance, that is, the way in which the fundamental frequency changes from syllable to syllable and even from segment to segment. Fundamental frequency can be affected by several factors, including the stress pattern of an utterance, tongue position of a vowel (high vowels have a higher f_0), and the speaker's emotional state.

Loudness

Loudness is related to sound intensity or to the amount of vocal effort that a speaker uses. Although loudness is ordinarily thought to be related to the amplitude or intensity of a sound, some evidence suggests that a listener's judgments of loudness of speech are related more directly to the perceived vocal effort, essentially the amount of work that a speaker does (Cavagna and Margaria, 1968). There is some evidence (Hixon, 1971; MacNeilage, 1972) that intensity variations in speech result mostly from respiratory activity, but variations of f_0 are easily accomplished at the level of the vocal folds.

Pitch Level

Pitch level is the average pitch of a speaker's voice and relates to the mean f_0 of an utterance. A speaker may be described as having a high, low, or medium pitch.

Juncture

Juncture, sometimes called "vocal punctuation," is a combination of intonation, pausing, and other suprasegmentals to mark special distinctions in speech or to express certain grammatical divisions. For example, the written sentence "Let's eat, Grandma," has a much different meaning than the same sentence without the comma, "Let's eat Grandma!" A speaker can mark a comma vocally with a short pause and an adjustment in intonation. Juncture is also used to make distinctions between similar articulations, such as between the word *nitrate* and the phrase *night rate*. Intonation and pausing enable a speaker to indicate which alternative he or she wants to express.

Speaking Rate

The rate of speaking is usually measured in words per second, syllables per second, or phonemes per second. As speaking rate increases, segment durations generally become shorter, with some segments affected more than others. The segments most vulnerable to contraction as a speaker talks more rapidly are pauses, vowels, and consonant segments involving a sustained articulation (like fricatives). Apparently, most speakers do not really increase the rate of individual articulatory movement as they increase their rate of speaking. Rather, they reduce the duration of some segments and reduce the overall range of articulatory movement (Lindblom, 1963). As a result, the articulatory positions normally assumed during a slow rate of speaking may be missed at a faster rate. The "missing" of articulatory positions as speaking rate increases is called *undershoot*. This is why a speaker's words are apt to sound less distinct to you as the rate of speaking increases.

Vowel Reduction

Vowels are particularly susceptible to articulatory change as speaking rate is increased or stress is decreased. Such articulatory alterations are termed *reduction* and are schematized in Figure 1.25. The arrows between pairs of vowels show directions of reduction; for example, /i/ reduces first to /ɪ/ and then to /ə/, the ultimate reduced vowel. The scheme shows that, with reduction, all vowels tend toward /ə/ or /ʌ/.

Clear versus Conversational Speech

There is considerable evidence to show that speakers alter their patterns of speech production depending on situation and listener. One variation is clear versus conversational speech.

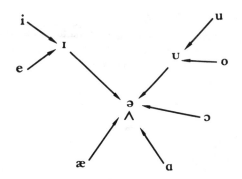

FIGURE 1.25   A scheme of vowel reduction. The arrows between vowel symbols show vowel changes resulting from reduction. For example, /i/ and /e/ reduce to /ɪ/, and /ɪ/ reduces to /ə/, which is the ultimate reduced vowel. Note that these changes occur within the quadrilateral defined by the corner vowels /i/, /æ/, /ɑ/, and /u/.

Clear speech is what speakers use when they are trying to be as intelligible as possible. Compared to more casual conversational speech, clear speech is (1) slower (with longer pauses between words and a lengthening of some speech sounds), (2) more likely to avoid modified or reduced forms of consonant and vowel segments (such as the vowel reduction described earlier), and (3) characterized by a greater intensity of obstruent sounds, particularly stop consonants (Picheny, Durlach, and Braida, 1986). When talkers want to be easily understood, they modify their speech to make it slower and more acoustically distinctive. Whereas vowels in conversational speech often are modified or reduced, therefore losing some of their acoustic distinctiveness, these sounds in clear speech are produced in distinctive forms. Similarly, word-final stops in conversational speech frequently are not released, so that the burst cue for their perception is eliminated. But in clear speech, stop consonants (and consonants in general) tend to be released and this feature enhances their perception.

These differences are central to a hypothesis proposed by Lindblom (1990) that speakers vary their speech output along a continuum from *hypospeech* to *hyperspeech* (the H&H hypothesis). The basic idea is that speakers adapt to the various circumstances of communication, to match their production patterns to communicative and situational factors. When a speaker believes that special care is required to be understood, he or she alters articulation accordingly. In Lindblom's view, clear speech (hyperspeech in his H&H hypothesis) is not simply loud speech but reflects an articulatory reorganization (Moon and Lindblom, 1989). Adams (1990), however, reported contrary evidence. He concluded from an X-ray micro-beam study of speech movements that changes in speech clarity did not seem to reflect a reorganization of speech motor control. Adams observed that in clear speech, articulatory movements tended to be both larger and faster but there was no general indication that the speech patterns were organized differently than in conversational speech. The important point for clinical purposes is that speech articulation can be controlled by a speaker to enhance intelligibility when conditions warrant such deliberate effort. The primary articulatory change appears to be in the magnitude and speed of movement.

New versus Given Information

New information in a discourse is information that the listener would not be expected to know from the previous conversation or from the situation. Given information is predictable, either from the previous discourse or from the general situation. New information often is highlighted prosodically. For example, Behne (1989) studied prosody in a mini-discourse such as the following:

"Someone painted the fence."
"Who painted the fence?"
"Pete painted the fence."

In this exchange, the new information ("Pete") is lengthened and produced with a higher fundamental frequency. In effect, the speaker uses prosody to highlight the new information.

Contrastive Stress in Discourse

Another discourse-related prosodic effect is *contrastive stress*. Such stress can be given to almost any word, phrase, or clause which the speaker considers to contradict or contrast with one that was previously expressed or implied. For instance, a speaker who wants to emphasize that she took the red ball rather than the green or blue one, might say, "I took the *red* ball" (where the italicized word receives contrastive stress). Contrastive stress is sometimes used clinically to give prosodic variation to an utterance or to elicit a stressed form of a target element.

Phrase-Final Lengthening

At the syntactic level, juncture and pause phenomena are used to mark multiword units. For example, in English, *phrase-final lengthening* operates to lengthen the last stressable syllable in a major syntactic phrase or clause. For example, if we contrast the following two sentences:

1. Red, green, and blue are my favorite colors.
2. Green, blue, and red are my favorite colors.

the word *blue* will be longer in (1) than in (2) because in the former this word is at the end of the subject noun phrase and is therefore subject to phrase-final lengthening. This regularity can be exploited clinically to obtain durational adjustments for a target word. In addition, Read and Schreiber (1982) showed that phrase-final lengthening is helpful to listeners in parsing (that is, to recognize the structure of) spoken sentences. They also suggested that children rely more on this cue than adults do, and, moreover, that prosody assists the language-learner by providing structural guides to the complex syntactic structures of language.

Declination

Another effect at the syntactic level is *declination*, or the effect in which the vocal fundamental frequency contour typically declines across clauses or comparable units. Why this tilt in the overall fundamental frequency pattern occurs is a matter of debate (Cohen, Collier, and t'Hart, 1982), but it is a robust feature of prosody at the sentence or clause level.

This pattern is helpful to listeners in recognizing the structure of discourse, such as in identifying sentence units.

Lexical Stress Effects

These effects operate at the level of the word. For example, English has many noun–verb pairs like *'import* versus *im'port*, or *'contrast* versus *con'trast*, in which the difference between the members of a pair is signaled primarily by stress pattern. Another common effect at the word level occurs with a distinction between compounds and phrases. For example, the compound noun *'blackbird* contrasts with the noun phrase *black 'bird* (a bird that is black).

Although the lay listener often thinks stress in English is just a matter of giving greater intensity to part of an utterance, laboratory studies have shown that stress is signaled by duration, intensity, fundamental frequency, and various phonetic effects (Fry, 1955). It is important to remember that stress affects segmental properties such as the articulation of vowels and consonants (Kent and Netsell, 1972; de Jong, 1991). Segments in stressed syllables tend to have larger and faster articulatory movements than similar segments in unstressed syllables. For this reason, stressed syllables often are favored in some phases of articulation therapy.

Toward a Unified Theory of Stress

The various stress effects summarized in the foregoing may appear to be a formidable collection of phenomena that the speaker somehow has to manage during the production of an utterance. Indeed, the list is imposing and belies the apparent ease with which most people can say something like, "But I didn't say *alveolar*, I said *velar* stop," which is produced with an overall pattern of declining fundamental frequency but with prosodic adjustments to place contrastive stress on the words *alveolar* and *velar*. The stressed words must be produced in accord with the lexical stress patterns, so that, for example, *velar* is spoken as *'velar* and not *ve'lar* or *'ve'lar*.

Some of the stress effects outlined in the previous section may be unified in a recent theory described by Beckman (1986) and Beckman and Edwards (1991). They propose a unified representation with four levels:

Level 1. Syllables with reduced nuclei, such as the second syllable in *vita*.

Level 2. Syllables similar to those above except that they have full vowels, e.g., *veto*.

Level 3. Syllables may be selectively given more stress by assigning to them a pitch accent.

Level 4. Syllables can receive a marking called *nuclear accent* (or *phrase accent*) in which the last accented item in a phonological grouping assumes the most prominent accent.

This proposal illustrates both the complexity of stress and a solution for its representation. Consider a speaker who wants to place pitch accent on the word *tuba*. The accent cannot be placed on the second syllable, which is a reduced nucleus. Rather, the accent must be placed on the stressed syllable. The levels discussed above help to show how various levels of the stress representation interact without destroying essential phonological patterns.

Because suprasegmentals like stress and speaking rate influence the nature of segmental articulation, some care should be taken to control suprasegmental variables in articulation tests and speech materials used in treatment. Vowels carry much of the suprasegmental information in speech, but stress, speaking rate, and other suprasegmentals can influence consonant articulation as well. The suprasegmental features of speech have been discussed by Crystal (1973), Lehiste (1970), and Lieberman (1967), and the reader is referred to these accounts for a more detailed consideration of this complex area.

Coarticulation: Interactions Among Sounds in Context

Convenient though it might be to consider phonemes as independent, invariant units that are simply linked together to produce speech, this simplistic approach does not really fit the facts. When sounds are put together to form syllables, words, phrases, and sentences, they interact in complex ways and sometimes appear to lose their separate identity. The influence that sounds exert on one another is called *coarticulation*, which means that the articulation of any one sound is influenced by a preceding or following sound. Coarticulation makes it impossible to divide the speech stream into neat segments that correspond to phonemes. Coarticulation implies nonsegmentation, or, at least, interaction of the presumed linguistic segments. Hockett (1955) provided a colorful illustration of the transformation from phoneme to articulation:

> Imagine a row of Easter eggs carried along a moving belt; the eggs are of various sizes, and variously colored, but not boiled. At a certain point, the belt carries the row of eggs between the two rollers of a wringer, which quite effectively smashes them and rubs them more or less into each other. The flow of eggs before the wringer represents the series of impulses from the phoneme source. The mess that emerges from the wringer represents the output of the speech transmitter (210).

Although this analogy makes the process of articulation sound completely disorganized, in fact the process must be quite well organized if it is to be used for communication. Phoneme-sized segments may not be carried intact into the various contractions of the speech muscles, but some highly systematic links between articulation and phonemes are maintained. Research on speech articulation has provided a clearer understanding of what the links are although the total process is far from being completely understood.

It often is possible to describe coarticulation in terms of articulatory characteristics that spread from one segment to another. Examine the following examples of coarticulation:

1a.	He sneezed	/h i s n i z d/ (unrounded /s/ and /s/)
1b.	He snoozed	/h i s n u z d/ (rounded /s/ and /n/)
2a.	He asked	/h i æ s k t/ (nonnasal /æ/)
2b.	He answered	/h i æ n s ɝ·d/ (nasal /æ/)

The only phonemic difference between the first two items is the appearance of the unrounded vowel /i/ in 1a and the appearance of the rounded vowel /u/ in 1b. The lip rounding for /u/ in *He snoozed* usually begins to form during the articulation of the /s/. You might be able to feel this anticipatory lip rounding as you alternately say *sneeze* and *snooze* with your finger lightly touching your lips. In articulatory terms, the feature of lip rounding for the vowel is assumed during the /sn/ consonant cluster as the consequence of anticipating the rounding. The contrast between *sneeze* and *snooze* shows that the /sn/ cluster acquires lip rounding only if it is followed by a rounded vowel. This example of sound interaction is termed *anticipatory lip rounding* because the articulatory feature of rounding is evident before the rounded vowel /u/ is fully articulated as a segment.

Another form of anticipatory coarticulation occurs in 2b. Perhaps you can detect a difference in the quality of the /æ/ vowel in the phrases *He asked* and *He answered*. You should be able to detect a nasal quality in the latter because the vowel tends to assume the nasal resonance required for the following nasal consonant /n/. In this case, we can say that the articulatory feature of velopharyngeal opening (required for nasal resonance) is anticipated during the vowel /æ/. Normally, of course, this vowel is not nasalized. The contrasts between 1a and 1b and between 2a and 2b illustrate a type of coarticulation called *anticipatory*. Another type, *retentive*, applies to situations in which an articulatory feature is retained after its required appearance. For example, in the word *me* the vowel /i/ tends to be nasalized because of a carry-over velopharyngeal opening from the nasal consonant /m/. The essential lesson to be learned is that coarticulation occurs frequently in speech, so frequently in fact that the study of articulation is largely a study of coarticulation.

Phonetic context is highly important in understanding allophonic variation. For example, you should be able to detect a difference in the location of linguavelar closure for the /k/ sounds in the two columns of words below.

keen	*coon*
kin	*cone*
can	*con*

The point of closure tends to be more to the front of the oral cavity for the words in the first column than it is for the words in the second column. This variation occurs because, in English, the velar stops /k/ and /g/ do not have a narrowly defined place of articulation; all that is required is that the dorsum, or back, of the tongue touch the ceiling of the mouth. Therefore, the tongue is simply elevated at the position needed for the following vowel. When the tongue is in the front of the mouth (note that the vowels in the left column are front vowels), the dorsal closure is made in the front of the mouth, and when the tongue is in the back of the mouth (as it would be for the vowels in the right column), the point of closure is to the back of the velar surface.

Coarticulation arises for different reasons, some having to do with the phonology of a particular language, some with the basic mechanical or physiological constraints of the speech apparatus. Hence, some coarticulations are learned and others are the inevitable consequences of muscles, ligaments, and bones of the speech apparatus that are linked together and unable to move with infinite speed. Consider, for example, the closing and opening of the velopharyngeal port. This articulatory gesture is rather sluggish (compared to movements of the tongue tip), so it is not surprising that the velopharyngeal opening for a nasal consonant carries over to a following vowel, as in the word *no*. The extent of this carryover nasalization, however, varies with the phonologic characteristics of a particular language. In French, vowel nasalization is phonemic (that is, it can make a difference in meaning), but in English, vowel nasalization is only allophonic. Some aspects of coarticulation reflect universal properties of the human speech mechanism and hence affect all languages. Other coarticulations are governed by the phonemic structure of a particular language and are therefore learned with that language. Many coarticulatory effects are assimilatory in that a feature from one segment is adopted by an adjacent segment. For example, the nasalization of vowels by neighboring nasal consonants is nasal assimilation. Such effects may make speech production easier and faster because articulatory movements can be adapted to a particular phonetic and motor sequence. Assimilation is a general process in spoken language and will be taken up later in discussions of phonology.

Another aspect of coarticulation is the overlapping of articulations for consonants in clusters. Quite often, the articulation for one consonant is made *before* the release of a preceding consonant in any two-consonant cluster. For example, in the word *spy* /spaɪ/, the bilabial closure for /p/ is accomplished shortly (about 10 to 20 msec) before the release of the constriction for /s/. This overlapping of consonant articulations makes the overall duration of the cluster shorter than the sum of the consonant durations as they occur singly; that is, the duration of /sp/ in *spy* is shorter than the sum of the durations of /s/ in *sigh* /s aɪ/ and /p/ in *pie* /p aɪ/. The overlapping of articulation contributes to the articulatory flow of speech by eliminating interruptions. The temporal structure of an /spr/ cluster, as in the word *spray*, is pictured schematically in Figure 1.26. Notice that the constrictions for /s/ and /p/ overlap by 10 to 20 milliseconds and that the closure for /p/ overlaps with the tongue position for /r/ by a similar amount. Because consonants in clusters frequently present special difficulties to children (and adults) with articulation disorders, clinicians must know how such clusters are formed. Because clusters have overlapping articulations of the constituent consonants, in general, the cluster is a tightly organized sequence of articulatory gestures. The articulation of clusters is further complicated by allophonic variations, such as those listed in Table 1.5. In English, unaspirated released stops occur only when stops follow /s/, as in the words *spy*, *stay*, and *ski*. Otherwise, released stops are aspirated, meaning that the release is followed by a brief interval of glottal frication (an /h/-like noise). Similarly, the

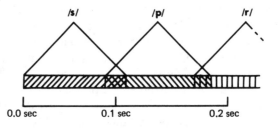

FIGURE 1.26   **Schematic drawing of the articulatory organization of a /spr/ consonant cluster (as in the word** *spray***), showing overlapping of consonantal articulations. Based on data from Kent and Moll (1975).**

devoiced /l/ and /r/ normally occur only after voiceless consonants, as in the words *play* and *try*.

The examples of context-dependent articulatory modifications in Table 1.5 show the variety of influences that sounds exert on adjacent sounds. For a given sound, place of articulation, duration, voicing, nasalization, and rounding may vary with phonetic context, and these variations are noted with the special marks shown in Table 1.5.

Some aspects of coarticulation can be understood by knowing the extent to which individual sounds restrict the positions of the various articulators. Table 1.6 summarizes degrees of restriction on lips, jaw, and parts of the tongue for the different places of consonant articulation. A strong restriction is indicated by an X, a slight to moderate restriction by a —, and a minimal restriction by an O. Because this table shows which parts of the vocal tract are free to vary during articulation of a given consonant, it can be used to predict certain aspects of coarticulation. For example, because bilabial sounds do not restrict the tongue as long as it does not close off the tract, Os are indicated for all parts of the tongue. Jaw position is shown as moderately restricted for most places of articulation because some degree of jaw closing usually aids consonant formation. The ability of jaw movement to aid tongue movement declines as place of articulation moves back in the mouth, so a velar consonant may not restrict jaw position as much as more frontal articulation (Kent and Moll, 1972). The only sound that allows essentially unrestricted coarticulation is the glottal /h/. Thus, /h/

TABLE 1.5   Examples of Context-Dependent Modifications of Phonetic Segments

Modification	Context Description
Nasalization of vowel	Vowel is preceded or followed by a nasal, e.g., [ɜ̃n]—*on* and [mǣn]—*man*
Rounding of consonant	Consonant precedes a rounded sound, e.g., [k̫win]—*queen* and [t̫ru]—*true*
Palatalization of consonant	Consonant precedes a palatal sound, e.g., [ki̯s ju]—*kiss you*
Devoicing of obstruent	Word-final position of voiced consonant, e.g., [dɔg̥]—*dog* and [liv̥]—*leave*
Devoicing of liquid	Liquid follows word-initial voiceless sound, e.g., [pl̥eɪ]—*play* and [tr̥i]—*tree*
Dentalization of coronal	Normally alveolar sound precedes a dental sound, e.g., [wɪd̪θ]—*width* and [naɪn̪θ]—*ninth*
Retroflexion of fricative	Fricative occurs in context of retroflex sounds, e.g., [har ʂ ɚ]—*harsher* and [pɝ˞ʂɚ]—*purser*
Devoicing of sound	Consonant or vowel in voiceless context, e.g., [sɪ̥stɚ]—*sister*
Lengthening of vowel	Vowel preceding voiced sound, especially in stressed syllable, e.g., [ni : d]—*need*
Reduction of vowel	Vowel in unstressed (weak) syllable, e.g., [t æ bjuleɪt] [t æ bjeleɪt]—*tabulate*
Voicing of sound	Voiceless in voiced context, e.g., [æbʂ̬ɝd]—*absurd*
Deaspiration of stop	Stop follows /s/, e.g., [sp = aɪ]—*spy* vs. [pʰaɪ]—*pie*

TABLE 1.6   Coarticulation Matrix, Showing for Each Place of Consonant Articulation Those Articulators That Have Strong Restrictions on Position (Marked with X), Those That Have Some Restriction on Position (Marked with —), and Those That Are Minimally Restricted (Marked with O). For Example, the Bilabials /b/, /p/, and /m/ Strongly Restrict the Lips, Moderately Restrict the Jaw, and Leave the Tongue Essentially Free to Vary. The Glides /w/ and /ʍ/ Are Not Included Because They Involve Secondary Articulations. Lip Rounding, as Often Occurs for /r/, Has Been Neglected.

			Tongue			
Place	Lip	Jaw	Tip	Blade	Dorsum	Body
Bilabial /bpm/	X	—	O	O	O	O
Labiodental /vf/	X	—	O	O	O	O
Interdental /ðθ/	O	—	X	X	—	—
Alveolar /dtzsln/	O	—	X	X	—	—
Palatal /ʃ ʒ dʒ tʃ j r/	O	—	—	X	X	X
Velar /gkŋ/	O	O	O	—	X	X
Glottal /h/	O	O	O	O	O	O

usually is made with a vocal-tract configuration adjusted to an adjacent sound, such as the following vowel in the words *he* /hi/, *who* /hu/, *ham* /hæm/, and *hop* /hɑp/.

Investigators of speech articulation (Daniloff and Moll, 1968; Moll and Daniloff, 1971; Kent and Minifie, 1977) have shown extensive overlapping of articulatory gestures across phoneme-sized segments, causing debate about the size of unit that governs behavior. Some investigators propose that the decision unit is an allophone, others argue for the phoneme, and still others for the syllable. A popular syllable-unit hypothesis is one based on CV (consonant-vowel) syllables, with allowance for consonant clustering (CCV, CCCV, and so on). This hypothesis states that articulatory movements are organized in sequences of the form CV, CCV, CCCV, and the like, so that a word like *construct* would be organized as the articulatory syllables /kɑ/ + /nstrʌkt/. Notice the odd assembly of the second syllable. This issue is of more than academic importance. Discovery of the basic decision unit would have implications for speech remediation; for example, enabling a speech clinician to choose the most efficient training and practice items for correcting an error sound. In addition, syllabic structures may explain certain features of speech and language development as discussed by Branigan (1976).

Coarticulation also has clinical relevance, in that a sound might be more easily learned or more easily produced correctly in one context than in others. In other words, the phonetic context of a sound can facilitate or even interfere with correct production of the sound. The effect of phonetic context could explain why misarticulations are often inconsistent, with correct production on certain occasions and incorrect productions on others. By judiciously selecting the phonetic context where an error sound is initially corrected, the clinician can sometimes enhance the efficiency of speech remediation. Such examples show why a thorough knowledge of articulatory phonetics is important to decisions in the management of articulation disorders.

There is considerable theoretical controversy about how speech is organized as a motor behavior. Figure 1.27, which illustrates the controversy, depicts three levels of speech organization. (Actually, some contributors to the debate do not agree that these three levels are required; however, since most writers recognize them, they are used here.) The highest level is a sequence of units. This sequence may take the form of a psychological network of conceptual dependencies, a surface-structure representation of words (as suggested by Chomsky), or a syntagma (a rhythmic organization of syllables).

Most experts (it is hard to think of an exception) recognize the existence of some basic speech unit, the second level of Figure 1.27, but they disagree about the nature of this unit.

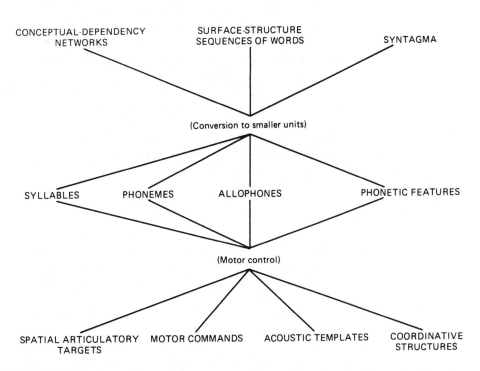

FIGURE 1.27   Some alternative representations at three levels of organization of speech production. The top level is one of networks or strings, the middle level refers to a basic unit of speech production, and the third level pertains to the direct motor control of speech.

Some prefer the syllable, others the phoneme, others the allophone, and still others the phonetic feature. Moreover, some think all of these units are involved in a hierarchical organization, with syllables branching into phonemes, phonemes into allophones, and allophones into features.

The third level is motor control—the level at which the basic unit described above is converted into instructions that tell the muscles of speech what to do. One candidate for this level is a spatial articulatory target, a kind of snapshot of what the total vocal tract configuration should be. A second candidate is the motor command, presumed to be identical for each occurrence of the basic control unit (whatever that may be!). For those experts who believe the speech system tries to produce patterns that fit the acoustic goals of speech, the third candidate is an acoustic template. And finally, a relatively recent view identifies this level as a coordinative structure, an assembly of elementary movements that defines a basic unit of action. Obviously, there is no lack of theory!

Aerodynamic Considerations in Speech Production

Because the production of speech depends on the supply and valving of air, a knowledge of air pressure, flow, and volume is essential to an understanding of both normal and disordered speech. Many abnormalities of speech production are caused by irregularities or deficiencies in the supply and valving of air, and a number of clinical assessment techniques rely on measures of air pressure, flow, or volume. To understand the regulation of air pressures and flows in speech, it is important to recognize that (1) air flows only in one direction—from a region of greater pressure to one of lesser pressure; and (2) whenever the vocal tract is closed at some point, the potential exists for the buildup of air pressure behind the closure.

English speech sounds are normally *regressive*, meaning that, in sound production, air flows from the inside (usually the lungs) to the outside (the air around us). The basic energy needed to produce sound is developed in the lungs. After air is inspired by enlargement of the lung cavity, the muscle activation changes so that the lung cavity returns to a smaller size. If the airway above is closed, the same volume of air is enclosed in a smaller space. Because the same amount of air is contained in a smaller cavity, the air pressure within the lungs increases. This overpressure (relative to atmosphere) in the lungs is the source of the regressive air flow for all speech sounds. It is a fact of clinical importance that the air flow requirements for speech are not much greater than the requirements for ordinary breathing; that is, the volume of air inspired and expired in speaking is not much different from that in quiet respiration.

The regulation of air pressure and flow for speech is diagrammed in Figure 1.28, a simple model of the vocal tract. This model, in the form of the letter F, shows the three general areas where constriction (narrowing or closure) can occur: the laryngeal, oral, and nasal sections. The first site of constriction for egressive air is in the larynx. If the vocal folds close tightly, no air can escape from the lungs. If the folds are maximally open, then air passes through the larynx readily. If the folds are closed with a moderate tension, then the buildup of air pressure beneath them eventually blows them apart, releasing a pulse of air. After the folds are blown apart, they quickly come together again through the action of var-

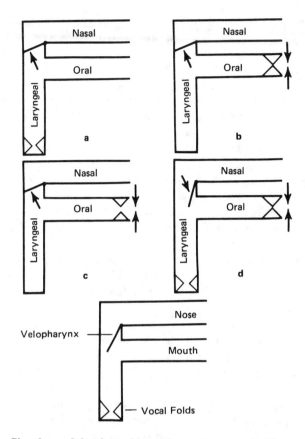

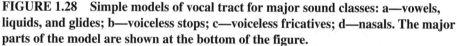

FIGURE 1.28 **Simple models of vocal tract for major sound classes: a—vowels, liquids, and glides; b—voiceless stops; c—voiceless fricatives; d—nasals. The major parts of the model are shown at the bottom of the figure.**

ious physical restoring forces. This alternation of closed and open states, occurring many times per second, is called voicing. Successive pulses of air from the vocal folds are a source of acoustic energy for all voiced sounds, such as vowels.

The F-shaped vocal tract model shown in Figure 1.28a illustrates the air flow for vowel sounds. The vocal folds are shown as being partly closed to represent the vibratory pattern of opening and closing. The nasal tube is tightly closed because vowels in English are nonnasal unless they precede or follow nasal consonants. The oral tube is widely open to represent the open oral cavity in vowel articulation. Because the nasal tube is closed, the acoustic energy from the vibrating vocal folds passes through the oral tube.

The configuration of the vocal tract for a voiceless stop like /p/, /t/, or /k/ is diagrammed in Figure 1.28b. The constriction at the larynx is shown as completely open because air from the lungs passes readily through the larynx and into the oral cavity. The constriction at the velopharynx is shown as closed to indicate that no air flows through the nasal tube. The oral constriction is closed to represent the period of stop closure. After this period, the oral constriction opens rapidly to allow a burst of air to escape from the oral pressure chamber. Assuming a stop closure of suitable duration, the air pressure developed within the oral cavity can be nearly equal to that in the lungs because the open vocal folds permit an equalization of air pressure in the airway reaching from the lungs up to the oral cavity. Therefore, voiceless stops have high intraoral air pressures. Also, it should be noted that children may use *greater* intraoral air pressures than adults (Subtelny, Worth, and Sakuda, 1966; Bernthal and Beukelman, 1978).

The model for voiceless fricatives in Figure 1.28c is like that for voiceless stops, but instead of a complete oral constriction, the model has a very narrow constriction, required for fricative noise. Because the velopharyngeal constriction is tightly closed and the laryngeal constriction is open, voiceless fricatives like /s/ and /ʃ/ have high intraoral air pressures. The voiceless stops and fricatives are sometimes called *pressure consonants*.

Voiced stops and fricatives differ from voiceless stops and fricatives in having vibrating vocal folds. Therefore, the models in Figures 1.28b and 1.28c would have a partial laryngeal constriction to represent voicing of these sounds. Because a certain amount of air pressure is lost in keeping the vocal folds vibrating (that is, pressure across the glottis drops), the voiced stops and fricatives have smaller intraoral air pressures than their voiceless cognates.

Finally, the model for nasal consonants is depicted in Figure 1.28d. A partial constriction at the larynx represents the vibrating vocal folds, and a complete oral constriction represents the stop-like closure in the oral section of the vocal tract. For nasal consonants, the acoustic energy of voicing is directed through the nasal cavity. Very little air pressure builds up within the oral chamber.

Liquids and glides can be modeled in essentially the same way as vowels (Figure 1.28a). Because the oral constriction for these sounds is only slightly greater than that for vowels, there is very little intraoral air pressure buildup.

Pressures and flows can be used to describe the function of many parts of the speech system. For example, a normal efficient operation of the larynx can often be distinguished from inefficient pathological states by the excessive air flow in the latter conditions. This excessive flow, or air wastage, may be heard as breathiness or hoarseness. Velopharyngeal incompetence can be identified by recording air flow from the nose during normally nonnasal segments. Frequently, velopharyngeal incompetence is signaled both by inappropriate nasal air flow (for example, air flow during stops or fricatives) and by reduced levels of intraoral air pressure. Sometimes, more than one pressure or flow must be recorded to identify the problem. For example, reduced levels of intraoral air pressure for consonants can be related to at least three factors: (1) respiratory weakness, resulting in insufficient air pressure; (2) velopharyngeal dysfunction, resulting in a loss of air through the nose; or (3) an inadequacy of the oral constriction, allowing excessive air to escape.

Clinically, aerodynamic assessment is especially important when dealing with a structural defect (such as cleft palate) or a physically based control problem (as in cerebral palsy, vocal fold paralysis, and other neurologic disorders). As noted above, young children may use greater intraoral air pressure than adults for consonant production, so normative pressure data obtained from adults should be used with caution in clinical evaluation of children. Moreover, the higher pressures in children's speech mean that children must close the velopharyngeal port even more tightly than adults to prevent nasal loss of air during stop or fricative consonants. Speech and language clinicians who do not possess equipment for aerodynamic recordings of speech should nonetheless be aware of the pressure and flow requirements in speech production. These requirements have important implications for the diagnosis and evaluation of communicative problems and for the design of remediation programs.

Acoustic Considerations of Speech

It is far beyond the scope of this chapter to consider in any detail the acoustic structure of speech sounds, but it is possible to draw here a few major conclusions about the acoustic signal of speech. Acoustic signals can be described in terms of three fundamental physical variables—frequency, amplitude, and duration. *Frequency* refers to the rate of vibration of a sound. Generally, the faster the rate of vibration, the higher the pitch heard. In other words, frequency is the most direct physical correlate of pitch. *Amplitude* refers to the strength or magnitude of vibration of a sound. The higher the magnitude of vibration, the louder the sound heard. Amplitude is the most direct physical correlate of loudness. Because the actual amplitude of vibration is minute and, therefore, difficult to measure, sound intensity or sound pressure level is used instead when making actual speech measurements. *Duration* refers to the total time over which a vibration continues. Duration is the most direct physical correlate of perceived length.

Virtually all naturally occurring sounds, speech included, have energy at more than a single frequency. A tuning fork is designed to vibrate at a single frequency and is one of the very few sound sources with this property. The human voice, musical instruments, and animal sounds all have energy at several frequencies. The particular pattern of energy over a frequency range is the *spectrum* of a sound. Speech sounds differ in their *spectra*, and these differences allow us to distinguish sounds perceptually.

Table 1.7 is a summary of the major acoustic properties of several phonetic classes. The table shows the relative sound intensity, the dominant energy region in the spectrum, and the relative sound duration for each class. Vowels are the most intense speech sounds, have most of their energy in the low to mid frequencies, and are longer in duration than other sounds (although the actual duration of vowel sounds may range from about 50 milliseconds to half a second). Because vowels are the most intense sounds, they typically determine the overall loudness of speech. The most intense vowels are the low vowels and the least intense, the high vowels.

The glides and liquids are somewhat less intense than the vowels and have most of their energy in the low to mid frequencies. The duration of the glides /w/ and /j/ tends to be longer than that of the liquids /l/ and /r/.

The strident fricatives and affricates (/s, z, ʃ, ʒ, tʃ, dʒ/) are more intense than other consonants but considerably weaker than vowels. The stridents have energy primarily at the high frequencies and, therefore, are vulnerable to high-frequency hearing loss. A good tape recording of the stridents requires a recorder with a wide frequency response. Stridents tend

TABLE 1.7   Summary of Acoustic Features for Six Phonetic Classes

Sound Class	Intensity	Spectrum	Duration
Vowels	Very strong	Low frequency dominance	Moderate to long
Glides and liquids	Strong	Low frequency dominance	Short to moderate
Strident fricatives and affricates	Moderate	High frequency dominance	Moderate
Nasals	Moderate	Very low frequency dominance	Short to moderate
Stops	Weak	Varies with place of articulation	Short
Nonstrident fricatives	Weak	Flat	Short to moderate

to be relatively long in duration, especially compared to other consonants, and fricatives typically are longer than affricates.

The nasals are sounds of moderate intensity, low-frequency energy, and brief to moderate duration. The nasals have more energy at very low frequencies than do other sounds.

The stops are relatively weak sounds of brief duration. The burst that results from release of a stop closure can be as short as 10 milliseconds. The primary energy for stops varies over a wide range of frequencies—from low to high; bilabials have relatively low-frequency energy, while velars and alveolars have most of their energy in, respectively, the mid and mid to high frequencies.

The nonstrident fricatives /f, v, θ, ð/ are weak sounds of typically moderate duration. They tend to have a flat spectrum, meaning that the noise energy is distributed fairly uniformly over the frequency range. Of all sounds, /θ/ usually is the weakest—so weak that it can barely be heard when produced in isolation at any distance from a listener.

Finally, two points should be made concerning acoustic implications for clinical assessment and management. First, the absolute frequency location of energy for speech sounds varies with speaker age and sex. Men have the lowest overall frequencies of sound energy, women somewhat higher frequencies, and young children the highest frequencies. This relationship follows from the acoustic principle that an object's resonance frequency is inversely related to its length. The longest pipe in a pipe organ has a low frequency (or low pitch) and the shortest pipe a high frequency (high pitch); similarly the adult male vocal tract is longer than a woman's or a child's and therefore has resonances of lower frequency. This difference has practical implications. Most acoustic data have been collected for men's speech; much less is known about women's or children's speech, and the data for men may not be directly applicable to either. Moreover, the recording and analysis of women's and children's speech requires a wider frequency range than that suitable for men's speech. This issue can be particularly important for fricatives and affricates.

Second, because speech sounds vary widely in intensity, dominant energy region, and duration, they are not equally discriminable under different listening situations. The acoustic differences summarized in Table 1.7 should be kept in mind when testing articulation or auditory discrimination.

Sensory Information in Speech Production

As speech is produced, a number of different kinds of sensory information is generated. The types of information include tactile (touch and pressure), proprioceptive (position sense), kinesthetic movement sense), and auditory. The total sensory information is genuinely plurimodal, that is, available in several modalities. Most authorities agree that the rich sensory information associated with speech production is particularly important in speech development and in the management of some speech disorders, as when a child must learn a new articulatory pattern. A clinician therefore should be knowledgeable about the kinds and characteristics of sensory, or afferent, information.

The major characteristics of the sensory systems in speech were reviewed by Hardcastle (1976) and more recently by Kent, Martin, and Sufit (1990). Tactile receptors, which consist of free nerve endings and complex endings (for example, Krause end-bulbs and Meissner corpuscles), supply information to the central nervous system on the nature of contact (including localization, pressure, and onset time) and direction of movement. Remarkably, the oral structures are among the most sensitive regions of the body. The tongue tip is particularly sensitive and can therefore supply detailed sensory information. Tactile receptors belong to a more general class of receptors called mechanoreceptors (which respond to mechanical stimulation). These receptors respond not only to physical contacts of articulatory structures but also to air pressures generated during speech.

The proprioceptive and kinesthetic receptors include the muscle spindles, Golgi tendon organs, and joint receptors. Muscle spindles provide rich information on the length of muscle fibers, degree and velocity of stretch, and the direction of movement of a muscle. Golgi receptors relay information on the change of stretch on a tendon caused by muscular contraction or by other influences, including passive movement. Joint receptors, located in the capsules of joints, inform the central nervous system on the rate, direction, and extent of joint movement. Even a relatively simple movement, such as closing the jaw and raising the tongue, supplies a variety of afference to the central nervous system.

The auditory system supplies information on the acoustic consequences of articulation. Because the purpose of speech is to produce an intelligible acoustic signal, auditory feedback is of particular importance in regulating the processes of articulation. Interestingly, when an adult suffers a sudden and severe loss of hearing, speech articulation usually does not deteriorate immediately, but only gradually. The other types of sensory information are probably sufficient to maintain the accuracy of articulation for some time.

Many tactile receptors are comparatively slow acting because the neural signals travel along relatively small fibers in a multisynaptic pathway (a pathway composed of several neurons). Much of the tactile information is available to the central nervous system after the event to which it pertains. This information is particularly important to articulations that involve contact between articulatory surfaces, such as stops and fricatives. Obviously, prolonging an articulation helps to reinforce its sensory accompaniment. When the mucosal surfaces of the articulators are anesthetized, one of the most disturbed class of sounds is the fricatives.

Proprioceptive and kinesthetic receptors tend to be faster because spindle afferent fibers are large, and neural transmission is monosynaptic (that is, a two-neuron pathway).

The relatively short latency of this afference means that some information can reach the central nervous system during the articulatory event.

The auditory system is slower than either the tactile or proprioceptive systems and provides most of its information after the corresponding articulatory event has occurred. Some current theories about sensory information in speech propose that this information is not sampled continuously but rather intermittently. Because speech is a highly rehearsed motor skill, it is not necessary to rely continuously on sensory information for its regulation. Instead, the process only samples the sensory feedback on an occasional basis to insure that the actual sensory information matches the expected sensory information.

Generative Phonology

Phonology has been defined as the part of linguistics concerned with "putting sounds together" or "putting sounds into words." Somewhat more precisely, Sloat, Taylor, and Hoard define phonology as "the science of speech sounds and sound patterns" (1978; 1). These authors note that each language has its own sound pattern, which is (1) the set of sounds used by a certain language, (2) the acceptable arrangement of these sounds to form words, and (3) the various processes by which sounds are added, deleted, or changed. Thus, the sound patterns of different languages can differ in the sounds available for use, the permissible ordering of these sounds, and the rules or processes that operate on the sounds. Phonological rules are prescriptions that convert abstract phonological representations into phonetic representations. An example from Hyman (1975) is the pronunciation of the verb *miss*. The word is pronounced /mis/ in the phrase *we miss it* but /mɪʂ/ in the phrase *we miss you*. In English, the /s/ often is palatalized when it is followed by a palatal /j/ (which itself may be deleted). Thus, the morpheme *miss* has these two pronunciations determined by the phonology of English.

Phonological processes are operations that affect sound change, both within individual language users and within the history of a particular language. Some examples of processes are cluster reduction: *snow* /snoʊ/ → /noʊ/; deletion of unstressed syllables: *baloney* /bəloʊnɪ/ → /bloʊnɪ/; and final consonant devoicing: *pig* /pɪg/ → /pɪk/. Other examples will be discussed later in this chapter and in other chapters of this book.

Although this chapter is not directly concerned with linguistics, the student should at least recognize the relevance of some phonological principles to the study of normal and disordered articulation. The study of phonology offers many important insights into the interactions among sound segments and the interactions between speech articulation and higher levels of linguistic organization. In a sense, phonological analysis is a key to the door between articulation and the various levels of language structure. Many aspects of articulation—such as the duration of constriction for an /s/, the duration of a vowel sound, the occurrence of palatalization for consonants, or the devoicing of a normally voiced segment—can be understood through the study of phonology.

Some of the interactions among units in the oral expression of language can be described and perhaps even explained through *phonological rules*. A phonological rule is a formal expression of a regularity that occurs in the phonology of a language or in the phonology of an individual speaker. These rules are either *context-free* or *context-sensitive*.

A context-free rule is not dependent on a specific context. For example, if a child always substitutes (replaces) stops for fricatives (e.g., *sees* /siz/ becomes /tid/), we can formulate a rule that states simply that fricatives become stops:

Fricative → Stop

In this example, the word *fricative* represents the category of fricatives and the word *stop* represents the category of stops and the arrow means "is replaced by." Thus, the rule means that a fricative unit is replaced by a stop unit. Because this change or replacement always occurs, it is not necessary to state any context restriction on its operation.

On the other hand, assume that a child replaces fricatives with stops only in the initial position of a syllable; for example /si/ (*see*) becomes /ti/ and /zu/ (*zoo*) becomes /du/. The restriction to syllable-initial position is a context restriction, or a constraint on the operation of the rule. To formalize this operation, the following rule can be used:

Fricative → Stop   /   #   ___

This rule states that a fricative unit is replaced by a stop unit if the fricative is in the context such that it initiates a syllable. The slash / means "in the environment such that," the # represents a syllable boundary, and the underline ___ indicates the location of the fricative segment. Hence, the slash-#-underline means that the fricative immediately follows the syllable boundary (that is, begins the syllable).

A general form of a phonological rule is the following:

$X \rightarrow Y$ / a ___ b

This rule expresses a modification in which X becomes Y whenever X occurs following a and preceding b. The rule structure is decomposed as follows:

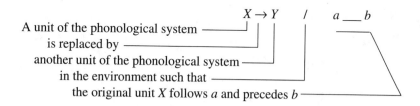

For example, imagine an allophonic modification in which a vowel is nasalized if it occurs between two nasal consonants (as in the word *man*). A rule of the form given above could be used to describe this change as follows:

Vowel → Nasal vowel   /   Nasal consonant ___ Nasal consonant

But a nasal consonant can be regarded as a sound having the features +nasal and +consonant. When features such as nasal and consonant apply together, it is convenient to place them in brackets so that the rule above becomes:

$$\text{Vowel} \rightarrow \begin{bmatrix} +\text{Nasal} \\ +\text{Vowel} \end{bmatrix} \quad / \quad \begin{bmatrix} +\text{Nasal} \\ +\text{Consonant} \end{bmatrix} \quad \underline{\qquad} \quad \begin{bmatrix} +\text{Nasal} \\ +\text{Consonant} \end{bmatrix}$$

Some additional examples of rules are given below. By studying these rules, the student should be able at least to interpret phonological rules, if not to devise them. The basic advantage of a phonological rule is that it expresses in a formal or mathematical fashion a regularity of the phonological system and allows for an accurate, compact description of various context dependencies.

Example of deletion rule: Consonants following nasal consonants are deleted.

$$C \longrightarrow \emptyset \quad / \quad \begin{bmatrix} +\text{Nasal} \\ C \end{bmatrix} \quad \underline{\qquad}$$

(Ex.: [ænt] $\longrightarrow$ [æn])

Explanation: As an abbreviatory convenience, *C* stands for consonant, and a nasal consonant is *C* with the feature +nasal. Deletion is represented by the null element ∅ so that the rule literally reads "a consonant is replaced by a null element (nothing) when the consonant follows a nasal consonant."

Example of insertion rule: A schwa vowel is inserted following syllable-final voiced stops.

$$\emptyset \longrightarrow /\text{ə}/ \quad / \quad \begin{bmatrix} +\text{Voiced} \\ +\text{Stop} \end{bmatrix} \quad \underline{\qquad} \# $$

(Ex.: [dɔg] $\longrightarrow$ [dɔgə])

Explanation: The rule literally reads "a null element (nothing) is replaced by a schwa vowel when the null element occurs at the end of a syllable following a voiced stop."

Example of feature-changing rule: Syllable-final voiced obstruents are devoiced.

$$\begin{bmatrix} -\text{Sonorant} \\ +\text{Voiced} \end{bmatrix} \longrightarrow [-\text{Voiced}] \quad / \quad \underline{\qquad} \# $$

(Ex.: [bɪg] $\longrightarrow$ [bɪk])

Explanation: Obstruents are stops, fricatives, and affricates, all of which are represented by the feature –sonorant. Thus, the rule states literally that "voiced nonsonorants (i.e., obstruents) are replaced by their voiceless counterparts at the end of syllables."

Example of feature-assimilation rule: A normally voiceless consonant is voiced when it occurs between two voiced sounds.

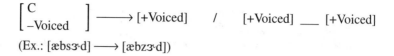

$$\begin{bmatrix} C \\ -\text{Voiced} \end{bmatrix} \longrightarrow [+\text{Voiced}] \quad / \quad [+\text{Voiced}] \underline{\quad} [+\text{Voiced}]$$

(Ex.: [æbsɜˑd] $\longrightarrow$ [æbzɜˑd])

Explanation: A voiceless consonant becomes voiced if the preceding and following segments are voiced.

Natural Phonology

A topic of considerable interest and importance in phonology is that of *naturalness*. A natural class, property, process, or rule is one that appears to be preferred or is frequently used in phonologic systems (Sloat, Taylor, and Hoard, 1978; Stampe, 1972; Ingram, 1976). Evidence of naturalness is generally taken from developmental studies (early appearance or acquisition in a child's language), from cross-linguistic studies (universality across languages), or from studies of sound change in a language. One phonological property is more natural than another if the first appears before the second in language development and if the first is attested to in a greater number of languages. *Markedness* is a term sometimes used in this connection. An *unmarked* sound is one that appears to be natural. Unmarked sounds are acquired earlier than marked sounds in children's language, tend to be established in a language before marked sounds can be added, and tend to occur in different languages more frequently than marked sounds. By these criteria, voiceless stops are an example of unmarked (more natural) sounds, whereas voiced obstruents are marked (less natural).

Studies of natural phonology have shown that certain *assimilatory* and *nonassimilatory* processes occur commonly enough to be regarded as natural (Sloat, Taylor, and Hoard, 1978). An assimilatory process is one in which a sound changes to assimilate (become similar) to another sound. A nonassimilatory process does not appear to be based on similarity between sounds.

Examples of Assimilatory Processes

Voicing changes. These are intervocalic voicing and voicing and devoicing of obstruents. In intervocalic voicing, an obstruent (stop, fricative, or affricate) becomes voiced when it occurs between two vowels (hence, intervocalic). For example, *puppy* /pʌpɪ/ becomes /pʌbɪ/. The voiceless obstruent is assimilated to the voiced elements that surround it. The pattern of obstruent voicing or devoicing varies with languages, but one common process is word-final devoicing, in which an obstruent loses its voicing when it occurs at the end of the word. This change sometimes is considered assimilatory because it is thought that the voiced segment is assimilated to the voiceless pause at the end of the word. For example, *dog* /dɔg/ becomes /dɔk/.

Nasalization. As already discussed in this chapter, vowels and, occasionally, other resonants are assimilated to nasal consonants by becoming nasal themselves. Thus, in the word *lamb* /læm/, the vowel often is nasalized.

Nasal assimilation. Nasal consonants tend to assume the place of articulation of a neighboring sound. In English, this process is amply illustrated by the large number of homorganic nasal-stop combinations: *impolite, imbue, improper, indelicate, unturned, endeared, anchor, anger, congress.*

Palatalization. Nonpalatal consonants become palatal when followed by a front vowel or a glide. For example, the /n/ in *news* and the /k/ in *cute* become palatalized when these words are produced with the glide + vowel /ju/ (/njuz/ and /kjut/). As mentioned above, /s/ often is palatalized when it is followed by the glide /j/ in phrases such as *miss you.*

Examples of Nonassimilatory Processes

Deletion or loss of segments. Sometimes a segment or number of segments at the end of a word are dropped in a process known as *apocope.* For example, in the Eastern dialect of English, speakers often drop the /r/ in words such as *car, store,* and *stair,* pronouncing *car* /kar/ as /ka:/. Young children also frequently delete the final consonants of words. Final consonant omission is noted by speech clinicians more often than initial consonant omission. When segments are lost at other than the end of a word, the process is sometimes called *syncope.* Apocope and syncope frequently simplify (or reduce) clusters; *extra,* for example, may become /ɛktrə/ and *asks* may become /æks/.

Insertion of segments. In one type of insertion process, called *prosthesis,* a segment is added in the initial position. In another type, called *epenthesis,* a segment is added elsewhere in the word. Children frequently will break up clusters by inserting vowels (often the schwa /ə/): *blue* becomes /bəlu/ and *clock* becomes /kəlak/.

Metathesis. The order of segments is reversed in this process. For example, a child may say /nets/ for *nest* /nɛst/ and /mjukis/ for *music* /mjusik/ (the second example also involves final-segment devoicing).

Breaking. By this process, long vowels become diphthongs, as in the examples *fast* /fæɪst/, *pass* /pæɪs/, *bag* /bæɪg/, and *cat* /kæɪt/. Breaking often may be heard in the speech of young children.

Natural phonology offers some valuable perspectives on the acquisition of phonology by children. Some authors believe that natural phonological processes are innate or are acquired early and rather easily by children and that whenever a natural process opposes a phonological property of the language the child is learning, some resistance may be expected. Stampe (1969) viewed natural processes as innate processes that simplify the adult target word. One interesting implication of naturalness is that children tend to exhibit strong biases or preferences in their sound formations and sound sequences. It has been proposed that some such preferences are based on phonetic grounds. For example, obstruent devoicing (or the tendency for stops, fricatives, and affricatives to be devoiced) may be related to the fact that it is difficult to maintain laryngeal vibrations during a period of vocal tract closure. To maintain voicing during closure of the tract, special measures must be taken to enable air flow to continue through the vocal folds. This can be done through an expansion of the oral air chamber (Perkell, 1969; Kent and Moll, 1969), accomplished by expanding the pharynx or by depressing the larynx. However, not all natural processes have a simple phonetic basis, and, most likely, other factors will have to be considered in reaching a full explanation. Whatever this explanation may be, it behooves the speech clinician to be aware that speech and language learning may be influenced by phonological forces that occur commonly enough to be called natural. Such preferences or predispositions in speech production may be a substrate for the process of acquisition. Furthermore, the maintenance of natural processes beyond their usual survival time in learning a particular phonological system could result in articulation disorders.

Nonlinear Phonology

Nonlinear phonology was developed as an alternative to linear generative phonology because the latter was perceived to have certain shortcomings. Some aspects of generative phonology (launched largely through the classic work, *The Sound Pattern of English* by Chomsky and Halle, 1968) were considered earlier. The basic goals of generative phonologies are to (1) describe phonological patterns in natural languages, (2) formulate the rules that account for these systems, and (3) identify universal principles that apply to phonological systems. A particular reason why nonlinear phonologies were introduced was to account for the influence of stress (as in weak and strong clusters in English stress systems) and the description of tone and stress features in levels of representation independent of the segmental representation. Linear generative phonology was regarded by some to be inadequate in dealing with prosodic effects in general. Early generative phonologies regarded phonological representation as "linear strings of segments with no hierarchical organization other than that provided by syntactic phrase structure" (Clements and Keyser, 1983; 1). This kind of generative phonology was characterized by rules that operated in a domain of linear strings of segments. But this approach encountered some difficulties in regard to the effects of stress and other prosodic variables. More generally, linear generative phonology failed to account satisfactorily for the relationships among various sizes of units because phonological operations were constrained to act on linear sequences.

There are several different versions of nonlinear phonology, but two particularly influential theories are autosegmental theory (Goldsmith, 1976, 1990; Hayes, 1988) and metrical theory (Goldsmith, 1990; Hayes, 1988). Autosegmental theory divides phonological features into parallel tiers of quasi-independent sequences. The tiers are like interconnected but independent levels. The term *autosegment* refers to a unit in a given tier. An autosegment can be realized in one or more ways; for example, a tonal tier may allow realizations such as high, mid, or low tones. The sequences in each tier are time-aligned with association lines that indicate simultaneity across tiers. In this way, stress and segmental representations are coordinated. A detailed discussion cannot be given here for this complex development in phonological theory, but the central idea is fairly simple: Phonological patterns evolve from connections across different representations, and not, as linear generative phonology maintained, from operations across a single linear sequence of phonological units. Nonlinear phonology is a significant break from an earlier theoretical view. It accommodates interactions across various sizes and types of phonological representation.

Metrical theory organizes phonological units into hierarchies, for example, feet, syllables, and segments. Unlike linear generative phonology, metrical theory gives a special definition to stress. Stress patterns arise from rhythm (an alternating prominence, such as strong–weak) and syllable weight. Stress assignments are made across the various levels of the hierarchy (such as syllables, feet, and words). This treatment of stress is very different from that of linear generative phonology.

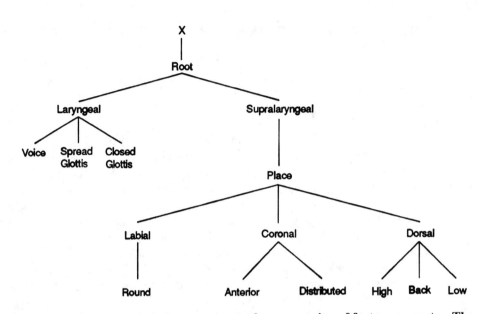

FIGURE 1.29   **Hierarchical tree structure for one version of feature geometry. The features under the supralaryngeal node have been defined previously. The features under the laryngeal node refer to vocal fold configurations.**

Hierarchy also is important to theories of feature geometry, another development in non-linear phonology. Two influential accounts of feature geometry are McCarthy (1988) and Sagey (1986). In systems such as that shown in Figure 1.29, syllable, consonant, and vowel appear as superordinate nodes that govern other nodes specifying laryngeal and supralaryngeal articulations. That is, the features are arranged hierarchically. Linear phonology, such as that of Chomsky and Halle (1968), typically specified features in a matrix where orthogonality or independence among features was desirable if not always attainable. In contrast, feature geometry exploits nonorthogonality among features. The hierarchical patterns implied by nonorthogonality become organizing principles in feature geometry.

The three phonological theories reviewed here—autosegmental theory, metrical theory and feature geometry—all represent major departures from what had been the standard phonological theory. Not surprisingly, these new theories are now being considered with respect to phonological development (Schwartz, 1992; Spencer, 1988) and phonological disorders in children (Bernhardt, 1990; Chiat, 1989; Chin and Dinnsen, 1991; Gandour, 1981; Spencer, 1984).

Summary of Levels of Organization of Speech

Various levels of organization of speech are shown in Table 1.8, beginning with the syllable and working down to the acoustic sequence that might be seen on a spectrogram or visual representation of sounds. Although *syllable integrity* is the highest level shown, the

TABLE 1.8   Levels of Organization of Speech

SYLLABIC INTEGRITY:	/p a/ SYL
PHONEMIC COMPOSITION:	/p/ + /a/
PHONETIC PROPERTIES: Note: stop /p/ is aspirated and vowel /a/ is lengthened	[pʰa:]
SEGMENTAL FEATURES:	[p] — +Stop +Labial +Consonantal –Nasal –Voice [a] — +Syllabic –Consonantal –Front +Low –Round –Nasal +Voice
ARTICULATORY SEQUENCE:	Closure of velopharynx Abduction of vocal folds Adjustment of tongue for /a/ Closure of lips Opening of lips and jaw Adduction of vocal folds Final abduction of vocal folds
ACOUSTIC SEQUENCE:	Silent period during /p/ closure Noise burst for /p/ release Aspiration period as folds close Voiced period after folds close, with distinct resonant shaping

table could have begun with an even higher level, such as a phrase or a sentence. However, for our purposes here, it is sufficient to consider only the levels presented in the table. The syllable is an organizational unit that consists of one or more phonemes; in this case, the syllable /pa/ includes the phonemes /p/ and /a/. Because phonemes are abstract, a phonemic description does not touch on a number of details of phonetic organization and speech behavior. Some of these details are shown in the level of *phonetic properties*. The phoneme /p/ has as its phonetic representation the aspirated [pʰ], and the phoneme /a/ has as its phonetic representation the lengthened [a:]. These phonetic representations are, of course, allophones of the /p/ and /a/ phonemes. The English phoneme /p/ is always aspirated in syllable-initial position, and the phoneme /a/ frequently is lengthened when uttered in an open monosyllable (that is, a CV syllable).

Segmental features comprise the next level of the table. These features are phonetic dimensions or attributes by which sounds may be described. For example, the consonant [p] is defined by its inclusion in the classes of *stops*, *labials*, and *consonantals* and by its exclusion from the classes of *nasals* and *voiced sounds*. These features are similar to the distinctive features discussed earlier in this chapter, but they are intended to be more phonetic in character. Even without rigorous definitions of the features suggested, it should be clear that each feature defines an articulatory property of the sound in question; for example, vowel [a] is a syllable nucleus, is not a consonant, is low-back and unrounded, and is a voiced nonnasal sound.

The features are less abstract than phonemes but still must be interpreted by the motor control system of the brain to provide proper neural instructions to the speech muscles; that is, the features listed for [p] and [a] must be translated into a pattern of muscle contractions that yields the *articulatory sequence* shown in the next to last level of the table. The *–nasal* feature of [p] requires that the velopharynx be closed, and the *–voice* feature of the same segment requires that the vocal folds be abducted (open). In this way, each feature requirement is given an articulatory interpretation, accomplished by the contraction of muscles.

Finally, as the consequence of muscle contractions, a series of speech sounds is uttered. In this *acoustic sequence*, the last level of the table, one can see acoustic segments of the kind visible on a spectrogram. Notice that one acoustic segment does not necessarily correspond to a single phoneme. The phoneme /p/ is associated with at least three acoustic segments: a silent period corresponding to the bilabial closure, a noise burst produced as the lips are rapidly opened, and an aspiration interval related to a gradual closure of the vocal folds in preparation for voicing the following vowel.

Although Table 1.8 is fairly detailed, it represents only part of the complexity of speech. In the linguistic-phonetic organization of speech behavior, we need to consider three major components: the segmental (or phonetic) component, the suprasegmental (*prosodic*) component, and the *paralinguistic* component. The first two already have been discussed in this chapter. The paralinguistic component is similar to the prosodic component in that it might be called nonsegmental. This component includes those aspects of speech represented by terms such as *emotion* and *attitude*. A speaker who plans an utterance must decide not only about phonetic sequencing but also about prosodic structure and emotional and attitudinal content (that is, the "tone of voice"). The segmental component includes words, syllables, phonemes, and features. The suprasegmental or prosodic component includes stress, intonation, juncture, rate, loudness, and pitch level. The paralinguistic component is made up of tension, voice quality, and voice qualifications (Crystal, 1969).

The complexity of speech behavior can be illustrated by listing the various types of information represented in the speech signal. A *partial* listing (mostly from Branigan, 1979) is

1. A set of articulatory targets or goals corresponding to the intended phonetic sequence
2. Assignment of stress to the syllables that make up the sequence
3. Adjustments of syllable duration to stress, phonetic composition, and position of the syllable in the utterance
4. Specification of junctural features, including transitions between elements and terminal juncture at the end of the utterance
5. Internal ordering of words as it reflects syntactic form to convey semantic intentions (meaning)
6. Determination of other prosodic features such as speaking rate, pitch, level, and loudness
7. Use of paralinguistic features to convey emotion or attitude

It is important to remember that even an apparently simple aspect of speech behavior can be influenced by a host of variables. For example, the duration of a vowel is determined by tongue height, tenseness or laxness, consonant context, stress pattern, frequency of occurrence of the word in which the vowel occurs, syntactic ordering of the word in which the vowel appears, and rate of speaking (Klatt, 1976).

Concluding Note on Implications for Speech Acquisition

Speech articulation has its early roots in the vocalizations of infants. Just how the coos and babbles of the first year of life relate to the development of speech is not well understood, but there is growing evidence that early vocalizations prepare the child for acquisition of a phonetic system. The syllable appears to be an important unit in early sound patterns, and the development of syllabic organization of sounds may be a major framework of speech development. If so, it is of interest to chart the way in which syllabic structures develop during the first year of life. The following account is based on several chapters in *Precursors of Early Speech Development*, edited by Bjorn Lindblom and Rolf Zetterström.

The major phases in syllable development are as follows: (1) Continuous phonation in a respiratory cycle provides the basic phonatory pattern from which refinements in articulation can develop; (2) intermittent phonation within a respiratory cycle breaks the basic pattern of continuous phonation and, thus, is a precursor of syllable units; (3) articulatory (supraglottal) movements interrupting or combined with phonation provide early experience in the control of co-occurring phonation and articulation; (4) marginal syllables (in isolation or in sequence) are early syllabic forms that, while lacking the detailed structure of adult syllables, prefigure the basic syllable shape; (5) canonical syllables (in isolation or in sequence) anticipate important structural properties of adult speech and may be particularly important in relating an infant's perceptions of adult speech with his or her own productive patterns; and (6) reduplicated babble (repeated syllable patterns) gives the infant experience with both prosody (especially rhythm) and sequences of articulations. It is on this vocal bedrock that speech develops. For a time, babbling and early words coexist, sharing some phonetic properties but, perhaps, differing in others.

The CV syllable, occurring in virtually all of the world's languages, has long been recognized as a preferred basic unit of speech articulation. It appears to be an optimal unit for learning perceptual discriminations in infancy. Infants younger than four months can discriminate segments contained in sequences of the form CV, CVC, VCV, and CVCV (Bertoncini and Mehler, 1981; Jusczyk and Thompson, 1978; Trehub, 1973); and an alternating CV pattern seems to enhance the infant's ability to discriminate variations in place, manner, and voicing. Since redundant syllable strings, such as [ba ba ba ba] (Goodsitt, Morse, and Ver Hoeve, 1984), further enhance this performance, we can conclude that the CV syllable train characterizing reduplicated babble is an excellent perceptual training ground for the infant.

The advantage of the CV syllable applies to production as well. This syllable form is one of the earliest syllables to be identified in infant vocalizations; the vocalizations of 1-year-olds are, predominantly, simple V or CV syllables and their elaborations, for example, VCV or CVCV (Kent and Bauer, 1985). Branigan (1976) regarded the CV sylla-ble as a training ground for consonant formation. Most consonants are produced first in the initial position of CV syllables and then, later, in postvocalic (e.g., VC) position.

The importance of the canonical CV syllable as a unit for perceptuomotor integration is indicated by its long-delayed appearance in the vocal development of hearing-impaired infants (Kent, Osberger, Netsell, and Hustedde, 1987; Oller, 1986). There is also evidence that early CV syllable production is linked, in a developmental chain, to the early word pro-duction and to the articulation of word-final consonants (Menyuk, Liebergott, and Schultz, 1986).

Speech acquisition is a complex process, one that involves learning a language (its syntax, semantics, and phonology)—a speech code that relates meaning to sound, and a motor skill by which the speech organs are controlled to produce rapid and overlapping movements. The layman often characterizes developing speech in the child by reference to frequently occurring substitutions (as when the child says *wabbit* for *rabbit* or *thee* for *see*) or other common misarticulations. But developing speech differs from adult speech in other ways.

First, children's speech generally is slower than adult speech. For example, McNeill (1974) reported speaking rates of slightly over 3 words per second for adults, about 2.5 words per second for 4- to 5-year-olds, and 1.6 words per second for children of about 2. Not surprisingly, then, the durations of individual segments are longer in children's speech (Naeser, 1970; Smith, 1978; Kent and Forner, 1980). Smith reported that the durations of nonsense utterances were 15 percent longer for 4-year-olds than for adults and 31 percent longer for 2-year-olds than for adults. Similarly, when Kent and Forner measured durations of phrases and short sentences, they found them to be 8 percent longer for 12-year-olds than for adults, 16 percent longer for 6-year-olds than for adults, and 33 percent longer for 4-year-olds than for adults. Some individual segments, such as the duration of stop closure, were observed by Kent and Forner to be twice as long in children's speech as in adult speech. The speaking rates of children have implications for both the production and per-ception of speech. It has been shown that children more successfully imitate sentences spo-ken at a rate nearer their own than at slower or faster rates (Bonvillian, Raeburn, and Horan, 1979).

Second, children's speech differs from adult speech in its variability. When children make the same utterance several times, the duration of individual segments varies more than for adults (Eguchi and Hirsh, 1969; Tingley and Allen, 1975; Kent and Forner, 1980). This difference in reliability of production may be an index of the child's linguistic and neuro-motor immaturity. In general, a young child's speech patterns are less well controlled than an adult's, and there is evidence that the control continues to improve until the child reaches puberty (Kent, 1976).

A third difference between the speech of children and adults is in patterns of coarticu-lation. Data on this difference are not abundant, but Thompson and Hixon (1979) reported that with increasing age, a greater proportion of their subjects showed nasal air flow begin-ning at the midpoint of the first vowel in /ini/. They interpreted this to mean that anticipa-tory coarticulation occurred earlier for progressively older subjects. In other words, more mature speakers show increased anticipation in producing a phonetic sequence.

In summary, young children differ from adults not only in their obvious misarticulations, but also in their slower speaking rates, greater variability (error) in production, and reduced anticipation in articulatory sequencing.

References

Adams, S. G., "Rate and clarity of speech: An x-ray microbeam study." Ph.D. dissertation, University of Wisconsin–Madison, 1990.

Beckman, M. E., "Stress and non-stress accent." *Netherlands Phonetic Archives 7.* Dordrecht: Foris, 1986.

Beckman, M. E., and J. Edwards, "Prosodic categories and duration control." *Journal of the Acoustical Society of America, 87,* Supplement 1 (1991): S65.

Behne, D., "Acoustic effects of focus and sentence position on stress in English and French." Ph.D. dissertation, University of Wisconsin–Madison, 1989.

Bernhardt, B., "Application of nonlinear phonology to intervention with six phonologically disordered children." Unpublished Ph.D. thesis, University of British Columbia, Vancouver, B.C., Canada, 1990.

Bernthal, J. E., and D. R. Beukelman, "Intraoral air pressures during the production of /p/ and /b/ by children, youths, and adults." *Journal of Speech and Hearing Research, 21* (1978): 361–371.

Bertoncini, J., and J. Mehler, "Syllables as units in infant speech perception." *Infant Behavior and Development, 4* (1981): 247–260.

Bock, J. K., "Toward a cognitive psychology of syntax: Information processing contributions to sentence formulation." *Psychological Review, 89* (1982): 1–47.

Bonvillian, J. D., V. P. Raeburn, and E. A. Horan, "Talking to children: The effects of rate, intonation, and length on children's sentence imitation." *Journal of Child Language, 6* (1979): 459–467.

Branigan, G., "Syllabic structure and the acquisition of consonants: The great conspiracy in word formation." *Journal of Psycholinguistic Research, 5* (1976): 117–133.

Branigan, G., "Some reasons why successive single word utterances are not." *Journal of Child Language, 6* (1979): 411–421.

Cavagna, G. A., and R. Margaria, "Airflow rates and efficiency changes during phonation." *Sound Production in Man, Annals of the New York Academy of Sciences, 155* (1968): 152–164.

Chiat, S., "The relation between prosodic structure, syllabification and segmental realization: Evidence from a child with fricative stopping." *Clinical Linguistics and Phonetics, 3* (1989): 223–242.

Chin, S. B., and D. A. Dinnsen, "Feature geometry in disordered phonologies." *Clinical Linguistics and Phonetics, 5* (1991): 329–337.

Chomsky, N., and M. Halle, *The Sound Pattern of English.* New York: Harper & Row, 1968.

Clements, G. N., and S. J. Keyser, *CV Phonology.* Cambridge, MA: M.I.T. Press, 1983.

Cohen, A., R. Collier, and J. t'Hart, "Declination: Construct or intrinsic feature of speech pitch?" *Phonetica, 39* (1982): 254–273.

Crystal, D., *Prosodic Systems and Intonation in English.* Cambridge (UK): Cambridge University Press, 1969.

Crystal, D., "Non-segmental phonology in language acquisition: A review of the issues." *Lingua, 32* (1973): 1–45.

Daniloff, R. G., and K. L. Moll, "Coarticulation of lip rounding." *Journal of Speech and Hearing Research, 11* (1968): 707–721.

Dewey, G., *Relative Frequency of English Speech Sounds.* Cambridge: Harvard University Press, 1923.

Eguchi, S., and I. J. Hirsh, "Development of speech sounds in children." *Acta Orolaryngologica,* Supplement No. 257 (1969).

Fry, D., "Duration and intensity as physical correlates of linguistic stress." *Journal of the Acoustical Society of America, 27* (1955): 765–768.

Gandour J., "The nondeviant nature of deviant

phonological systems." *Journal of Communication Disorders, 14* (1981): 11–29.

Giles, S. B., "A study of articulatory characteristics of /l/ allophones in English." Ph.D. dissertation, University of Iowa, 1971.

Goldsmith, J., "Autosegmental phonology." Ph.D. dissertation, Massachusetts Institute of Technology, 1976 (published by Garland Press, 1979).

Goldsmith, J. A., *Autosegmental and Metrical Phonology*. Oxford: Basil Blackwell, 1990.

Goodsitt, J., P. Morse, and J. Ver Hoeve, "Infant speech recognition in multisyllabic contexts." *Child Development, 55* (1984): 903–910.

Hardcastle, W. J., *Physiology of Speech Production*. London: Academic Press, 1976.

Hayes, B., "Metrics and phonological theory" (pp. 220–249). In F. Newmeyer (Ed.), *Linguistics: The Cambridge Survey. II. Linguistic Theory: Extensions and Implications*. Cambridge (UK): Cambridge University Press, 1988.

Hixon, T. J., "Mechanical aspects of speech production." Paper read at Annual Convention of the American Speech and Hearing Association, Chicago, November 17–20, 1971.

Hockett, C. F., "A manual of phonology." In *International Journal of American Linguistics (Memoir II)*. Baltimore: Waverly Press, 1955.

Hyman, L. M., *Phonology: Theory and Analysis*. New York: Holt, Rinehart and Winston, 1975.

Ingram, D., *Phonological Disability in Children*. New York: Elsevier, 1976.

Jong, K. J. de, "The oral articulation of English stress accent." Ph.D. dissertation, Ohio State University, Columbus, Ohio, 1991.

Jusczyk, P., and E. Thompson, "Perception of phonetic contrasts in multisyllabic utterances by 2 month old infants." *Perception and Psychophysics, 23* (1978): 105–109.

Kantner, C. E., and R. West, *Phonetics*. New York: Harper & Row, 1960.

Kent, R. D., "Anatomical and neuromuscular maturation of the speech mechanism: Evidence from acoustic studies." *Journal of Speech and Hearing Research, 19* (1976): 421–447.

Kent, R. D., and H. R. Bauer, "Vocalizations of one year olds." *Journal of Child Language, 12* (1985): 491–526.

Kent, R. D., and L. L. Forner, "Speech segment durations in sentence recitations by children and adults." *Journal of Phonetics, 8* (1980): 157–168.

Kent, R. D., R. E. Martin, and R. L. Sufit, "Oral sensation: A review and clinical prospective" (pp. 135–191). In H. Winitz (Ed.), *Human Communication and Its Disorders: A Review—1990*. Norwood, NJ: Ablex, 1990.

Kent, R. D., and F. D. Minifie, "Coarticulation in recent speech production models." *Journal of Phonetics, 5* (1977): 115–133.

Kent, R. D., and K. L. Moll, "Vocal-tract characteristics of the stop cognates." *Journal of the Acoustical Society of America, 46* (1969): 1549–1555.

Kent, R. D., and K. L. Moll, "Cinefluorographic analyses of selected lingual consonants." *Journal of Speech and Hearing Research, 15* (1972): 453–473.

Kent, R. D., and K. L. Moll, "Articulatory timing in selected consonant sequences." *Brain and Language, 2* (1975): 304–323.

Kent, R. D., and R. Netsell, "Effects of stress contrasts on certain articulatory parameters." *Phonetica, 24* (1972): 23–44.

Kent, R. D., M. J. Osberger, R. Netsell, and C. G. Hustedde, "Phonetic development in identical twins differing in auditory function." *Journal of Speech and Hearing Disorders, 52* (1987): 64–75.

Klatt, D. H., "Linguistic uses of segmental duration in English: Acoustic and perceptual evidence." *Journal of the Acoustical Society of America, 59* (1976): 1208–1221.

Ladefoged, P., *Preliminaries to Linguistic Phonetics*. Chicago: University of Chicago Press, 1971.

Ladefoged, P., *A Course in Phonetics*. New York: Harcourt Brace Jovanovich, 1975.

Lehiste, I., *Suprasegmentals*. Cambridge, MA: M.I.T. Press, 1970.

Lieberman, P., *Intonation, Perception and Language*. Cambridge, MA: M.I.T. Press, 1967.

Lindblom, B. E. F., "Spectrographic study of vowel reduction." *Journal of the Acoustical Society of America, 35* (1963): 1773–1781.

Lindblom, B., "Explaining phonetic variation: A sketch of the H&H theory" (pp. 403–439). In W. J. Hardcastle and A. Marchal (Eds.), *Speech Production and Speech Modelling*. Amsterdam, The Netherlands: Kluwer, 1990.

Lindblom, B., and R. Zetterström (Eds.), *Precursors of Early Speech Development*. New York: Stockton, 1986.

McCarthy, L., "Feature geometry and dependency: A review." *Journal of Phonetics, 43* (1988): 84–108.

MacNeilage, P. F., "Speech physiology" (pp. 1–72). In H. H. Gilbert (Ed.), *Speech and Cortical Functioning*. New York: Academic Press, 1972.

McNeill, D., "The two-fold way for speech." In *Problèmes Actuels en Psycholinguistique*. Paris: Editions du Centre National de la Recherche Scientifique, 1974.

Menyuk, P., J. Liebergott, and M. Schultz, "Predicting phonological development" (pp. 79–93). In B. Lindblom and R. Zetterström (Eds.), *Precursors of Early Speech*. Basingstoke, Hampshire (UK): MacMillan, 1986.

Moll, K. L., and R. G. Daniloff, "Investigation of the timing of velar movements during speech." *Journal of the Acoustical Society of America, 50* (1971): 678–684.

Moon, S. J., and B. Lindblom, "Formant undershoot in clear and citation-form speech: A second progress report." *Royal Institute of Technology (Stockholm, Sweden) Speech Transmission Laboratory, Quarterly Progress and Status Reports, 1* (1989): 121–123.

Naeser, M. A., "The American child's acquisition of differential vowel duration." Technical Report No. 144, Wisconsin Research and Development Center for Cognitive Learning, University of Wisconsin, Madison, 1970.

Oller, D. K., "Metaphonology of infant vocalizations" (pp. 21–35). In B. Lindblom and R. Zetterström (Eds.), *Precursors of Early Speech*. Basingstoke, Hampshire (UK): MacMillan, 1986.

Parker, F., "Distinctive features in speech pathology: Phonology or phonemics?" *Journal of Speech and Hearing Disorders, 41* (1976): 23–39.

Perkell, J. S., *Physiology of Speech Production*. Cambridge, MA: M.I.T. Press, 1969.

Picheny, M. A., N. I. Durlach, and L. D. Braida, "Speaking clearly for the hard of hearing. II: Acoustic characteristics of clear and conversational speech." *Journal of Speech and Hearing Research, 29* (1986): 434–446.

Rabiner, L., H. Levitt, and A. Rosenberg, "Investigation of stress patterns for speech synthesis by rule." *Journal of the Acoustical Society of America, 45* (1969): 92–101.

Read, C., and P. A. Schreiber, "Why short subjects are harder to find than long ones." In E. Wanner and L. Gleitman (Eds.), *Language Acquisition: The State of the Art*. Cambridge (UK): Cambridge University Press, 1982.

Sagey, E., "The representation of features and relations in non-linear phonology." Unpublished Ph.D. thesis, Massachusetts Institute of Technology, Cambridge, Massachusetts, 1986.

Schwartz, R. G., "Nonlinear phonology as a framework for phonological acquisition." In R. S. Chapman (Ed.), *Processes in Language Acquisition and Disorders*. Chicago: Mosby-Year Book, 1992.

Sloat, C., S. H. Taylor, and J. E. Hoard, *Introduction to Phonology*. Englewood Cliffs, NJ: Prentice Hall, 1978.

Smith, B. L., "Temporal aspects of English speech production: A developmental perspective." *Journal of Phonetics, 6* (1978): 37–68.

Spencer, A., "A nonlinear analysis of phonological disability." *Journal of Communication Disorders, 17* (1984): 325–348.

Spencer, A., "A phonological theory of phonological development" (pp. 115–151). In M. J. Ball (Ed.), *Theoretical Linguistics and Disordered Language*. London: Croon Helm, 1988.

Stampe, D., "The acquisition of phonetic representation" (pp. 443–453). In R. I. Binnick et al. (Eds.), *Papers from the Fifth Regional Meeting of the Chicago Linguistics Society*. Chicago: Chicago Linguistics Society, 1969.

Stampe, D., "A dissertation of natural phonology." Ph.D. dissertation, University of Chicago, 1972.

Subtelny, J., J. Worth, and M. Sakuda, "Intraoral

pressure and rate of flow during speech." *Journal of Speech and Hearing Research, 9* (1966): 498–518.

Thompson, A. E., and T. J. Hixon, "Nasal air flow during speech production." *Cleft Palate Journal, 16* (1979): 412–420.

Tingley, B. M., and G. D. Allen, "Development of speech timing control in children." *Child Development, 46* (1975): 186–194.

Trehub, S., "Infants' sensitivity to vowel and tonal contrasts." *Developmental Psychology, 9* (1973): 91–96.

Walsh, H., "On certain practical inadequacies of distinctive feature systems." *Journal of Speech and Hearing Disorders, 39* (1974): 32–43.

Wise, C. M., *Introduction to Phonetics*. Englewood Cliffs, NJ: Prentice Hall, 1957a.

Wise, C. M., *Applied Phonetics*. Englewood Cliffs, NJ: Prentice Hall, 1957b.

Chapter 2

Early Phonological Development

MARILYN MAY VIHMAN
University of Wales–Bangor

As a prelude to our discussion of normal phonological development, let us consider what a child accomplishes in a mere three or four years of exposure to language. At the outset of adultlike vocal production, sometimes called the babbling period, the vocalizations of children exposed to different languages are virtually indistinguishable (Atkinson, MacWhinney, and Stoel, 1968). Babies learning languages as different as English and Spanish (Thevenin, Eilers, Oller, and LaVoie, 1985) or French and Chinese (Boysson-Bardies, Sagart, and Durand, 1984) cannot be reliably distinguished, based on tape recordings, by adult judges speaking one of these languages. Francescato suggested that "two hypotheses are possible: Either all children, of all languages, at the beginning of their linguistic activity share the 'same' language, or every child, of every language, speaks from the beginning its own language" (1968: 152f.). Today, the consensus seems to be that both hypotheses are true. Children in different language environments draw on the same "universal" repertoire of syllable shapes and sounds. At the same time, it seems that each child creates, out of these universal syllable shapes and sounds, a unique subset of sound preferences and patterns as he or she develops a phonological and communicative system of his or her own. Gradually, these unique or idiosyncratic patterns accommodate to and, finally, are replaced by the adult system to which the child is exposed.

In a remarkably short time most children develop intelligible speech. In fact, they even come to articulate well enough so that people outside the immediate family can understand what they are saying. At that point, the child can already be recognized as a member of a specific language community by his or her speech patterns; that is, he or she will have acquired the incidental phonetically distinguishing features as well as the system of contrasting sounds of the specific language spoken in his or her environment. In other words, in learning the phonology of, for example, American English, the infant also will have learned to pronounce like an American from Kansas or California or New Jersey. How do such profound changes take place in such a short time? The challenge of research in phonological development is to arrive at a better understanding of this process.

Models of Phonological Development: The Child as an Active Learner

Linguists and psychologists have long sought to explain how children learn to distinguish and produce the sound patterns of the adult language. Not surprisingly, the earliest studies were largely *diary studies* or descriptions of the investigator's own child; several detailed studies of this sort were available by the 1940s. The first well-articulated model of phonological development—namely, Jakobson's structuralist model—was formulated at that time. Although it continues to be influential today, a number of other models, based on different perspectives and assumptions, have since been proposed (cf. Ferguson and Garnica, 1975; Ferguson, Menn, and Stoel-Gammon, 1992). In the past 20 years, there has been a notable increase in available data, due, in part, to the advent of tape recording as a common observational procedure, and, at the same time, there has been a shift in thinking about other areas of language acquisition. The earlier structuralist model presupposed little initiative on the part of the learner. Today, however, most investigators agree that the child, whose goal is to "sound like the adults around her" (Menn, 1981; 131), is an active participant in the learning process.

Behaviorist Model

In the United States, the prevailing view from the 1950s to the early 1970s was the behaviorist model associated with Mowrer (1960) and Olmsted (1971). This model applied a psychological theory of learning to the human infant and emphasized the role of contingent reinforcement in speech acquisition. The child's babbling was held to be gradually "shaped," through classical conditioning principles, into forms appropriate for the adult speech community in question. Specifically, it was held that, in the course of the daily caretaking routines of feeding and changing, the infant comes to associate the vocalizations of the caretaker, usually the mother, with "primary reinforcement," such as food and comfort; thus, the adult's vocalizations acquire the value of "secondary reinforcement." The child's own vocalizations acquire secondary reinforcing value as well, by virtue of their similarity to the caretaker's vocalizations. The speech sound repertoire is further refined as the caretaker selectively reinforces sounds that resemble those used in the adult language and as the child is "self-reinforced" for producing sounds that match those in the environment.

Structuralist Model

In contrast to the behaviorists, who drew on psychological theory for their assumptions about learning, Jakobson (1941/68) drew on the linguists' structuralist theory of language to account for the observed phenomena of babbling and early speech. Jakobson postulated that phonological development follows a universal and innate order of acquisition. The distinctive features, arranged in a hierarchy, "unfold" in a predictable order as the child produces phonemic contrasts embodying them. The child was thought to start with two maximally contrasting sounds: a bilabial stop, /p/, and a low vowel, /a/. The child then begins to differentiate the consonant system by acquiring the contrast between nasal and oral: /p/ (oral) versus /m/ (nasal). The next feature contrast divides both oral and nasal consonants into a labial (/p/, /m/) and a dental pair (/t/, /n/). Jakobson proposed that the child's consonant and vowel systems continue to diversify and differentiate, step by step, as the child learns new feature contrasts. Features needed to differentiate stops, nasals, bilabials, and dentals were held to be acquired earlier than those needed to differentiate fricatives, affricates, and liquids. It should be pointed out that for Jakobson, babbling was a random activity which had little, if anything, to do with the development of the sound system of language.

Comment on the Behaviorist and Structuralist Models

Both the behaviorist and structuralist models concentrated on the relation between babbling and early speech. The behaviorists emphasized **continuity** between these two kinds of early vocalization. The structuralists, on the other hand, insisted on a **discontinuity** between the two, a view which followed from their conception of language as an autonomous structured system. The behaviorist paradigm is no longer widely accepted today as a model for language acquisition, primarily because it fails to account for the infinite capacity to produce *new patterns* that is the hallmark of human language (cf. Chomsky's [1959] critique of B. F. Skinner's *Verbal Behavior*): With specific reference to phonology, there is little evidence that caretakers selectively reward (or "shape") the child's sound productions in the prelinguistic period.

Though Jakobson's views provided a vital stimulus to research and are still widely cited, recent data have tended to weaken several aspects of his position. For one thing, the existence of regularities in prelinguistic (or babbling) vocal patterns has now been clearly demonstrated (cf., e.g., Ferguson and Macken, 1983) as has the gradual emergence of adult-based word shapes from the babble vocalizations (Vihman, Macken, Miller, Simmons, and Miller, 1985). Thus, the hypothesis of discontinuity between babble and speech appears to be unfounded.

A more basic difficulty is Jakobson's postulation of phonemic contrast as the basis of phonological development in the earliest stages. As Kiparsky and Menn (1977) pointed out, the corpus of words a child begins with is typically too small to provide clear evidence for or against the hypothesized sequence of **phonemic oppositions**. No set order of use of consonants is evident in the early words of the many different children whose data have been carefully recorded and analyzed. More importantly, the order of emergence of phonemic oppositions (nasal vs. oral, labial vs. dental) is extremely difficult to ascertain, as this requires an evaluation of the child's system based on the adult phonemes attempted as well as on the phonemic patterns used by the child. The undertaking is further complicated since many children seem to selectively **avoid** attempting words that include certain consonants. In fact, the child is now widely thought to be targeting *whole-word shapes* rather than individual segments or phonemes (Ferguson and Farwell, 1975). Furthermore, in light of the great *variability* found to be characteristic of early child forms, the issue of a universal order of acquisition of phonemes has lost much of its original interest.

Natural Phonology Model

The natural phonology model proposed by Stampe also emphasizes the universal and maturational aspect of phonological acquisition (Stampe, 1969; Donegan and Stampe, 1979). According to Stampe, the child comes innately equipped with a universal set of phonological processes—operations which change or delete phonological units—that reflect the natural limitations and capacities of human vocal production and perception. The innate processes correspond to the phonological regularities found in the languages of the world; the child's task is to suppress those processes which do not occur in the particular adult language to which he or she is exposed. For example, a child may be expected to devoice word-final obstruents (i.e., at first, the English-speaking child would pronounce *bad* as [bæt]), since this is a phonetically natural process found in many languages. In German, where *Hund* ('dog') is pronounced [hunt], the devoicing process accurately reflects adult phonology, and thus, the German-speaking child need not "suppress" it; however, the English-speaking child must suppress the process to match adult pronunciation (eventually producing *bad* as [bæd]).

Generative Phonology Model

Another influential model was developed in the 1970s by Smith (1973). Smith presented a lengthy formal description of the phonology of his son Amahl, from age 2 to 4. He described the child's phonology in terms of two distinct models: (1) a mapping of the adult forms into the child's, using "re-write rules" (e.g., "/f, v/ become [w] prevocalically," or in other words, "rewrite /f/ or /v/ as [w] . . ." to account for *feet* → [wi:t], *fork* → [wɔ:k], etc.); and (2) an account of the child's system viewed in its own right, with the functional units and their interrelations defined and organized differently than in the adult system. Smith concluded that there is no psychological reality to the child's system; that is, he found no evidence that the system which seemed to underlie the child's forms, irrespective of the latter's relationship to the adult models, was productive. It did not bear upon the child's response to unfamiliar adult forms, his or her phonological treatment of new forms, or his or her reorganization of older forms under the influence of new patterns. Smith postulated a set of ordered universal tendencies, such as the use of consonant and vowel harmony and cluster reduction, that he considered to be either innate or learned very early.

Comment on the Natural Phonology and Generative Phonology Models

In recent years, the natural phonology and generative phonology models have been influential in clinical practice by disordered speakers. The models of Stampe and Smith agree in several respects. Both reject the possibility of the child having a system of his or her own. Both insist on the "innate" or universal status of child phonological rules or processes—a position which remains highly controversial, though use of the term *process* and of the rewrite or realization rule format has become general in the fields of normal and disordered child phonology (cf. Ingram, 1976; Grunwell, 1981; Edwards and Shriberg, 1983). Finally, both assume full, accurate perception from the earliest stages of speech production; that is, the child is assumed to perceive and store or *represent* speech forms correctly. According to this position, it is the innate constraints on the child's *production* that lead to simplification in the child's output forms.

Prosodic Model

Waterson's (1971, 1981) prosodic model is rooted in the linguistic theory developed by J. R. Firth. Firth's prosodic linguistics differs sharply from traditional (especially American) linguistic practice, which has emphasized rules affecting individual segments. Waterson, like other Firthian linguists, focuses on the *word* rather than the segment as a basic unit of phonological structure. She describes groups of early words as schemata that share certain overall features derived from the adult form, such as intonation pattern, syllable structure, nasality, continuance (presence of fricatives), or voicing. In Waterson's view, the child's perception of the phonetic features of adult words is incomplete or partial at first. For Waterson and others (e.g., Braine, 1976; Maxwell, 1984), both child perception and production are likely to involve imperfect matches with the adult model at first, and therefore, both must undergo development and change before the child can arrive at an adult-like system.

Cognitive Model

Another widely adopted perspective is the "cognitive" or "problem-solving" model (Menn, 1983; Macken and Ferguson, 1983; Ferguson, 1978, 1986). In this view, the child encounters and eventually masters a series of challenges in acquiring the phonological system of the adult language. Individual strategies vary considerably across children, probably depending on their natural predispositions as well as on a number of external factors (such as the child's birth order and the interactional style of the primary caretakers).

Longitudinal studies have provided converging evidence for the view that active hypothesis testing and problem solving play an important role in phonological acquisition. Some of the major types of evidence follow.

Selectivity in Early Word Choice

In their earliest word productions, children have been found to begin by targeting adult words of certain shapes while avoiding sounds or sound patterns which are outside their repertoire. For example, one child initially used only two-syllable words with open syllables beginning with a stop or nasal (*daddy, mommy, doggy, patty(-cake)*), and *bye-bye:* Ferguson, Peizer, and Weeks, 1973). Different children begin by mastering different articulatory patterns and, accordingly, by attempting different (identifiable) adult words.

Unique Reduction Devices

Children use unique reduction devices to produce long words (Ferguson, 1978). For example, Priestly (1977) described the use by his son Christopher of the pattern [CVjVC] to produce a number of polysyllabic words—for example, *Panda* → [pajan], *berries* → [bɛjas], and *tiger* → [tajak]. Though these "exploratory forms" fail to match the adult forms in segmental terms, they accurately, if idiosyncratically, capture the correct syllable count.

"Phonological Idioms" and Regression

A child may first produce a complex adult word in a relatively advanced form (e.g., *pretty*, pronounced [prəti]) and only later revert to a simplified form which conforms more closely to the other forms in his or her productive vocabulary (e.g., *pretty* → [bɪdi]; Leopold, 1947). In such cases, the child apparently takes a step backward or regresses since the new form is farther from the adult model. On the other hand, the new form fits into the child's own emerging **phonological system**. Thus, the **regression** seems to reflect systematization on the child's part, suggesting that the child's own system has psychological validity of some sort.

Comment on the Prosodic and Cognitive Models

Waterson's approach provides a useful complement to the phonological process-based (segmental) analysis, which was most widespread in the 1970s. In particular, Waterson is able to capture the "gestalt" or the "canonical form" underlying certain child productions that are highly irregular in terms of segment-by-segment comparison with the adult model. Waterson also differs with Stampe and Smith in her position regarding perception in the period of early words.

Like Waterson, the cognitive model focuses primarily on the earliest period of word production, when the child appears to be targeting whole words rather than segments (Ferguson and Farwell, 1975; Menyuk, Menn, and Silber, 1986). Although Waterson did not frame her findings in those terms, her prosodic analyses of child language data provide rich illustrations of the characteristic **individuality** of early phonological development later emphasized by the cognitive model. In fact, that model may be criticized for overemphasizing the individual creative aspects of phonological acquisition. Within the framework of the biologically possible, the child is seen as having considerable space for active exploration, hypothesis-formation, and systematization. Little attention is paid to the **constraints** on learning which may result from maturation, both physiological and psychological, or from the structure of language in general and also from the particular language of the child's environment.

Biological Model

Locke (1983, 1990; Locke and Pearson, 1992) has proposed a biological model of the origins of phonological system in the child (cf. also Kent, 1992). He suggests that innate perceptual biases and dispositions to certain motor action are at the root of phonological acquisition. In babbling, the child's phonetic repertoire is essentially universal, being constrained by biological factors such as the size and shape of the infant vocal tract and the relative complexity of neuromotor control required for various articulations. For example, simply raising and lowering the jaw can result in alveolar stop production at a time when independent manipulation of the tongue has not yet come under voluntary control (Locke, 1993; see also Davis and MacNeilage, 1990; MacNeilage and Davis, 1990). Babbling is critical in that it allows the child to construct auditory-kinesthetic links which can serve as a phonetic guidance system for acquiring language (Fry, 1966; Vihman, 1991).

Influence from the language of the child's environment is thought to emerge only with the production of first words, and is based on the storage and retrieval of some relatively stable perceived forms of the language. However, constraints on production remain basically unchanged until the child has a larger vocabulary (by about 18 months), and begins to deviate from the biologically given babbling production patterns to produce forms that reflect specific phonetic characteristics of the target adult language. At this point the child manifests the developmental mechanisms of **maintenance** (of babbling production patterns which occur in the adult language as well), **learning** (of patterns of the adult language not found in babbling), and **loss** (of patterns not found in the adult language).

Self-Organizing Model

Biological and linguistic approaches to vocal development have converged in the idea of self-organizing principles (Lindblom, 1992). According to his view, phonetic forms in all languages have evolved to meet the complementary needs of the two participants in vocal communication, the *listener* and the *speaker*. The needs of the listener are met when a language uses vowels such as /i/, /a/, and /u/, which are maximally distant from one another and thus *easy to discriminate*. On the other hand, the needs of the speaker are met when a language uses consonant-vowel sequences which require little tongue movement and are thus *easy to articulate*, such as apico-dental /t/ followed by a front (or "apical") vowel (/i/), or velar /k/ followed by a back vowel (/u/). The compromise between these two sets of **performance constraints** leads to phonetic universals, specifying "core" segments used in most languages and "exotic" segments which occur only in languages with large phonetic inventories.

In the case of the child learning to speak, a small number of articulatory gestures are used over and over in different combinations to produce word patterns, or articulatory **motor scores** corresponding to **unitary acoustic patterns**. The overlapping use of the same articulatory gestures to produce different word patterns or syllables (/ti/, /tu/, /ki/, /ku/) will eventually lead to the emergence of a network of phonologically contrastive segments (/t/, /k/, /i/, /u/) by "self-segmentation."

Comment on the Biological and Self-Organizing Models

Despite the evidence that problem solving plays a role in phonology, as in other areas of learning, universal biologically or linguistically based constraints undoubtedly set the parameters within which acquisition must occur. Beyond this, both **maturation** (natural biological development and change) and **practice** may be said to influence learning. Both Locke's and Lindblom's models are similar to Jakobson's in their emphasis on the *universal* aspects of early speech. However, neither model accepts the notion of *discontinuity* between babbling and speech.

An apparent difficulty for Locke's view is the extent of **individual differences** that have been reported among children from a single language background in the babbling stage (Vihman, Ferguson and Elbert, 1986). If the earliest period of linguistic development is under relatively strict biological or maturational control, one might expect greater uniformity across infants at this stage. However, genetic variation across individual members of a species is the rule in developmental biology and may account for the early differences in phonetic production (Locke, 1988). On the other hand, some global influence of the specific ambient language has been detected in infant vocalizations as early as 10 months (cf. Boysson-Bardies, Hallé, Sagart and Durand, 1989; cf. Boysson-Bardies and Vihman, 1991), suggesting that phonetic "learning" must begin in the pre-lexical period.

The basis of the principle of self-organization is that neither genetic specification nor linguistic input is sufficient to account for the development of a phonological system, but that the *interaction* of the two promotes novelty and complexity in the child's emergent system.

Nonlinear Phonology

In the 1980s a new type of formal model of adult phonology gained widespread attention and acceptance. The term **nonlinear phonology** is sometimes used to cover this entire family of formal models of somewhat different types, since they have in common a deemphasis on rules or processes, with their associated (linear) segmental strings, and a new focus on prosodic phenomena. The term *prosodic* must be understood to refer to two different kinds of phenomena, neither of them identifiable at the level of the individual segment: (1) so-called **suprasegmental phenomena**, such as word-accent involving stress or tone, which take at least a whole word or syllable as their domain, and (2) other whole-word-based phenomena, formerly understood by the term *phonotactics* or arrangements of sounds, such as the permissibility of particular consonant sequences, vowel sequences, or syllable-final consonants (recall Waterson's prosodic model). In these new models, representations are regarded

> less as a sequence of segmental "beads on a string" than as analogous to an orchestral score in which the synchronization of each instrument with the other instruments is as much a part of the score as the actual notes each is to play. In phonological terms, the "instruments" are the various separable components of the speech apparatus. (Anderson, 1985, 348)

Some of the new modes which fit under the general rubric **nonlinear** are autosegmental, metrical and lexical phonology (Goldsmith, 1990), prosodic phonology (Nespor and Vogel, 1986—not to be confused with Waterson's earlier model), and articulatory phonology (Browman and Goldstein, 1992). A promising recent outgrowth of this perspective is optimality theory, in which rules are dispensed with entirely, being replaced by permissible patterns or constraints (Paradis, 1988).

Nonlinear models offer important advantages in accounting for developmental data. As Menn (1978) pointed out, two properties of autosegmental formalism are particularly well suited to the description of children's phonological systems: (1) the possibility of specifying domains of application for phonetic features which extend beyond the segment, such as the syllable or the word; and (2) the freedom from sequential ordering of features which results from placing them on separate tiers, or levels of organization (see Figure 2.1). The separate specification of features that affect only or mainly consonants (glottalization, retroflexion)

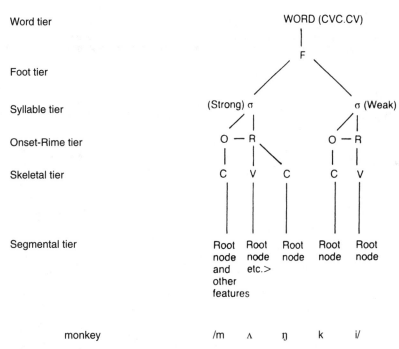

Word tier   WORD (CVC.CV)

Foot tier

Syllable tier   (Strong) σ   σ (Weak)

Onset-Rime tier   O — R   O — R

Skeletal tier   C   V   C   C   V

Segmental tier   Root Root Root   Root Root
                                                       node node node   node node
                                                       and   etc.>
                                                       other
                                                       features

              monkey   /m   ʌ   ŋ   k   i/

Key   F = Foot. This is composed of a strong and weak syllable.
      σ = Syllable.
      O = Onset. This includes all prevocalic consonants (C) in a syllable.
      R = Rhyme/Rime. This includes the vowel (V) and postvocalic consonants
          in a syllable

FIGURE 2.1   Nonlinear representation of the word *monkey*.

Source: Bernhardt and Stoel-Gammon (1994), reprinted by permission of the American Speech-Language-Hearing Association.

or only vowels (vowel harmony, nasalization) in adult language provides a natural format for dealing with consonant harmony, a very common pattern in child phonology that is rarely encountered in adult languages. The reordering of adult segments, or apparent metathesis, is also often reflected in child forms. The notion of specifying different features on different tiers provides a useful account for the reordering of heterogeneous segments.

Later applications of nonlinear models to child data have made bolder departures from the generative model. For example, Velleman (1992) suggested that whole levels of representation may be lacking in the initial stages of phonological organization, notably skeletal (CV) or segmental levels (see Figure 2.2). Similarly, the child's representation may lack branching, either at the word level (if only monosyllabic words are produced: see Figure 2.2, 14 and 15 mos.) or at the syllable level (no clusters, diphthongs, or syllable-final consonants are produced: contrast the first and second syllables of *monkey* in Figure 2.1).

The notion of planar segregation has proven highly useful for analyzing child data. The idea is that features can spread only within a plane or tier, so that consonants affect

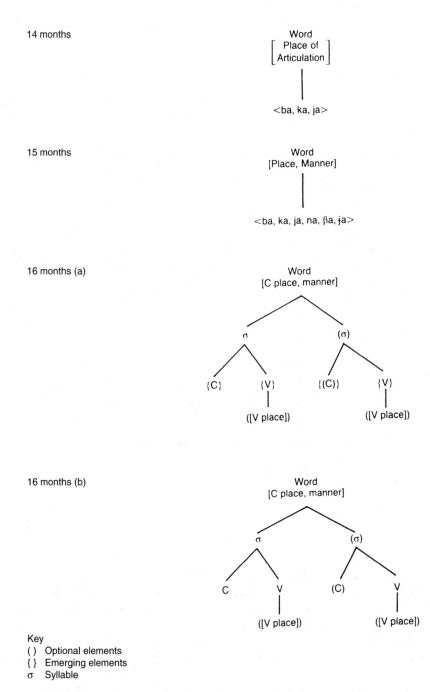

14 months

Word
[Place of
Articulation]

<ba, ka, ja>

15 months

Word
[Place, Manner]

<ba, ka, ja, na, βa, ɟa>

16 months (a)

Word
[C place, manner]

σ   (σ)

{C}   {V}   {(C)}   {V}

([V place])   ([V place])

16 months (b)

Word
[C place, manner]

σ   (σ)

C   V   (C)   V

([V place])   ([V place])

Key
( ) Optional elements
{ } Emerging elements
σ   Syllable

FIGURE 2.2   Development of a lexical representation.

Source: Vihman, M.M., Vellman, S., and McCune, L., 1994. In Yavas (Ed.), *First and Second Language Phonology*. Reprinted with the permission of Singular Publishing Group.

consonants or vowels affect vowels (resulting in consonant or vowel harmony, respectively), with no concomitant C to V or V to C effects. Underspecification of features and the inclusion in lexical representation of default features also play a role in these models, though the interpretation of particular data as motivating one or another of these accounts remains controversial (Spencer, 1986; Iverson and Wheeler, 1987; Stemberger and Stoel-Gammon, 1991). In short, planar segregation, underspecification of features and default features are all ways of expressing a relative lack of complexity in the child's initial representations.

Nonlinear models are, in principle, equally compatible with nativist and functionalist development approaches to the acquisition of phonology. Following Chomsky's (1981) parameter-setting model of language acquisition, Bernhardt (1994) has proposed a nativist interpretation:

> If a child comes to the language-learning situation with a representational framework and a set of universal principles, "templates" are then available to utilize for decoding and encoding. . . . Exposure to the input language(s) will both confirm the universally-determined representation (e.g., that, as expected, the language has CV units and stop consonants) and also result in "setting" of parameters where options are available (e.g., that the language has final consonants and that stress is syllable-initial in a given language) . . . (161) [See also the excellent tutorial in nonlinear phonology and its application to phonological disorders: Bernhardt and Stoel-Gammon, 1994.]

An alternative functionalist interpretation of the establishment of the expectation of CV syllables and stop consonants is equally plausible and follows quite naturally from the character of vocal development in the first year (see below). However,

> whether these options are available to all children, specified by innate parameters, determined by some characteristics of the language to which the child is exposed, "chosen" by the child based on idiosyncratic perceptual, physiological, or cognitive biases, or some combination of the above is an open and widely debated question. In any case, the course of phonological development includes the addition of complexity to any or all of these aspects of the representation. (Vihman, Velleman, and McCune, 1994, 20)

Summary

The earlier behaviorist and structuralist models developed out of the prevailing American and European linguistic schools of the midcentury and were, to a great extent, deductive rather than empirically based. Extensive analysis of the vocal productions of children in the past two decades has led to rejection, for the most part, of both these views. More controversial currently are the remaining models. Stampe and Smith emphasize universal constraints and a systematic, smooth progression toward the adult model; both explicitly deny any reality to the child's own system, and both posit accurate perception of the adult forms from the start. Waterson, on the other hand, allows for individual or idiosyncratic child systems, based on imperfect perception of adult forms. Ferguson, Macken, and Menn emphasize the active role of the child, involving individual strategies, hypothesis-formation, and problem-solving. The work of Locke, Kent, and Lindblom complements rather than competes with the prosodic and cognitive models, reflecting current renewed interest in the biological roots of language in mankind as well as in the individual child. Finally, the more recent formal models of adult phonology, nonlinear models, provide a new perspective on developing structure which is better adapted to child phonology than were earlier, segmentally-based generative models.

Infant Perception: Breaking into the Code

Having reviewed the main theories of normal phonological development, we will now present a chronological account of infant perception and production. We begin with speech perception by infants, since perception of the sounds of the adult language would logically seem to precede adultlike sound production. Perception and production are thought to develop in parallel but to interact with each other. Perception and production are treated separately here for expository purposes only.

The study of infant perception is a relatively new field of inquiry, dating back to the early 1970s. Nevertheless, research findings in this area are abundant. The data base is sufficient to establish that very young infants are capable of differentiating most of the sounds used in speech. In attempting to construct a picture of the child's phonological acquisition, we start with these findings since they afford a clue to the perceptual capacities with which the infant first begins to attend to the "blooming buzzing confusion" around him.

Problems Facing the Child

At the outset of our inquiry, we must ask how the child gets started on the difficult task of "learning to pronounce." To begin with, what do we know about how the child hears the sounds of language? The stream of speech is not naturally segmented into separate sounds, but rather consists of a continuous flow of overlapping sounds. This presents a **segmentation** problem for the infant. The adult listener applies his or her knowledge of the language to pick out contrasting syllables and segments as well as words and phrases. But what of the naive ear of the infant? How does the child pick out the sound units of language?

Equally problematic is the question of **perceptual constancy**. How does the child listening to speech decide what counts as the "same sound," despite differences in the physical features of the sound? The acoustic signals produced by males, females, and children are quite different due to significant differences in vocal tract size and configuration. Equally important acoustic differences result from differences in phonetic context (e.g., consonant before /i/ versus /u/), positional context (e.g., word-initial versus word-final), and rate (e.g., the rapid, fluent speech of "small talk" versus the slower, more hesitant production of carefully considered discourse). How does the child recognize as the "same sound" variations associated with different speakers, different contexts, and different rates of speech?

Research Methodology Used to Study Infant Perception

A considerable body of evidence concerning the perceptual abilities of infants is available as a result of the ingenious research methodologies developed in the past two decades.

These methodologies are based on a simple observation: Infants like older people, react to *changes* they perceive in their environment and become bored by ("habituate to") repetitions of the same event.

In 1971, Eimas, Siqueland, Jusczyk, and Vigorito reported a procedure known as the **high-amplitude sucking** paradigm to test infants' discrimination of voiced and voiceless and aspirated and unaspirated stops. This procedure has been used to obtain data on the discriminatory skills of infants from birth to 3 or 4 months of age. It allows the infant to control the presentation of a speech stimulus by the rate of sucking on a pacifier attached to a pressure transducer. Once the infant's baseline sucking rate has been established, a repeating speech stimulus such as [pa pa pa] is presented. The frequency of repetition of the sound is controlled by the infant's sucking rate. The presentation of the speech sound is presumed to serve as "contingent reinforcement" for the infant; increased sucking is interpreted as an expression of awareness of, and interest in, the sound stimulus. After several minutes, the infant's sucking rate typically levels off (reaches asymptote) and then decreases. Decreased sucking is taken to indicate that the infant has habituated and is no longer interested in the stimulus. The stimulus is then changed for the experimental group of infants, who hear a different repeated syllable (e.g., [ba ba ba]), while the infants in the control group continue to hear the sound stimulus first presented.

The sucking responses of the experimental group during this changed-stimulus condition are compared with those of the control group, which receives only a single stimulus throughout the experiment. If, following presentation of the second stimulus, the experimental group increases its sucking response while the control group maintains or slows its sucking rate, it is inferred that the experimental subjects perceive the difference between the two stimuli.

The other procedure most often used to test infant perception is the **visually reinforced head turn**, which is most appropriate for older infants (aged 6 to 12 months). Originally developed for assessing audiometric thresholds, this localization technique typically presents a repeated background sound for a time, follows it with a minimally different stimulus for a few seconds, and then repeats the original background stimulus. A head turn toward the sound source when the second sound is introduced is reinforced with the presentation of a lighted, animated toy that "rewards" the infant for discriminating the new sound from the old. If the infant turns his or her head during **change** trials (in which a new sound is introduced) but not during **control** trials (in which the same sound continues to be presented), it is concluded that the infant is able to discriminate the two contrasting sounds.

There are difficulties in the use of each of these procedures. In particular, since not all infants will habituate, large numbers of subjects must be tested to obtain statistically meaningful results. Nevertheless, several of the findings have been replicated many times over, in different laboratories by different investigators, so the results appear to be robust.

Categorical Perception

The acoustic cues relevant to speech sounds—such as the cues associated with voicing and aspiration or with place of articulation—may vary along a continuous parameter, but adults respond to these acoustic signals as if sharp boundaries were present at specific points along the continuum. For example, in producing the syllable /pa/ or /ba/, the speaker completely closes off the flow of air through the vocal tract (by bringing his or her lips together) and then releases the closure (by opening his or her mouth) in order to produce the following vowel. The difference between /p/ and /b/ is determined by the timing of the opening of the lips and the onset of vocal-cord vibration for vowel production. If the vocal cords begin to vibrate *before* the release of the oral closure, the stop is "pre-voiced," as in French word-initial /b/ or English intervocalic /b/. If the vocal cords begin to vibrate *at about the same time* that the lips are opened, an English (word-initial) /b/ is heard, but if the vibration of the vocal cords is *delayed*, English (word-initial) /p/ (aspirated [pʰ]) is heard. The parameter just described is referred to as *voice onset time*, or VOT.

A continuum of VOT possibilities exists beyond those associated with English "pre-voiced" (intervocalic) /b/, word-initial /b/, and word-initial /p/, although most languages seem to make use of one or more of these three in their phonemic system. Using **speech synthesis** (the artificial production of speech sounds), investigators have tested adult perception of the acoustic cues corresponding to the VOT continuum (Lisker and Abramson, 1964). Presented with a series of synthetic speech-like sounds resembling a range of different VOT values, adults generally perceive the stimuli as belonging to one of the phonemic categories distinguished in their own language. Thus, English-speakers hear virtually all stimuli as either /ba/ or /pa/, as if a sharp boundary divided the two; this is known as **categorical perception**. For some years, these findings were assumed to reflect adults' experience with the categories of their language. However, research with infants led to the surprising finding that 2- to 4-month-old babies also hear in terms of categories—despite their inexperience with the sounds of any language. The infants do not discriminate between acoustically different stimuli *within* the adult categories, but they are able to discriminate similar acoustic differences *between* categories.

English /b/ versus /p/ are discriminated by infants as if the two phonemic categories were known to them. This finding was initially attributed to an *innate mechanism* in humans for the recognition of speech categories. Later research has shown that not only human infants but also chinchillas and monkeys can distinguish this categorical boundary (Kuhl, 1987). So the argument for an innate human mechanism *specialized for speech perceptions* lacks strong supporting evidence. It is more likely that the phonetic boundary between the English language categories of voiceless and voiced stops happens to correspond to a *naturally salient physical boundary* distinguished by infants, whether or not they have been exposed to English, and also by certain mammals possessing auditory biases similar to those of humans.

The human auditory system seems to be especially attuned to **abrupt discontinuities**, or natural breaks, in the acoustic stream, like those created by stop consonants. Such a phonetic predisposition, together with the ability to discriminate continuous acoustic signals in a categorical way, may be crucial in enabling the child to solve the segmentation problem; that is, to break into a code based on overlapping sounds embedded in an ongoing speech stream.

Universal Perception: Early Abilities

Using the various procedures described earlier, investigators have been able to demonstrate infant discrimination of a wide range of phonetic contrasts used in adult languages, regardless of the language of the child's environment (for overviews, see Eilers, 1980; Kuhl, 1987). Thus, children as young as 2 to 3 months of age can discriminate **place of articulation** in syllable-initial [b], [d], and [g]. Two-month-old infants can also discriminate [d] versus [g] in medial and final position. Only the distinction between contrasting unreleased (C)VC syllables (e.g., *bat* [bæt] and *back* [bæk]), which are not always easily identified by adults (Householder, 1956), were found to exceed infants' perceptual abilities. Investigation of **manner of articulation** contrasts has shown that infants can discriminate stops from nasals and glides and [ra] and [la].

Furthermore, 1- to 4-month-old infants have been found to discriminate the three vowels most commonly contrasted in languages ([a] vs. [i] vs. [u]). Embedding the vowels in a syllable ([pa] vs. [pi]) did not impede discrimination. In addition, infants of this age raised in an English-speaking environment were able to distinguish **oral** versus **nasal** vowels ([pa] vs. [põ]), even though the oral-nasal contrast is not used phonemically in English vowels (Trehub, 1976). (It does function phonemically in French and Hindi.) Finally, Kuhl (1987) reviewed a number of studies in which she and her colleagues tested 1- to 4-month-old infants for perceptual constancy by presenting tokens of the vowels [a] and [i], each produced on monotone and rise-fall **pitches**, with the different pitch-tokens varied randomly. The children were able to discriminate the vowels and disregarded the differences in pitch. However, when the reverse situation was tested, contrasting the two pitch contours with random shifting between [a] and [i] as the vowel carrying the pitch, the infants failed to discriminate the pitch contrast. Thus, infants showed perceptual constancy with respect to the vowel-color dimension (i.e., [a] vs. [i]), which appeared to be more salient to them than the pitch-contour dimension (monotone vs. rise-fall). Similar testing of vowel contrasts produced by adult male versus female and child talkers showed that infants easily discriminate even the acoustically similar vowels /a/ and /ɔ/ regardless of changes in the speaker.

A few contrasts have been reported to resist discrimination in the early months and thus to require learning by the child. These include contrasts of voicing and place in fricatives, for example ([sa] vs. [za], [fa] vs. [θa], [fi] vs. [θi]: Eilers and Minifie (1975); Eilers, 1977). These results are interesting because the /f/ versus /θ/ distinction is a notoriously difficult one for children, even as late as age 3 or 4 (cf., e.g., Locke, 1980b); and, under less than ideal listening conditions, it can prove difficult for adults as well. However, other studies have shown that when computer-synthesized tokens are used instead of naturally produced syllables, 2- to 3-month-olds can discriminate [fa] versus [θa] (Jusczyk, Murray, and Bayly, 1979).

Another type of discrimination that may exceed infants' perceptual capacities is that between different stops embedded in multisyllabic vocalizations with relatively short syllables (less than 300 milliseconds: [ataba] vs. [atapa]: Trehub, 1973). This observation is interesting in light of children's use of syllable deletion and unique reduction devices well into the third year, which reflects the difficulty that the production of multisyllabic words poses for them. These production problems may result from perceptual as well as articulatory difficulties; that is, the relatively shorter syllables embedded in long words may continue to be difficult to perceive and store in sufficient segmental detail even when the child is successfully producing one- and two-syllable words. Later studies have shown that the difficulty of making discriminations within a "long word" context can be attenuated by adding exaggerated stress to the contrasting syllable, as caretakers typically do in speaking to children (Fernald and Simon, 1984; Karzon, 1985).

In summary, in the first few months of life, infants are capable of distinguishing between consonants that differ in place and manner of articulation, and also between some vowels. Distinguishing among certain fricatives and between stops embedded in longer, multisyllabic vocalizations is more problematic for young children.

The Role of Linguistic Experience

Some investigators have suggested that *linguistic experience* within the first six months of life may influence the child's perceptual capacities, particularly with respect to voicing and aspiration contrasts in stops. Children exposed to Spanish (Eilers, Gavin, and Wilson, 1979) or Kikuyu (Streeter, 1976) were found to discriminate pre-voiced from voiced (unaspirated) stops, whereas infants exposed only to English did not make this discrimination. Since the pre-voiced/voiced stop distinction is phonemic in Spanish and Kikuyu but not in English, it was inferred that the phonemic contrasts used in the adult language to which the child is exposed may affect the child's ability to discriminate phonetic categories within the first few months of life. Interpretation of the findings, however, has been criticized on both logical and methodological grounds. In particular, exposure to the speech of a given language does not ensure that a specific **phonemic category** or contrast will be perceived (MacKain, 1982). Recall that pre-voiced stops do occur in English, though only in intervocalic position. Thus, the child exposed to English does "experience" pre-voiced stops, though they are not contrastive. It is unclear how the young child's exposure to the phonetic realization of different phonemic categories in particular languages could lead to differential categorical perception of speech at this stage of development.

The Role of Prosody

The most recent line of research on infant perceptual capacities has focused on larger speech units (sequences of sentences, clauses, and phrases rather than isolated syllables) and on other influences affecting infant attention to the speech signal (own mother or own language vs. other mother, other language; speech directed to infants, or "motherese", vs. speech directed to adults). Such studies have provided evidence that infants are strongly attracted to the sound of their own language, especially when spoken by the mother and especially when she uses the wide pitch contours characteristic of motherese. The attraction of prosodically varied speech is thought to be related to its emotional tone; it is part of the process of bonding between mother and infant. In addition, the infant's close attention to the caretaker's speech most likely plays an important facilitory role in beginning to identify the relevant **units** of the adult language. Specifically, infants appear to be sensitive to the perceptual unity of **clauses** by 6 months of age; **phrasal** units (subject noun, predicate verb) appear to be detectable by 9 months. It has been argued that the salience of prosodic cues reflects an **innately guided learning process**, like the tendency for goslings to follow the mother shortly after hatching or for the sparrow to attend to and learn the song typical of its species (Jusczyk and Bertoncini, 1988).

Summary

What perceptual capabilities are infants born with? How do they break into the acoustic flow of speech? And which capabilities develop with age and exposure to the sounds of the language used around them? Researchers report that during the first months of life, infants respond differentially to different speech stimuli and treat some sounds varied along a continuum as if they belonged to categories of sounds used in the adult language. These discriminations probably reflect inherent biases in the auditory systems of mammals, including humans. Certain natural boundaries between sounds appear to be universally salient to infants, whether or not the natural boundary is matched by a phonemic contrast in the adult language to which the child is exposed. These built-in biases make it possible for the infant to begin finding recognizable patterns in the stream of overlapping sounds that constitute speech.

Many contrasts used in language are discriminable from an early age, including the differences among place of consonant articulation (labial/dental/velar) or manner of articulation (stops vs. nasals or glides, and /ra/ vs. /la/); other contrasts, especially distinctions among different fricatives, unreleased final stops, and those embedded in multisyllabic utterances, may be discriminated only later, as they require maturation and increased exposure to language. Attempts to demonstrate the effects of experience with different phonemic systems during the first few months of life remain controversial and the potential effects unclear.

Prosodic characteristics of speech play an important role in language acquisition, although only limited data are available at this time and the role of prosody is not yet well understood.

Infant Production: Interaction of Maturation and Experience

The problem facing the infant learning to produce speech sounds can be broken down into a series of increasingly complex tasks, ranging from vocal production per se to communicative use, in context, of adult-based sound patterns, or *words* (Menyuk, Menn, and Silber, 1986). These tasks include (1) learning to produce a variety of vocal sounds, (2) matching sound patterns produced by adults to some of the well-practiced vocal patterns already in the infant's repertoire, (3) associating certain adult sound patterns with situations where they are often produced (the basis for situation-bound word use), (4) achieving the understanding that sound-pattern production can be used as a means to share a focus of attention or to make a request, and (5) marshaling adult-based words to serve communicative goals in novel settings (the referential and symbolic use of words).

The task analysis outlined above identifies the cognitive challenges in learning to speak. Mastery of the articulatory gestures alone will take five years or more; perceptual development presumably plays a role in this process as well. When the process is barely underway, however, the child has already begun work on other aspects of communicative development, including the problem of apprehending the significance of regular and recurrent form-meaning correspondences (i.e., developing comprehension of words and of communicative gestures, such as pointing, clapping, or waving). As outlined above, the

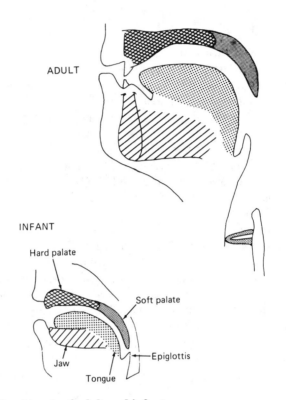

FIGURE 2.3   Vocal tracts of adult and infant.

From R. D. Kent and A. D. Murray, "Acoustic Features of Infant Vocalic Utterances at 3, 6, and 9 Months."
JASA, 72 (1982): 353–365. Used with permission.

cognitive problems for the would-be language user involve matching his or her own productive capacities to the sound patterns of the adult language, developing the ability to access them at will, and developing the skills to use language to refer to events outside the
immediate situational context. These tasks are largely encountered and mastered in the
course of what is called "the transition period"; that is, the phase of development which reflects the transition from babbling to speech. We begin our account of vocal production with
the first task, learning to produce a variety of vocal sounds.

Learning to Produce a Variety of Vocal Sounds

It is important to note that the infant's vocal tract is not simply a miniature or smaller version of the adult's (see Figure 2.3). Differences include: (1) a much shorter vocal tract; (2) a
relatively shorter pharyngeal cavity; (3) a tongue mass placed relatively farther forward in
the oral cavity; (4) a gradual, rather than a right-angle, bend in the oropharyngeal channel;
(5) a high larynx; and (6) a close approximation of the velopharynx and epiglottis (Kent and
Murray, 1982). The differences in anatomical structure affect the nature of infant vocal pro-

ductions. For example, the close relationship of laryngeal and velopharyngeal cavities leads to nasal breathing and early nasal vocalizations by the infant; it is only after the velum and epiglottis grow farther apart, when the infant is about 4 to 6 months old, that nonnasal vocal sounds first appear in significant quantities.

Early Stages of Production

Oller (1980) and Stark (1980) have provided compatible descriptions of vocal production over the first year of life (cf. also Roug, Landberg, and Lundberg, 1989, who offer a similar description for Swedish infants). **Reflexive** vocalizations (i.e., vocalizations arising as automatic responses to internal or external stimulation, such as hunger or discomfort) have typically been set aside in the literature on infant vocal production from the perspective of speech and language. One of these should be mentioned here, however, as it appears to be of some consequence in the transition to language. This is the "grunt," a brief glottal-initial sound with no supraglottal constriction that first occurs as the product of physiological changes associated with effort (McCune, Vihman, Roug-Hellichius, Delery, and Gogate, 1996). Stark (1993) has described such grunts in the context of communication, as a result of the physical effort involved for the infant in maintaining the head erect. The same involuntary vocal production has been noted in association with other postural adjustments, such as reaching (Trevarthan and Hubley, 1978) or crawling (Stark, Bernstein, and Demorest, 1993). This then can be seen as a foundational sound-meaning link in production, though it is neither intentional, communicative, nor arbitrary.

Oller (1980) divides the first six months into three sequential stages, which he terms the *phonation stage,* the *cooing stage,* and the *expansion stage.* He also identifies two stages, in the second half of the first year, of *canonical* and *variegated babbling.* There is considerable overlap between stages, and the ages assigned to each stage are only approximations. Furthermore, although the appearance of canonical babbling is a landmark event, variegated babbling has been found to be difficult to distinguish as a chronologically separate "stage."

1. In the **phonation** stage (0–1 month), speechlike sounds are rare. The largest number of nonreflexive, nondistress sounds are the "quasi-resonant nuclei," which Oller (1980) characterizes as vocalizations with normal phonation but limited resonance, produced with a closed or nearly closed mouth. These elements give the auditory impression of a syllabic nasal.
2. In the **goo** or cooing stage (2–3 months), velar consonantlike sounds are produced with some frequency and "primitive syllabification" may be detected (Zlatin, 1975), but the rhythmic properties of adult syllables and the timing of the articulatory gestures for adult consonants have not yet been mastered. Acoustically, the cooing sounds are similar to rounded back vowels such as [u].
3. In the **expansion** stage (4–6 months), the child appears to gain increasing control of both laryngeal and oral articulatory mechanisms. He or she explores the vocal mechanism through the playful use of squealing, growling, yelling, and "raspberry" vocalizations (bilabial trills). "Fully resonant nuclei" (adultlike vowels) begin to be produced in this period, as does "marginal babbling," in which consonantlike and vowellike

features occur but lack the mature regular-syllable timing characteristics of canonical babbling.

Stark (1978) emphasized the interrelationship of earlier and later vocal behaviors in the first six months of life. The emergence of cooing is dependent on increased control over voicing, which is first found only in crying. The new co-occurrence of voicing, egressive breath direction, and consonantlike closures results from the overlap between the maturation in voluntary laryngeal control and continuing reflexive activity of the vocal tract. The acquisition of control over this new behavioral combination is probably derived from the interaction of maturation and the experience of exercising the new behavior. The modified combination is then ready to begin to form new combinations with other more primitive behaviors. Thus, cooing or comfort sounds are expanded through the use of vocal play, which allows the infant to gain greater control over the activity of the tongue, lips, and jaw.

Beginnings of Adultlike Production: The Emergence of Consonants

The first probable evidence of adult language influence on production is manifested by the emergence of canonical babbling (Oller's Stage 4; also known as reduplicated babbling), typically at about 6 to 8 months. The sudden appearance of genuine syllabic production involving a true consonant and a "fully resonant nucleus" or vowel, often (though not exclusively) chained in repeated sequences such as [bababa], [dadada], or [mamama], constitutes the chief production milestone in the first year. The onset of this stage is easily recognized by parents, who report the child to be babbling or even "talking," although few, if any, consistent sound-meaning relations are likely to be observed.

Canonical babbling has been viewed primarily as the outgrowth of physiological maturation, uninfluenced by exposure to the adult language. However, Oller and his colleagues have reported that deaf children do not produce canonical babbling within the first year (Oller and Eilers, 1988; cf. also Stoel-Gammon and Otomo, 1986), whereas such babbling typically occurs in hearing babies by 10 months at the latest. These recent findings suggest that canonical babbling depends on auditory exposure and, thus, may reflect the influence of the adult language as well as physiological maturation.

The onset of canonical babbling may be viewed as a production discontinuity since it represents the first use of true consonantal articulation. The fact that stops (and nasals, or stops articulated with a lowered velum) are the earliest true consonants to be produced may be related to the natural perceptual salience of syllables with a stop onset. Stops present the sharpest possible contrast with vowels and provide the most obtrusive break in the acoustic stream of speech sounds. On the other hand, stop production is also relatively undemanding: syllables such as [ba], [da], [na] may be articulated through mandibular action alone (Kent, 1992). It is likely that this production milestone represents an advance in: (1) the motoric control, which is maturational or tied to natural physiological development in the first year, (2) the (experience-based) integration of visual and auditory perception of adult sequences of open/closed mouth and voice/silence alternation, and (3) the expression of the precept of adult vocalization through global imitation. In other words, children see as well as hear stop consonants in adult speech, produce such sounds themselves, and engage in repetitive vocal production or sound play, recreating their impression of adult speech.

Variegated Babbling and Universal Production Patterns

The last babbling stage (Oller's Stage 5) is **variegated babbling**, in which continued use of adult-like syllables is supplemented by the use of increasingly varied consonants and vowels within a single vocalization (e.g., from the babbling of a 9-month old girl, [ʔzmae:h], [w'tU], [te:koe], [h'tapa]: Vihman, Ferguson, and Elbert, 1986). Elbers (1982) has traced the development from reduplicated to variegated babbling in the speech of one child, between 6 and 12 months of age. Elbers (1982) views babbling in this period as "a systematic, continuous and largely self-directed process of exploration," in which the child constructs a phonetic "spring-board" to speech (45). Variegated babbling may emerge very soon after the onset of canonical babbling (Smith, Brown-Sweeney, and Stoel-Gammon, 1989; Mitchell and Kent, 1990). A number of studies have looked at the sound **repertoire** found in the variegated babbling of children learning different languages. These segmental repertoires are virtually indistinguishable. Locke (1983) cited the babbling repertoires for infants (aged 9 to 15 months) acquiring one of 15 languages each. He found that stops and nasals formed the base of each inventory, with a relatively low incidence for most other sounds. However, direct cross-linguistic comparisons of sound production frequencies in babbling vocalizations, examined through both instrumental analysis (of vowels) and phonetic transcription (of consonants), have revealed the first language-specific differences at 10 months, when word production is barely underway or has not yet begun (Boysson-Bardies and Vihman, 1991).

Vowel Production in the First Year

So far, we have concentrated mainly on early development of consonants since it is the onset of true consonant use that seems to mark the beginning of adultlike vocal production. However, it is vowel production that dominates infant vocalization throughout the first year. Vowels have been less extensively investigated, primarily because they are particularly difficult to transcribe reliably and thus difficult to characterize. For example, Lieberman (1980) reported inter-transcriber reliability of 73 percent for the vowels produced by children aged about 3 to 14 months. He reported frequencies only for vowels identified as belonging to the English repertoire. Lieberman's findings for a single child are summarized below, but the relatively low reliability figure should be kept in mind.

Lieberman used spectrographic analysis as a supplement to phonetic transcription and reported little change in average formant frequency values over the period investigated. However, the various vowels transcribed for 4 months showed considerable acoustic overlap in formant frequencies. A month later, spectrographic analysis yielded identification of a rudimentary vowel triangle. The gradual differentiation in the acoustic vowel space could be seen to continue (based on data from other subjects) until age 3.

The vowels most often perceived over the entire period were lax—[ɛ, ɪ, æ, ʌ, ʊ]—and were already present at the earliest session. [ɛ] was heard most frequently (33 percent of all the vowels transcribed), and the remaining lax vowels each accounted for 11 percent (17 percent of the data). The remaining (tense) vowels each accounted for no more than 5 percent, with the back rounded [o] and [u] least frequent (1 percent each).

Kent and Murray (1982) investigated the acoustic features of vocalic utterances at 3, 6, and 9 months (seven infants at each age). Their findings were similar to those reported by Lieberman. The range of F_1 and F_2 frequencies increased somewhat across each age interval, but the majority of the vowels used by the 9-month-old infants showed roughly the same formant pattern as did the vowels of the younger subjects. Given the anatomical differences between adults and infants, it is not surprising that the range of possible infant vowel productions should be more restricted than those of adults. The formant patterns of infant vowels fit within the range of mid-front or central adult vowels (Figure 2.4).

In a study of 10-month-old infant vowel productions drawn from four linguistic communities—Arabic, Chinese, English, and French—Boysson-Bardies and her colleagues (1989) found that the categories of **front-low** and **mid-central** vowels accounted for the vast majority of vowels from all four groups. Acoustic analysis revealed characteristic patterns of vowel production for each group within those limits, however, with more high front

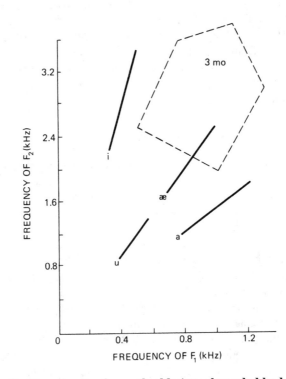

FIGURE 2.4 **F_1–F_2 region for 3-month-olds (area bounded by broken line) compared to isovowel lines for /i æ o u/.**

From R. D. Kent and A. D. Murray, "Acoustic Features of Infant Vocal Utterances at 3, 6, and 9 months." *JASA*, 72 (1982): 353–365. Used with permission.

vowels for English, for example, and more low back vowels for Chinese. The investigators interpreted these differences in vowel production as showing that infants begin to position their lips and tongue in a manner specific to the language of their environment even before they produce word-forms modeled on adult speech.

Prosodic Development in Early Vocal Production

The development of the intonational patterns of language has received considerably less attention than has the development of segments and segmental contrasts. This reflects, in part, the fact that the prosodic properties of adult languages are also less well understood. Nevertheless, the literature points to a few conclusions. Acoustic analysis of infant vocalizations across the first year of life shows that falling pitch is the most common contour during this period (Delack and Fowlow, 1978; Kent and Murray, 1982). Kent and Murray offer a physiological explanation, suggesting that a falling fundamental frequency, or **pitch contour**, is the natural result of a decline in subglottal pressure in the course of a vocalization. A reduction of vocal fold length and tension as the muscles of the larynx relax at the end of a vocalization could also lead to a falling pitch contour. A rising pitch contour requires an increase in vocal fold length or tension at the end of the vocalization, or an increase in subglottal pressure, or both. It seems natural, then, that the development of contrastive, rising pitch contours should develop later than falling pitch contours. It appears that this sequence is a general one, regardless of the language being acquired.

Once the variegated babbling stage has been reached, the child may also produce jargon. This phenomenon, which Oller (1980) calls "gibberish," results when adultlike pitch movement and rhythm are imposed on rapidly produced multisyllabic strings of variegated babble. In children acquiring English, multisyllabic jargon strings of this kind typically end with a relatively low pitch on the next-to-last syllable followed by a shift to a mid or mid-falling pitch on the last syllable. Notice that a phrase-final shift in pitch is a characteristic adult English intonation pattern. Jargon seems to represent the child's attempts to reproduce the surface impression of longer strings of speech, that is, of phrases or sentences instead of isolated words; the result often impresses the adult listener as conversation without words (cf. Menn, 1976; Boysson-Bardies, Bacri, Sagart, and Poizat, 1981; Vihman and Miller, 1988).

Summary

Young children face a series of production tasks on their way to learning the language of their environment. To begin with, they must gain control of laryngeal and articulatory gestures to develop the precision necessary to produce the sounds of language at will. Developing such control involves both maturation of the laryngeal, articulatory, and perceptual mechanisms and accommodation to the sound patterns of the specific language spoken to the child. Thus, phonological development in the young child involves the interaction of physical maturation and social experience.

During the first six months of life, three stages of voluntary vocal behavior can be distinguished: the phonation stage, the cooing stage, and the expansion stage. Acquisition of control over each new behavioral combination is the result of the interaction of maturation and experience or practice in using the new motor behavior.

Between age 6 and 10 months, canonical babbling begins to be produced. This constitutes the main discontinuity, or sharp qualitative change, in infant production in the first year, and it provides the first concrete evidence of the influence of auditory experience with an adult language. In the last babbling stage, variegated babbling, the child prepares the phonetic ground for his or her first attempts at adult words. At this stage, infant consonantal repertoires are largely indistinguishable across languages, but consonant and vowel production frequencies begin to reflect differences in the child's linguistic experience.

During the first year, infant vowel production shows little change. Adult transcribers typically perceive the primitive vowels as mid-front or central. Falling pitch contours predominate in the children's productions in the first year, perhaps for (universal) physiological reasons. Once the child has begun producing variegated babble, adultlike stress patterns and intonation contours may also be used, giving the surface effect of adult language, but without content or meaning.

The Transition Period: From Babble to Speech

We have reviewed the infant's perception and production of speech during the first year of life. The infant manifests impressive discriminatory abilities for speech sounds at a very early age. However, we have yet to consider how these abilities serve the child in linguistic perception, in identifying and remembering meaningful sound patterns of the adult language. The child also faces a series of tasks in learning to produce meaningful speech. So far, we have only discussed the first of these tasks—learning to produce a variety of vocal sounds. By the end of the first year, the child is babbling or, in other words, producing adultlike sequences of syllables that include a range of different consonants and vowels. Furthermore, the child is no longer restricted to a single consonant or vowel type per vocalization. Some use of rising pitch contours may occur alongside the more common falling pitch.

We turn now to the transition period, when the babbler becomes a talker. The critical development in this period is the linking of sound patterns with meaning, first in comprehension, then in word production. Sporadic signs of understanding may occur in the middle of the first year, so we will have to backtrack slightly in our chronological account to pick up the trail of the child's first steps in the use of meaning and communication.

The transition period is best defined by certain developmental events. It begins with the onset of comprehension of the adult language, and it closes when word use begins to dominate babble, typically when the child is using about 50 different words spontaneously. The age range in which these developments occur is extremely variable. Some normally developing children fail to produce many recognizable words before the age of 2, although they will show evidence of good language comprehension long before this time. For many, and perhaps most, children, the transition to speech will occur during the period from about 9 to 18 months.

Relating Sound Patterns to Meanings

When the child first begins to respond differentially to particular words or phrases of the adult language—that is, begins to show comprehension—he or she has begun to match discriminable differences in sound patterns with differences in the use or function of those patterns. The first reports of language comprehension, found in the diary records kept by linguist parents, noted earliest signs of comprehension at age 4 or 5 months. At 20 weeks, Hans Lindner responded to *Tick-tack* (German for *tick-tock*) by looking toward the large, loudly ticking wall clock that had often been pointed out to him (Lindner, 1898, reported in Ferguson, 1978). At 6 months, Deville's daughter responded to *bravo* by clapping her hands, and at 7 months she would respond to French *chut* (*quiet!*) by refraining from touching an item of interest (Deville, 1890, 1891, reported in Lewis, 1936). Lewis observed his child's first responses to words at 8 or 9 months: a smile for *Cuckoo!* "uttered in a special tone of voice," recoil from a movement for *No!* and a wave for *Say goodbye!* (Lewis, 1936; 107). In each case, the child had heard the word repeatedly in context, and the expected behavior (e.g., the appropriate gesture for routines involving clapping or waving) had been made clear on numerous occasions. The earliest signs of word recognition may be isolated occurrences. By 10 or 11 months, there is generally considerable evidence of language comprehension although it is difficult to determine precisely how much the child understands from words alone and how much involves familiarity with the situational contexts in which words are used.

Perception in the Transition Period: Entry into the Native Language

The beginnings of comprehension of the adult language, combined with production of the first learned gestures (e.g., clapping, waving), mark a significant new step in the child's development. We assume that at this point children have begun to develop a repertoire of familiar phonetic patterns drawn from the adult language and linked with specific meanings. Unfortunately, there has been little direct testing of perception of word-patterns or phonemic contrasts (linguistic perception) in this period. It would be of great interest to know whether certain meaningful sound patterns are more easily distinguished than others. For example, do children distinguish between words or phrases on the basis of pitch or rhythm before they make a distinction between words differing only in their segmental properties, as anecdotal accounts suggest (Lewis, 1936)? Are differences carried by syllable shape (e.g., presence or absence of a final consonant) easier to recognize than differences carried by specific segments, or do children vary in this regard? Is there a relationship between the patterns most consistently recognized by a given child and the patterns in that child's babbling? Reliable experimental results regarding the relationship between perception and production would be helpful in deciding between the views espoused, on the one hand, by Smith (1973) and Stampe (1969), who posit complete, accurate representation of the adult language from the earliest period of word production and, on the other hand, by Waterson (1971), who presupposes imperfect perception as the source of production constraints on early words (cf. also Schwartz and Leonard, 1982; Menn, 1983).

Recent investigations of infant perception at the end of the first year have revealed an important shift whose timing coincides with the beginnings of word recognition—or at least with early comprehension of language in well-established contexts. Werker and her colleagues (Werker, Gilbert, Humphrey, and Tees, 1981; Werker and Tees, 1983) set out to discover the point at which the infant's broad capacities for discrimination of phonemic contrasts are replaced by the adult's language-specific responses to speech sounds (see

Trehub, 1976). They tested adults and 4-, 8-, and 12-year-old children on two contrasts which are phonemic in Hindi but unfamiliar to English-speakers: place of articulation (dental /t/ vs. retroflex /t/) and voice-onset time (voiceless aspirated /th/ vs. breathy voiced /dh/). In addition, they tested a contrast used in an Interior Salish Northwest Indian language, glottalized velar /k'/ versus glottalized uvular /q'/. Less than half of the adults and children aged 4 or over were able to discriminate these foreign contrasts, whereas most of the 6- to 8-month-old infants tested showed evidence of discrimination. In a critical study, Werker and Tees (1984) tested infants in age groups spanning the last half of the first year (6–8, 8–10, and 10–12 months) on the Hindi and Salishan place of articulation contrasts. The youngest group again showed discrimination, while the oldest group did not. The 8–10-month-olds were relatively successful with the Hindi contrast but most of them did not discriminate the Salishan contrast.

The apparent decline in "universal" perceptual capacity at the end of the first year is intriguing and has aroused a good deal of controversy. Have infants "entered into" the phonemic system of the language to which they are exposed at this time (Werker, 1991), when they are just beginning to attend to language with some sign of understanding of the (arbitrary) association of verbal sounds and (situation-based) meanings? It is difficult to see how the child could have structured perceptual information to that extent at this early stage. Furthermore, the child's earliest word production appears to reveal a broad or holistic phonological base rather than a full-blown set of phonemic (segmental) contrasts. One hypothesis for the apparent reorganization of perception at the onset to speech is that it is mediated by the child's emerging productive (articulatory) abilities (Locke, 1990; Vihman, 1991, 1993). As the child develops articulatory control and familiarity, through self-monitoring, with the sound as well as the feel of a few well-practiced articulatory gestures, we may suppose that certain salient sound patterns of the adult language begin to "stand out" perceptually, since they appear to match those familiar vocal patterns that the child has been repeatedly producing. Since influence from the particular language of the child's environment has just begun to affect the child's babbling at this age, it is possible that such an articulatory filter may serve to alter the child's initial "unbiased" response to speech sounds, replacing the "universal" readiness for any language by a more finely tuned readiness for the language of the child's caretakers (Werker and Pegg, 1992).

Protowords

The child develops intentional communication at the same time that he or she is improving articulatory control and increasing in capacity to recognize adult sound patterns. Thus, a child may communicate meaning with gestures before doing so consistently with adultlike words. A number of observers of infants in this age range have noted the use of **protowords** (or **invented words**), consistent vocal forms with no apparent adult model with the same or similar range of uses (Dore, Franklin, Miller, and Ramer, 1976; Ferguson, 1978; see also the review in Vihman, 1996). Generally, the forms are simple CV shapes, with glottals, [ʔ] and [h], or stops filling the consonant slot. Meanings are simple as well: broad markers of focus of attention or attempts to share interest or make a request; also expressions of affect—excitement, disgust—or accompaniments to the child's activity (another kind of focus), or simply conversational fillers (Vihman and Miller, 1988). Recently, it has been observed that grunts commonly occur early in this period during moments of focused attention, involving quieting of the body, concentrated visual and manual exploration of an object or looking toward an event (McCune et al., 1996). These minimal vocal expressions—brief monosyllables of the form [ʔV], typically with a neutral vowel, ['], or a syllabic nasal—are produced quietly, with no apparent communicative intent at first; they appear to be related to the effort grunts observed contemporaneously as well as earlier, and may reflect the "effort of attention" (Porges, 1992; Richards and Casey, 1992; compare the "attentional grunt" we as adults unconsciously produce when something we are reading or listening to suddenly arouses our interest).

Between about 14 and 16 months a new function may be observed, typically first expressed by grunts or other simple glottal-initial vocalizations (such as [ha], [aha], or [haha]). The new function involves the sharing of a focus of attention or interest; a related function is that of request (for an adult to do something for the child or provide something). The child may vocalize and point or show an object, all the while looking at an adult. These simple communicative forms reflect an important shift in the child's understanding of vocal function: Now meanings can be expressed by vocal forms—though the grunt form is not fully arbitrary, since it has its origin in the effort of movement and, secondarily, the effort of attention. Such a shift in understanding appears to be one of the prerequisites for adult-like word use, or the generalized use of words across a range of different situational contexts. Even children who already have a sizable conventional vocabulary may continue to use communicative grunts for some months, frequently together with pointing.

Phonetic Characteristics of Late Babbling and Early Words

Vocalization at the end of the first year has just begun to be affected by the phonetic makeup of the specific language of the child's environment and is not markedly different when an adult word is intended. What are the phonetic characteristics of the vocalizations typically used in the period when word use is first being established? How similar are these vocalizations across infants learning the same language?

Several detailed reports are available on the phonetic characteristics of vocalizations during this period. Kent and Bauer (1985) described the syllable structures, vowel- and consonantlike segments, and intonation contours used by five 13-month-old children. Vihman and her colleagues (1986) focused on vocalization length, syllable shape, and consonants in a longitudinal study of ten children, aged 9 to 17 months. These studies addressed the same phenomena for children of approximately the same age and reported similar findings. Boysson-Bardies and Vihman (1991) extended the study by Vihman and her colleagues (1986) to three more languages, French, Japanese, and Swedish (five subjects each), and reported both similarities and differences across the four languages. For English learners, monosyllabic (one-syllable) vocalizations were the most common form of vocalization, followed by disyllables (or two-syllable productions), while disyllables predominated in the other three language groups studied. Of the consonants used, stops were by far the most common for all the infants, followed by nasals and fricatives.

Kent and Bauer (1985) noted a difference in consonant use in vocalizations of different structures. Although stops dominated consonant use in CV vocalizations, they made up less than half of the consonants in VCV vocalizations and were greatly exceeded by fricatives and nasals in VC vocalizations. Bilabial and apical consonants were used the most often. Consonant clusters were very rare. Kent and Bauer (1985) found that the basic consonant-vowel contrast was primarily learned within the framework of the CV syllable, and concluded that such a syllable, which is found in all languages, may be viewed as "a simplest form . . . or a kind of atom in the formulation of speech" (517).

Kent and Bauer found that the most common vowels used were central, mid-front, and low-front ([ʌ, ɛ, æ]), while high vowels ([i, u]) were rare. Of the various intonation contours used, the fall and rise-fall accounted for over 75 percent of all vocalizations; a simple rising contour accounted for 10 percent more. Kent and Bauer stressed the fact that in all these respects, the vocalizations of 13-month-olds were continuous with the vocalizations of both younger children and children in the second year of life.

Davis and MacNeilage (1990), who described vowel production for one child learning English (14 to 20 months), were less impressed than Kent and Bauer by the evidence of continuity between babbling and early words. Although they found the expected predominance of relatively low, lax vowels, especially in babbling production, they also found high use of [l], especially in the second syllable of word productions. Finally, they noted that the vowels of babbling were not produced more correctly in speech, but did tend to be used as substitutions for other vowels. In other words, the well-established vowels of babbling were overused in speech production, but a vowel less often used in babbling—[i]—appeared frequently in the child's words, reflecting the influence of the adult language.

Another major finding of the Davis and MacNeilage (1990) study was the interaction of consonant and vowel productions. High front vowels were found to occur most frequently following alveolars, high back vowels (when used at all) after velars, and central vowels after labials. In a replication of this analysis based on 23 subjects learning four languages—English, French, Japanese, and Swedish—Vihman (1992) reported some of the same associations. Velars and back vowels were rare but were produced together when they did occur. Labials were typically followed by central vowels in the vocalizations of several children. Alveolars were not significantly associated with front vowels. Davis and MacNeilage (1990) suggested that the alveolars and velars may each tend to be followed by the high vowel closest in articulatory space for mechanical reasons, reflecting a lack of differentiation of articulatory gestures. However, Vihman reported a tendency for these C-V associations to reflect the influence of different adult languages (e.g., /(alveolar) Ci/ is a common sequence in English—*daddy, pretty, lady, dolly, while* /ko/ occurs in many Japanese words used by the children), and suggests that reliance on such sequences may be a strategy particular to word production. Only the labial/central vowel association appears to reflect an early physiological basis, in which the tongue remains in a neutral, resting position while the lip gesture is actively recruited for articulation. A later controlled study of nine children acquiring English at 18, 21, and 24 months of age found little evidence of C-V interactions in word production, although velar words with back vowels tended to be preferentially selected, and back vowels tended to be accurately produced after velars (Tyler and Langsdale, 1996).

Common Tendencies

Vihman and her colleagues have investigated the extent of common tendencies vs. individual differences in early vocalizations, both across children learning the same language and across different languages (Vihman et al., 1986; Vihman and Greenlee, 1987; Boysson-Bardies and Vihman, 1991; Vihman, 1993). To assess variability across subjects at comparable stages of development, they defined sampling points on the basis of lexical use. Two early points reflected the beginnings of word use (ages ranged from 8 to 15 months), and two later points were taken from half-hour sessions in which 15 or more different words were used spontaneously (in this later period, the children had cumulative vocabularies, as reported by their mothers, of about 30 to 50 words; ages ranged from 12 to 23 months).

These studies found that variability in the phonetic categories analyzed was greatest at the earlier stages; a trend toward uniformity across subjects learning the same language was detected as the children's productive vocabularies increased. The strongest finding for the early lexical period was the considerable differences across subjects learning the same language, both in specific phonetic choices and in the degree of stability of phonetic preferences over time.

We can see the growing influence of the adult language in various ways during the transition period. A trend toward increased use of consonants begins for all infants with the onset of canonical babbling (Kent and Murray, 1982), although this trend levels off toward the end of the first year if lexical acquisition is proceeding slowly. Once lexical acquisition is underway, early words are considerably more likely to include a true consonant (stop, nasal, fricative or liquid) than are babble vocalizations. This finding suggests that increasing knowledge of the adult language plays a significant role in the continued shift toward the use of consonants in this period.

The use of labials is highly variable in the earlier lexical stages, when the children have 10-word vocabularies at most. In the later stages, however, labials account for over a third of all consonant productions. Labial use is more characteristic of words than of babble, yet a study of mothers' speech in English, French, and Swedish showed that alveolars were more frequently used than labials in all three groups (Vihman, Kay, Boysson–Bardies, Durand, and Sundberg, 1994), so that the source of heavy labial use is not the child's greater exposure to such use by adults. Instead, the disproportionate production of labials in words might be ascribed, at least in part, to the visibility of labial articulation. Since one can see the articulatory movement involved in producing the *b* of words like *baby* or *bottle*, it may well be easier for the child to gain control of the production of labials than of other consonants. Interestingly, this "overuse" of labials is not found in the early lexicon of blind children (Mulford, 1988) but is particularly characteristic of the vocalizations of the deaf (Stoel-Gammon and Otomo, 1986). We can expect the sighted and normally hearing child's preference for labials to gradually diminish as he or she gains greater control over articulatory production.

In summary, then, by the end of the transition period, when the child has a cumulative vocabulary of about 50 words, there are several signs of the influence of the adult language on the segmental shape of the child's vocalizations. Some of the characteristics of the child's vocal patterns reflect characteristics of all adult language, such as the dominance of true consonants. The preference for producing words with labials is also detectable in a range of languages, but it probably reflects characteristics of the learning process—mastering an articulation for which visible as well as auditory cues are available—rather than the form of adult languages. On the other hand, some early signs of the influence of the specific language environment are also evident by this point. For example, some children learning English, a language particularly rich in word-final consonants, begin to make use of final consonants in babble and especially in words by the end of the transition period (Vihman and Boysson-Bardies, 1994), whereas children learning languages with fewer final consonants make negligible use of them.

Prosodic Advances

Cross-linguistic study of the transition period has revealed the beginnings of prosodic organization by the time the child has produced 50 words or more (at about 17–18 months, typically). Hallé, Boysson-Bardies, and Vihman (1991) compared the disyllabic vocalizations (both words and babble) of four children each learning French and Japanese. The French infants showed a predominance of rising pitch contours, typical of adult French speech, as well as lengthening of final syllables, which is a near-universal in the world's languages (Cruttenden, 1986). The Japanese infants used more falling pitch contours and failed to show longer second than first syllable rimes. Abrupt final-syllable endings (closure with glottal stop) typified the Japanese infant productions, but not the French. Just one of the Japanese children lacked the abrupt offset; that child was the only Japanese subject to show lengthening of the final syllable. These findings were interpreted as supporting the idea of a physiological basis to final lengthening (Robb and Saxman, 1990), with a learned suppression of natural lengthening in the case of children learning the abrupt glottal offset of Japanese.

Summary

The changes that occur in infant perception and production during the transition from babbling to speech have been reviewed. By the beginning of the transition period (ca. age 9 to 18 months), the child has begun to demonstrate understanding of a variety of words, even if only in narrow or routine contexts. At this time children express their growing communicative abilities through the use of gestures, grunts and idiosyncractic word forms to express attention to and interest in familiar objects and events. By the end of the transition period, the child's experience with a particular language is reflected in both production and perception. Once the child has begun to make intentional efforts to communicate with particular adult sound patterns (form) associated with particular situations (meaning), phonological organization can begin.

The sounds which occur most commonly in a child's babbling are likely to be the sounds the child uses in early words. Both words and babble are characterized at this time by a high proportion of mono- and disyllabic forms, stops, and open syllables. Use of consonants increases with knowledge of the adult language, and relatively extensive use of labials is particularly characteristic of early words. Language-specific phonotactic features, such as final consonants in English, and prosodic features, such as rising pitch for French and abrupt offset for Japanese, also emerge over this period.

The bulk of phonological development takes place over the age range one to three years, at a time when the child is also experiencing an extraordinary growth of word knowledge and embarking on the acquisition of syntax. Yet it seems fair to say that the biggest hurdle of all—that of "getting the idea" of what language is all about, apprehending form-meaning correspondences, and learning to match, store, and reproduce them at will—has already been surmounted.

Individual Differences: Profile of Two One-Year-Old Girls

Although a general sequence of vocal development can be identified for the first year and a half of life, the extent of individual variability is striking. For one thing, children differ greatly in amount of vocalization during this period. In one study, for example, the average number of vocalizations produced by nine infants ranged from 97 to 265 per half-hour session (the children's interaction with their mothers was sampled at monthly intervals: Vihman et al., 1985).

Individual differences are also apparent in other aspects of phonological development. Infants vary in the sounds they produce (*phonetic preferences*) and in the stability of these sound preferences. Finally, infants may differ in the organization of their phonological systems and in their approaches to learning phonology. These differences can be identified as early as the period of transition from babbling to speech. We will illustrate differences in phonetic preferences and in phonological organization in this period by describing the development of two girls.

Phonetic Preferences and Word Selection

Molly and Deborah are both first-born daughters of well-educated parents with a strong interest in their children's development. Both girls are naturally "talkative" (in fact, they ranked first and third in amount of vocalization among the nine children studied by Vihman et al., 1985), and both developed large vocabularies by the end of the study (50 words or more, at 16 months).

Although Molly and Deborah were similar in many respects, they differed substantially in their phonetic preferences, word selection, and stability of their word shapes (Vihman, Ferguson, and Elbert, 1986; Vihman and Greenlee, 1987). In the early lexical period, Molly showed a striking preference for labials (66 percent: mean use for the group, 44 percent) and nasals (41 percent: group mean, 16 percent), while Deborah more closely resembled the other nine children sampled. In the later period, Molly developed a strong focus on final consonants (23 percent: mean use for the group, 12 percent), while Deborah began using an unexpectedly large proportion of fricatives (26 percent against a mean of 10 percent).

Children select their early words at least partly on phonetic grounds (Ferguson and Farwell, 1975; Schwartz and Leonard, 1982). The word-initial consonant is most likely to be the child's target in deciding to attempt a word (cf. Shibamoto and Olmsted, 1978), although overall word shape, prosody, and vowel pattern undoubtedly play some role in the selection of early words (cf. Stoel-Gammon and Cooper, 1984; Davis and MacNeilage, 1990). Deborah's preference for fricatives is reflected in the words she attempts, which tend to include the sounds [s] and [t]: *scratchy* [t i:t i], *Sesame Street* [si:si] (14 months), while Molly selects an unusually large number of words with final nasals (*bang, down, name, around*: Vihman and Velleman, 1989).

The two girls also differed in phonological organization. Although Molly gradually increased the number of different consonants she would attempt, she largely restricted herself to stops and nasals throughout this period of early word use. Even in a session in which she used over 20 different words (at 15 months), she still did not attempt any words with sibilants or liquids. Deborah, on the other hand, used a broad array of consonants from the beginning. By the end of this period she had greatly expanded her repertoire by attempting words with interdentals as well as sibilants. In general, Deborah seemed to advance in an exploratory way, whereas Molly's progress was more systematic.

Finally, the two girls differed in the extent of variability in their productions of different tokens of a single word. Molly's word production was highly repetitive (i.e., she produced many tokens of a single word type), with remarkably little variation across the different tokens or productions of a single word. In contrast, Deborah produced a different shape for almost every token of a given word. This appeared to result, in part from her inclusion of extra syllables at the beginning of a word, perhaps as a tentative effort to reproduce the sound of the English articles *a* and *the* and the possessive pronoun *my* (*a baby, my baby, the glasses*: cf. Ramer's [1976] discussion of *presyntactic forms*). Here again, Molly's highly stable word production seems to reflect a systematic approach to the learning of phonology, whereas Deborah appears to be exploring new forms before she has a good grasp of their function. The difference between the two girls appears to illustrate Ferguson's (1979) distinction between a cautious, analytic (systematic) style and an unanalytic, risk-taking (exploratory) style.

In summary, these two children differed widely in the phonetic preferences they displayed during babbling although they were matched for sex, socioeconomic status, amount of vocalization, and relative rate of lexical development. These same individual phonetic preferences appeared to carry over to the children's choices of early words. We see the beginnings of phonological structure as each child gradually expanded her range of phonetic segments and attempted increasingly complex syllable shapes.

Summary

We have suggested that differences in approach to learning can be discerned among children early in their language acquisition. We provided evidence of individual differences in phonetic preferences, word selection, and stability or variability of word shapes. One child showed a cautious, systematic approach, while the other made bold leaps from one point to another in word selection, with exploration of a wide range of sounds in both babble and first words. In both cases, the child's phonetic preferences were found to influence her choice of early words.

Linguistic Perception: Representing Speech Sounds

We began our account of the origins of phonological development by asking what perceptual abilities or natural biases the infant brings to the task of learning to pronounce. Before reviewing phonological development beyond the transition period, we will consider what is known about perceptual development during the period of rapid phonological advancement, from the transition to speech through the mastery of the sound system. Current theories of phonological development differ crucially on the issue of the timing of perceptual development. Some scholars view linguistic perception, or the ability to identify and represent or store the sound pattern of lexical items, as essentially complete even before the child has acquired a small lexicon of 50 words or so. From this perspective, the child's production errors may be largely ascribed to difficulties in motor control and phonological organization. Other scholars believe linguistic perception continues to develop during the preschool period and even beyond, and thus, some production errors may be due to perception-based differences between the adult word and the sound pattern the child is targeting—that is, to inaccuracies and gaps in the child's perception and consequent internal representation of the adult word.

It is important to note that the term *linguistic perception* refers not only to the auditory perception or identification of contrast between different sounds but also to the *storing and accessing for recognition* of the particular sound patterns that constitute words and phrases in the language being acquired. Previously, we dealt with the child's auditory capacities. Here, we are concerned with the child's use of those capacities in constructing a repertoire of word forms and extrapolating from there a store of phonological knowledge—knowledge of the sound system of his or her language.

In our account of infant perception, we stressed that infants in the first few months of life seem to respond to graduated differences in the acoustic signal in a categorical way and, furthermore, that these categorical responses resemble adult responses, which are based on knowledge of phonemic (meaning-bearing) contrasts in the language. We ascribed the infants' surprising discriminatory ability to natural biases in the auditory structure of humans (and other mammals). Given the wide range of phonemic differences to which infants have been found to be sensitive, it is easy to see why some scholars have concluded that perception of speech patterns can be assumed to be completely accurate by the time children begin to produce lexical items on their own. It is important, however, to bear in mind the distinction between the nonlinguistic sensory *capacity* (the ability to make same-different distinctions) tested in studies of infant perception and the *use* of that discriminatory capacity to distinguish different meaningful lexical items, as well as to store or remember them (**internal representation**). Infant perception tasks used in research investigations involve an essentially **passive response** to change in the signal, which indicates auditory sensitivity to the change. But perception of sound patterns as a basis for language use involves **active attention** to contrasting speech sounds and sequences in order to identify, store, and recognize distinct lexical items (Ferguson, 1975). Furthermore, discrimination between phonemes involves a learned response to a range of different and variable acoustic signals in terms of a single (abstract) linguistic category. With respect to the child who is beginning to speak, we shift our focus from the perception of differences between sounds per se to the perception of phonemic contrasts and the use of that perception to recognize different words and, thus, to understand language. This shift in focus naturally leads to a shift in the methods used to investigate linguistic perception.

We cannot directly observe a child's perception of speech sounds. Instead, tasks must be devised requiring the child to respond in a way that reveals something about his or her perceptions. As Locke (1980a) has pointed out, this is a formidable challenge since both linguistic perception itself and the required behavioral responses are complex processes involving several steps. First, the salient features of the speech sound stimuli must be *heard* ("go in the ear of the subject") and then *registered* and *interpreted* by the child ("reach and reside briefly in the brain": Locke, 1980a; 433). In other words, the child's perception of a speech sound involves receiving the auditory stimulus and identifying the auditory cues in terms of the phonemic system, or the speech sound categories, of the adult language. Secondly, in order for the observer to judge the "accuracy" of the child's perception, or the extent to which it agrees with that of adults from the child's linguistic community, the perception must be *translated* into an interpretable behavioral response. Considerable ingenuity is required to devise satisfactory tasks since they not only must be within the child's conceptual capacities and repertoire of behavioral responses but also require the child to make a comparison of an adult surface form with his or her own internal representation. Additional ingenuity is needed to determine the critical acoustic cues leading to the child's response.

The difference between two speech sounds may depend on any combination of multiple acoustic cues (cf., e.g., Lisker, 1978). This built-in redundancy helps to make speech intelligible even in noisy or otherwise distracting surroundings. For example, the difference between voiced and voiceless final stops in English is cued by the length of a preceding vowel (which is greater before voiced consonants), by the voicing of the voiced stop, and by differences in the release, if any, of the voiced versus the voiceless stop. The discrimination of contrasting sounds, then, involves *knowledge of a particular phonemic system* as well as discrimination per se. Fluent users of a language disregard some sound-differences that are irrelevant to the phonemic categories of their language (recall the earlier discussion of categorical perception). In the case of children, auditory discrimination is subject to multiple interpretations; we do not necessarily know which cues the child is attending to; for example, vowel lengthening or voicing or release burst in the discrimination of the voicing contrast (cf. Greenlee, 1978).

Methodological Considerations

Over the past quarter century, many experiments have been conducted to test the speech sound discrimination abilities of children. The experiments have originated in such diverse fields as speech perception, child development, linguistics, and speech-language pathology, and their specific goals have ranged from the establishment of a universal order of acquisition for the perception of phonemic contrasts to the establishment of norms for preschool- or school-age children. Subjects have ranged in age from under one to adolescence. Methods have been accordingly diverse; both live or recorded real speech and synthetic stimuli have been used, and tasks have included naming nonsense objects after extensive training as well as picture-naming. We will review here some of the major methodological factors that may affect the interpretation of findings and thus, our conception of perceptual development. We will then describe a few selected studies.

Natural versus Synthetic Stimuli
In general, two conflicting demands must be weighed in making methodological choices. On the one hand, we are usually interested in "real world" behavior, or speech discrimination under everyday circumstances. From this point of view, live presentation of real speech

has an obvious advantage. On the other hand, we must be concerned to carefully control the experiment to be sure that we are actually testing the ability of interest. As regards presentation, a live speech test is much more difficult to control than a recorded one. The experimenter may inadvertently cue the child by emphasizing a contrasting sound, looking toward the object the child is expected to choose, or simply allowing the child to see the experimenter's face as he or she pronounces a labial versus a dental, so it becomes unclear whether the task is testing visual or auditory discrimination or both. The greatest control is achieved in the use of synthetic stimuli designed to differ along a particular criterial acoustic dimension. Compared with real-life discrimination tasks this method is unnaturally simplified. Specifically, the child is not required to selectively attend to the criterial dimensions while ignoring irrelevant variations as is necessary in the case of natural speech. Furthermore, the perceptual weighting of the various cues may differ markedly from live speech.

Meaningful versus Nonsense Stimuli

There are advantages and disadvantages to both real and nonsense words as stimuli. Setting out to determine the age at which children can discriminate the phonemic contrasts of English, one soon discovers that some contrasts are relatively rare, and the minimal pairs that do occur may be difficult to illustrate clearly or are likely to be unfamiliar to young children. For example, the contrast between /f/ and /θ/ minimally distinguishes relatively few common word-pairs (such as *fin-thin*). Thus, there is an advantage in inventing (nonsense) speech sound sequences that are ideally suited for testing the contrasts of interest.

The use of nonsense words, however, gives rise to other difficulties, in particular, the problem of assuring that the child's internal representation of speech sounds is consulted. If we are interested in the child's knowledge of speech sounds and mental representation of the forms of words, as well as in the purely auditory ability to distinguish sounds, we must somehow contrive to tap his or her internal lexicon. When nonsense syllables are used, the child is often asked to decide whether two stimuli are the same or different. A purely auditory comparison of the two stimuli, without reference to any internal representation, is therefore possible; *linguistic* perception is not necessarily involved at all. On the other hand, when real words are used, the child is typically asked to look at two pictures representing similar sounding words while one of the words is named (e.g., *rake* vs. *lake*). In order to decide which of the two pictures goes best with the sound pattern just heard, the child must refer to some internal representation of the relevant words.

But words unfamiliar to the child are, in effect, no different from nonsense words. If the child is unfamiliar with a word, he or she may develop a strategy, for example, of always responding with the familiar picture, thereby avoidng entirely the intended discrimination task (Clumeck, 1982). When word familiarity has been controlled, error scores have been found to be higher for contrasts involving a relatively unfamiliar word (Barton, 1976; Clumeck, 1982; Smit and Bernthal, 1983).

Research with Young Children

Methodological difficulties are the most acute with younger children. By the age of 10 or 12 months, children are beginning to understand and produce language and, thus, have already internalized a certain number of meaningful sound patterns. It would be of great interest to determine if children's internal representations of words conform more completely with adult models than do the word patterns they are able to produce. At this age, however, the child's cognitive capacities (e.g., attention span) and repertoire of behavioral responses are limited, and it is difficult to obtain on command consistent responses, such as pointing to a named picture or fetching a named object, from a child under the age of 2 or 3. Considerable ingenuity has gone into the development of experiments usable with children under 3, but the results remain disappointingly ambiguous.

Full versus Partial Linguistic Perception

In an effort to test the idea that full perception is achieved very early, Barton (1976) developed two procedures, one for use with children aged 2;3 to 2;11, the second adapted for use with younger children. In the first case, after assessing each child's ability to identify a given set of pictures and training them on unfamiliar labels, Barton repeatedly presented two cards at a time—each pair representing a minimal contrast, while a recorded voice instructed the child to point to one of the pictures. A wide range of contrasts was tested, including differences in voicing, nasality, and place of articulation, as well as /l/ versus /r/, /w/ versus /r/, and /tr/ versus /tʃ/. Overall discrimination was 80 percent; errors primarily occurred when one of the pictures was initially unfamiliar to the child.

In his second study, Barton used just two minimal pairs (*pear–bear* and *coat–goat*), focusing on the contrast in voicing, which Shvachkin (1948/1973) and Garnica (1973) had reported to be a late or difficult discrimination. He began with teaching sessions in which the children played various games with small objects that represented each of the words but with no need to discriminate the minimal contrasts. After checking familiarity with the object names at least a day later, he tested the children on the minimal contrasts by repeatedly asking them to take different objects out of a bag or to place them back in it. Eight out of 10 subjects (aged 1;8 to 2;0) succeeded in making one or both discriminations. Failures of discrimination due to task difficulty could not be clearly differentiated from failures due to difficulty with the linguistic discrimination of interest. Despite the methodological difficulties, Barton (1976) interpreted his data as evidence for the position that full perception occurs at an early age. He concluded that discrimination was less difficult for 2-year-olds than had been reported in some earlier work.

The significance of the effect of word familiarity on the child's discrimination should not be overlooked. If children make more errors in discriminating contrasts in *new words*, then it may be wrong to assume that they are typically able to draw on accurate internal representations of surface forms when they produce words. Instead, it seems likely that children's internal representations continue to change for some years. When first attempting a word, the child may be operating with a partially correct internal representation. In time, this representation becomes more accurate as the child profits from additional exposure to the adult form. But the child may fail to notice the discrepancy between his or her initial internal representation and the adult surface form and could then persist in the perception-based error for some time.

Examples of such changing internal representations are difficult to obtain in any systematic or experimental way but may be revealed by careful analysis of longitudinal data (cf. Macken, 1980). Specifically, when a child begins to produce a new adult sound (such as /θ/) for which he or she formerly produced a substitute sound (such as /f/), we can look to see if the change seems to occur "across the board" (Smith, 1973), in all and only the words containing the relevant phoneme. If so, we can assume that the words were correctly represented although they were not yet correctly produced. On the other hand, if the child begins to use the new sound (/θ/) in words that were formerly correctly produced with the substituting sound (*wife, frosty* as /waiθ/, /θrɔsti/), we conclude that /θ/ words had formerly been mistakenly represented with /f/, and the child is now faced with the problem of sorting out which are actually /θ/ words and which are /f/ words. This process may take a matter of months or even years (cf. Vihman, 1982, for a fuller account of just such an error).

Interaction of Perception and Production

To resolve the question of whether or not internal representations may be assumed to reflect adult surface forms accurately from the earliest stages of lexical acquisition, data are needed on both production and perception from the same subjects. Several studies of this kind have been reported for normal children.

Eilers and Oller (1976) specifically expected to find a relation between ease of perception of a contrast and frequency of production errors involving the contrast. They adapted a technique of Vincent-Smith, Bricker, and Bricker (1974), using both real and nonsense words, to test 14 two-year-old children. Eilers and Oller combined familiar objects, such as fish, with nonsense toys given minimally contrasting names, such as /θi/f/. To test discrimination, the child was told to choose a specific toy; a reward was hidden under the object named. The pairs were of three types: (1) pairs in which the second element typically substitutes for the first in child production of the pairs: [kʰ]–[k], [pl]–[p], [θ]–[f], [Vŋk]–[Vk], and [r]–[w]; (2) pairs of elements not typically involved in such a substitution relationship: [pʰ]–[tʰ] and [pl]–[pʰ]; and (3) non-minimal pairs. Eilers and Oller reasoned that if the substitutions were motivated by perceptual confusions, type (1) pairs should prove more difficult for children to discriminate than type (2) or (3) pairs. The hypothesis was partially confirmed. Some of the type (1) pairs were not discriminated by any of the children ([θ]–[f], [Ṽŋk]–[Vk]), but one was unexpectedly discriminated by most of the children ([kʰ]–[k]). The type (3) pair was the easiest, as predicted. Transcription of the children's productions of each of the test pairs showed that the type (1) pairs were the least well distinguished, as predicted. In short, Eilers and Oller showed that some production errors may derive from perceptual difficulties although others (e.g., the contrast in voicing or aspiration) are more likely to relate to motor constraints.

Strange and Broen (1980) conducted a careful test of both the production and the perception of word-initial /w/, /r/, and /l/ by 21 children aged 2;11 to 3;5. Production was examined through the use of an imitation task and transcription of the child's forms; each phoneme was scored for each child as a "correct" production, a distortion, a substitution by another approximant, or a substitution by a segment outside the class of approximants. The children made virtually no errors on /w/; responses with /r/ and /l/ fell into three groups: (1) mastery, (2) few errors, and (3) many errors. Perception was tested through the use of live voice, recorded, and synthetic stimuli for the pairs *rake–lake, wake–rake*, and (as a control), *wake–bake*. The acoustic stimuli were designed to differ in not just one, but several, of the criterial dimensions that distinguish the target phonemes, but they had identical rhyming portions (*-ake*). The children were asked to point to one of two pictures. They proceeded from live voice to recorded to synthetic pairs.

Overall accuracy was over 90 percent; /w/–/r/ was the most difficult contrast, /w/–/b/ the easiest. The synthetic stimuli gave rise to more errors for some pairs, but there was no consistent overall pattern of errors in relation to type of stimulus. Identification accuracy was clearly related to /r/ and /l/ production ability, with far more errors made by the eight children in group (3), who had made the most production errors. However, there was a great deal of variability in performance among those subjects, and all showed better than chance identification of all three contrasts on one or more tests. Strange and Broen tentatively concluded that both perception and production of phoneme contrasts develop gradually and that perception of a contrast normally precedes its production. However, they emphasized that their test situation was highly constrained; it involved only two response alternatives and a long series of tests using the same stimuli, which could serve as training on the contrast. Thus, the study does not reflect "intentional, coordinated perception," such as ordinary life requires, in which the child-listener is actively involved in extracting the relevant phonetic cues from a complex set of stimuli in order to determine which words were intended by the speaker.

Locke (1980b) has argued that evaluation of a child's perception of speech sounds should be based on the child's patterns of sound substitutions, with attention paid to the **particular phonetic contexts** that give rise to the child's production errors. He developed a *speech production-perception task* in which the perceptual stimuli used are based on a preliminary test of the child's productions. The child is tested on the sounds he or she misarticulated (the *stimulus phoneme*), on the substituting sound (the *response phoneme*), and on a perceptually similar control sound. The different stimulus types are presented six times each in a live-voice object or picture identification task ("Is this X?"), with the tester seated beside the child. For more detail and a copy of the test form, see Chapter 6.

Locke reported that of 131 children tested, ranging in age from 3 to 9 (mean age 5;3), most had speech substitutions, but they did not necessarily have speech disorders. About one third of the contrasts misproduced were also misperceived. However, misperception was not equally likely to be involved in all production errors. Specifically, only 49 percent of those errors consisted of the substitution of one voiceless fricative for another, yet this type of substitution accounted for fully 89 percent of the misperceived contrasts. The pair that accounted for the largest number of perception errors was /f/–/θ/ (67 percent incidence of misperception). Of 52 children who substituted /f/ for /θ/ in production, the 26 younger subjects (mean age 3;7) were much more likely also to misperceive the contrast than were the older subjects (mean age 6;2).

Finally, Velleman (1988) designed a study to test the hypothesis that some English phonemes typically involved in production errors (e.g., /s/) are easy to perceive, so late acquisition is likely to be due to articulatory difficulty. She predicted that in the case of /s/, poor production would occur in the *absence* of poor perception. For other phonemes, the production problem might be related to a perceptual problem; specifically, the articulation of /θ/ and /f/ yields signals that are relatively weak and can be confused with one another. Velleman predicted that in this case, production would be dependent on perception: "Only children with high perception scores would also have high production scores" (223).

Velleman tested 12 English-speaking children aged 3 to 5. She sampled production in free speech as well as in picture- and toy-naming and imitation of nonsense syllables. Initial fricatives were judged on the basis of three independent transcriptions and were then subjected to detailed acoustic analysis. To test perception, Velleman first assessed word familiarity and then used a live-voice, real-word picture-identification task. The pairs of interest were *thumb–some, thumb–fum* (as in *fee, fi, fo, _____*), and *some–fum*.

Velleman's results confirmed her hypotheses. Perception and production of /s/ showed no correlation. Some children with poor /s/ production had good perception of contrasts involving /s/, and in general, perception errors with /s/ were rare. In contrast, perception and production of /θ/ were highly correlated, with production of /θ/ better for children with perception scores of over 80 percent. More errors were made in both perception and production in the case of /θ/ than in the case of /s/.

In summary, the results of the few studies examining production and perception in the same children all point to an identical conclusion: Some phonemic contrasts remain difficult to discriminate perceptually as late as age 3 or older (e.g., /θ/–/f/, /r/–/w/), and production errors involving these pairs typically continue to occur in the later preschool period. It should be mentioned that the /f/–/θ/ contrast in particular is notoriously difficult for adults as well. Other production errors show no evident relation to perception (voicing in stops at age 2, /s/ at age 3 to 5).

Internal Representations

We can now reconsider the question raised earlier regarding internal representations. Note, first of all, that linguistic perception has not yet been successfully tested in the earliest period of lexical production (age 12 to 18 months). Anecdotal data are available from diary studies, but they are sparse, often based on once-only occurrences, and difficult to evaluate in the absence of transcriber reliability or other statistical procedures. Based on production data from this period, a bias toward perception and/or storage in terms of the favored shapes of the babbling period (e.g., CV syllables) seems likely (Locke, 1983; Vihman, 1991). By about age 2, when the child has a sizable lexicon but many production errors, we can assume that the child is perceiving words in a shape that closely resembles the adult surface forms. For some elements (e.g., fricatives, clusters, and /r/), however, nonadultlike perception may still be the rule, and it is precisely those sound classes that continue to give rise to production difficulties for many children into the later preschool and early school years. It is possible, then, that some children persist in misproducing a few sounds because they are inaccurately storing the adult form. Such errors may arise in an early period, when the child is unable to either produce the relevant articulatory gestures or *represent* (store) the relevant distinction. The production error may persist long after the child's motoric or articulatory difficulty has been resolved, due to the child's lack of self-monitoring or lack of attention to the difference between his or her inaccurately stored form and the adult form.

The possible effect on the child's phonology of the child's perception of his or her *own* output forms has received little attention. Straight (1980), who insists on a sharp dichotomy between auditory and articulatory processes, suggested that, in some cases, the child's own simplified or otherwise distorted output may lead to a radically inaccurate internal representation that then underlies the child's subsequent spontaneous productions. Vihman (1982) offered two possible illustrations of such "feedback" from the child's own productions to his or her internal representations. For a discussion of the complex interrelation between children's perceptions, misarticulations, and self-monitoring on the phonetic and phonemic level, see Locke, 1979.

Summary

Infants have been found to respond differentially to a wide range of contrasting speech sounds. Linguistic perception, however, requires active attention to speech sound contrasts, in order to identify, store, and recognize distinct lexical items. Given a variety of potential acoustic cues to speech sound contrasts, the child must be able to select and integrate the relevant cues while disregarding those that play no contrastive role in the phonemic system of the language in question.

Testing linguistic perception in children presents many methodological challenges. For example, the investigator must balance the need for *control* to ensure a valid test against the need for *naturalistic* data. As a result, studies of young children have used both real and nonsense words, live-voice, recorded, and synthesized stimuli. It has also proven important to test children on words that are familiar to them since more errors are made in the identification of relatively unfamiliar words.

The question of whether or not a child's perception of lexical items is fully accurate from the beginning of speech production is currently of considerable theoretical interest. Attempts to test children younger than age 2 have been limited and not entirely successful. Nevertheless, the role of word familiarity has proven to be highly significant, suggesting that some production errors may derive from perceptual misinterpretations, that is, internal representations that fail to match the adult model, since initial attempts at a new word inevitably reflect an internal representation based on perception of a relatively unfamiliar word. The results of studies of production and perception in the same children support the idea that imperfect perception is involved in production errors with respect to certain contrasts, such as /f/ versus /θ/ and /w/ versus /r/. The production errors that appear to be related to perceptual difficulties are errors that typically persist into the later preschool or even early school-age years.

Systematization and Reorganization: From Word to Segment

It has been suggested that the earliest units the child targets for production are whole-word patterns rather than segments or even syllables (cf. Ferguson and Farwell, 1975). At least three different kinds of evidence have been adduced to support this view. The first kind involves variation in the child's production across different target words, the second, the relation of particular child word shapes to their adult models, and the third, the interrelation of child forms at a given point in time.

Lexical Idiosyncrasy

Individual segments vary across words, even in similar phonetic contexts. For example, *baby* may be realized with initial [d], while *bye-bye* has initial [b] in the child's forms. Similarly, some words are relatively stable in form from the beginning (e.g., Hildegard Leopold's *papa*: [papa~baba]), while others vary widely from one attempt to another (e.g.,

Hildegard's *mama*: [mama-ma~bama~maba]). Data of this sort suggest that the child does not target word-initial /b/ or /m/ in isolation from the particular adult word patterns in which the consonants occur.

Prosodic Phenomena

In some cases, the child's form seems to match the adult word as a whole, but with no evident sequential segment-to-segment correspondence. Ferguson and Farwell provide two examples: *shoe*: [gutçi], [gutʃidi]; *feet* [ˈfi ʔ] (cf. also, e.g., Waterson, 1971). This strongly suggests that the child is targeting a whole gestalt, not a sequence of individual segments.

Phonological Idioms

It has been noted (cf. especially Moskowitz, 1973) that some early words may occur in surprisingly advanced form, for example, with consonant clusters produced as in the adult model. The best-known instance is Hildegard's first permanent word, *pretty* pronounced [prəti], at 10 months. This represents a relatively rare case of an unusually good reproduction of a difficult adult form, but it is unlikely to have been planned and produced segment by segment. Several months later, Hildegard simplified the form to [pɪti] and [bɪdi], structures that conformed more closely with her other word forms. These later productions seem to be integrated into Hildegard's phonological system at that stage of development and may be viewed as at least partially analyzed (into two syllables, say) prior to production. The more complex early form seems to be extra-systemic or "pre-systemic," since it is unrelated to other sound patterns in Hildegard's own repertoire.

As the child begins to acquire new vocabulary at an accelerated pace, typically after accumulating 50 words or more, there is pressure to "systematize" the phonological representations and production routines to allow smoother functioning of word production (cf. Chiat, 1979; Menn, 1983). The changes that occur at this time reflect a process of internal reorganization, like that shown to occur in other domains of language acquisition, such as syntax and semantics (cf., e.g., Slobin, 1973; Bowerman, 1982). The classic examples come from English morphology. Although the child at first produces apparently correct (irregular as well as regular) plural and past tense forms (*shoes, feet, walked, broke*), at a later point, he or she will begin to apply the regular inflectional endings to words that happen to have irregular plural or past tense forms in English (*foots, breaked*). This is generally taken as evidence that the child has "analyzed out" or "discovered" the productive inflectional suffixes marking regular plural and past tense forms. The "overregularized" forms thus reflect new knowledge and reorganization. Only much later will the child again begin to use the correct irregular forms, which, at that point, have a new status as known exceptions to the general morphological rule.

Evidence for phonological reorganization is indirect and thus difficult to trace in terms of specific stages. Nevertheless, there are data from a range of children learning difficult languages that suggest that such reorganization, based on internal analysis and systematization, does occur (see Vihman, Velleman, and McCune, 1994). This reorganization will affect the basic unit of the child's phonological system. While the primary unit at the earliest stage appears to be the word, reanalysis will allow the child to operate with a more efficient, segment-based system. We will consider three characteristics of the process of reorganization and, at the same time, illustrate different children's responses to phonological challenges.

Apparent Regression

Hildegard Leopold's production of *pretty*, first in a more complex, adultlike form and only later in a simplified form, is a good example of apparent regression; that is, a step backward for an individual lexical form in the service of greater progress or coherence for the child's phonological system as a whole. The extensive data available on the phonological development of Hildegard, who was raised as a bilingual speaker of English and German, provides a fuller illustration of this process as it pertains to the acquisition of /l/ (Leopold, 1947; our account is based on the analysis in Ferguson and Farwell, 1975). The word *hello* appeared in the form [ʔəlɔ] at 1;5 and showed no change until 1;10, when Hildegard began to produce it as [jojo], a superficially more primitive form. The substitution of the palatal glide [j] for /l/ affected some, but not all, of the /l/ words Hildegard attempted (see Table 2.1). In its original form, *hello* could be considered a phonological idiom. It showed no evidence of analysis below the word level, whereas [jojo] appears to reflect the "discovery" of the medial *l*, a troublesome segment for Hildegard, and the consequent application of the gliding rule, which began to play a role in Hildegard's phonology only after the time of her first use of *hello*. This is a classic example of "regression," or "nonlinear progression," in which early attempts at systematization—themselves a sign of progress toward a more sophisticated phonology—result in a more primitive child form of a word formerly pronounced in an adultlike way.

Creative Strategies

Virve Vihman acquired Estonian as her first language although she was exposed to some English as well (see Vihman, 1978). Multisyllabic forms were difficult for her. Among her first 50 words, only two had adult models longer than two syllables. At 17 months, her first trisyllabic form appeared: /ˈapːelsin/ → [ˈapːɛsi] 'orange'. Within the same month, the child began to make use of an idiosyncratic long-word production strategy. Starting from a three-syllable adult model, she would produce a three-syllable form in which the last two (unstressed) syllables were always identical. She maintained the syllable count and overall

Table 2.1   Development of the Lateral /l/ in H's Speech during the Second Year

	hello	alle "all"	bottle	lie	Loch "hole"	Löscher "eraser"
1;5	ʔəlɔ					
1;6			ba:I			
1;7		ʔatə	ba:I			
1;8		ʔajə	baIu			
1;9			balu			
1;10	jojo	ʔalə	baju		lok'/jok'	
1;11	jojo		balu	jal		loko/joke

Source: From Vihman, M. M., C. A., Ferguson, and M. Elbert, "Phonological Development from Babbling to Speech: Common Tendencies and Individual Differences." *Applied Psycholinguistics,* Vol. 7 (1986), 3–40, © Cambridge University Press. Used with permission.

syllabic structure of the adult word, but she abandoned any attempt at segmental fidelity for all three syllables. Instead, her choice of segments seemed to reflect a prosodic approach, in which certain features of the adult word were adopted and spread over more than one syllable, while other segments or features were disregarded. For example:

/'takasi/ → ['tasisi] "(to go, take) back" (1;5)
/'len:uk:it:/ → ['nanunu] "airplane (obj.)" (1;6)
/'porkanit:/ → ['ponini] "carrot (obj.)" (1;6)
/'ra:mat:ut:/ → ['ma:nunu] "book (obj.)" (1;6)

Virve continued to produce new long words according to her invented pattern for five months. Ferguson (1978) has used the term *unique reduction device* to describe such creative strategies for coping with words of greater complexity than the child's production system can handle. Here again, the use of an adultlike form (['ap:əsi]) was followed by a more primitive type of production (e.g., ['tasisi]); the latter, however, reflects hypothesis-formation or system-building and, therefore, can be viewed as a step toward a more complex phonology.

Changing Hypotheses

Macken's (1979) description of the phonology of a Spanish-speaking child, Si, demonstrates the development from a word-based to a segment-based system. The child was recorded weekly from 1;7 to 2;5. For the first six months of the study, Si had a strong preference for a CVCV word pattern consisting of an initial labial consonant followed by a medial dental. Subpatterns developed during this period through the expansion of earlier patterns; as a new word pattern became dominant, some words would change patterns. Most strikingly, in order to achieve an output form which agreed with the preferred pattern "labial–dental," the child would restructure different adult models in different ways, selectively deleting the initial syllable(s) of *Ramon* and *elefante* ("elephant"), for example, but the medial syllable of *manzana* ("apple") and *Fernando*.

manzana → [mən‿na] ("apple') (1;7)
Fernando → [man‿nə - wan‿no o- nan‿no] (1;8)
Ramon → [mən] (1;8)
elefante → [bat‿te] ("elephant") (1;9)

Si gradually increased her repertoire of sounds and syllable shapes over a six-month period while maintaining some control over the range of complexity she had to handle in terms of contrasting consonants in a single word. Any attempt to match Si's forms segment-for-segment to the adult model, as in a strict phonemic analysis like the one Smith (1973) provides to account for his son's development, would prove extremely difficult since Si's output depended heavily on her own current repertoire of word patterns. In the last four months of data collection, Si's phonemic system quickly grew to include most of the phonemes of adult Spanish, and the unusual substitution patterns of the earlier period disappeared, along with the constraints on co-occurrence of consonants that had motivated those patterns.

Summary

The first units targeted in the earliest period of adult-based word production appear to be whole-word patterns rather than segments. This is suggested by the variation typically found in the treatment of individual segments across different words, by the gestaltlike match of early child forms to adult models, and by the occasional occurrence of extrasystemic forms or phonological idioms. After this early period, the pressure of a rapidly growing lexicon leads to gradual reorganization. Indirect evidence of this process may be found in the phenomenon of non-linear progression, in which superficially more advanced forms are later produced in a less adultlike form—but one that is integrated into the child's repertoire of phonological forms and appears to reflect the operation of regular phonological processes.

References

Anderson, S. R., *Phonology in the Twentieth Century: Theories of Rules and Theories of Representation.* Chicago: University of Chicago Press, 1985.

Atkinson, F., B. MacWhinney, and C. Stoel. "An experiment on the recognition of babbling." *Language Behavior Research Laboratory Working Paper, 14.* Berkeley: University of California, 1968.

Barton, D., "The role of perception in the acquisition of phonology." Ph.D. thesis, University of London, 1976. (Reprinted by the Indiana University Linguistics Club, 1978).

Bernhardt, B., and C. Stoel-Gammon, "Nonlinear phonology: Introduction and clinical application." *Journal of Speech and Hearing Research, 37* (1994): 123–143.

Bernhardt, G., "The prosodic tier and phonological disorders." In M. Yavas (Ed.), *First and Second Language Pathonology.* San Diego: Singular Publishing Group, 1994.

Bowerman, M., "Reorganizational processes in lexical and syntactic development." In E. Wanner and L. R. Gleitman (Eds.), *Language Acquisition: The State of the Art.* Cambridge (UK): Cambridge University Press, 1982.

Boysson-Bardies, B., de, N. Bacri, L. Sagart, and M. Poizat, "Timing in late babbling." *Journal of Child Language, 8* (1981): 525–539.

Boysson-Bardies, B., de, P. Hallé, L. Sagart, and C. Durand, "A crosslinguistic investigation of vowel formants in babbling." *Journal of Child Language, 16* (1989): 1–17.

Boysson-Bardies, B., de, L. Sagart, and C. Durand, "Discernible differences in the babbling of infants according to target language." *Journal of Child Language, 11* (1984): 1–15.

Boysson-Bardies, B., de, and M. M. Vihman, "Adaptation to language." *Language, 61* (1991): 297–319.

Braine, M. D. S., "Review of N. V. Smith, *The Acquisition of Phonology: A Case Study.*" *Language, 52* (1976): 489–498.

Browman, C. P., and L. Goldstein, "Articulatory phonology: An overview." *Phonetica, 49* (1992): 155–180.

Chiat, S., "The role of the word in phonological development." *Linguistics, 17* (1979): 591–610.

Chomsky, N., "A review of B. F. Skinner's *Verbal Behavior*" (New York: Appleton-Century-Crofts, 1957). *Language, 35* (1959): 26–58.

Chomsky, N., *Lectures on Government and Binding.* New York: Foris Publications, 1981.

Clumeck, H., "The effects of word-familiarity on phonemic recognition in children aged 3 to 5 years." In C. E. Johnson and C. L. Thew (Eds.), *Proceedings of the Second International Congress for the Study of Child Language*, Vol. 1. Lanham, MD: University Press of America, 1982.

Cruttenden, A., *Intonation.* Cambridge: Cambridge University Press, 1986.

Davis, B. L., and P. F. MacNeilage, "Acquisition of correct vowel production: A quantitative case study." *Journal of Speech and Hearing Research, 33* (1990): 16–27.

Delack, J. B., and P. J. Fowlow, "The ontogenesis of differential vocalization: Development of prosodic contrastivity during the first year of life." In N. Waterson and C. Snow (Eds.), *The Development of Communication.* New York: John Wiley, 1978.

Deville, G., "Notes sur le développement de l'enfant." *Revue de Linguistique, 23* (1890): 330–343; *24* (1891): 10–42, 128–143, 242–257, 300–320.

Donegan, P., and D. Stampe, "The study of natural phonology." In D. Dinnsen (Ed.), *Current Approaches to Phonological Theory.* Bloomington: Indiana University Press, 1979.

Dore, J., M. B. Franklin, R. T. Miller, and A. L. H. Ramer, "Transitional phenomena in early language acquisition." *Journal of Child Language, 3* (1976): 13–28.

Edwards, M. L., and L. D. Shriberg, *Phonology: Applications in Communicative Disorders.* San Diego, Calif.: College-Hill, 1983.

Eilers, R. E., "Context-sensitive perception of naturally produced stop and fricative consonants by infants." *Journal of the Acoustical Society of America, 61* (1977): 1321–1336.

Eilers, R. E., "Infant speech perception: History and mystery." In G. Yeni-Komshian, J. Kavanagh, and C. A. Ferguson (Eds.), *Child Phonology*, Vol. 2. *Perception.* New York: Academic Press, 1980.

Eilers, R. E., W. Gavin, and W. R. Wilson, "Linguistic experience and phonemic perception in infancy: A cross-linguistic study." *Child Development, 50* (1979): 14–18.

Eilers, R. E., and F. D. Minifie, "Fricative discrimination in early infancy." *Journal of Speech and Hearing Research, 18* (1975): 158–167.

Eilers, R. E., and D. K. Oller, "The role of speech discrimination in developmental sound substitutions." *Journal of Child Language, 3* (1976): 319–329.

Eimas, P., E. Siqueland, P. Jusczyk, and J. Vigorito, "Speech perception in infants." *Science, 171* (1971): 303–306.

Elbers, L., "Operating principles in repetitive babbling: A cognitive continuity approach." *Cognition, 12* (1982): 45–63.

Ferguson, C. A., "Sound patterns in language acquisition." In D. P. Dato (Ed.), *Developmental Psycholinguistics: Theory and Application.* Georgetown University Roundtable, 1–16. Washington, DC: Georgetown University Press, 1975.

Ferguson, C. A., "Learning to pronounce: The earliest stages of phonological development in the child." In F. D. Minifie and L. L. Lloyd (Eds.), *Communicative and Cognitive Abilities—Early Behavioral Assessment.* Baltimore: University Park Press, 1978.

Ferguson, C. A., "Phonology as an individual access system: Some data from language acquisition." In C. J. Fillmore, D. Kempler, and W. S.-Y. Wang (Eds.), *Individual Differences in Language Ability and Language Behavior.* New York: Academic Press, 1979.

Ferguson, C. A., "Discovering sound units and constructing sound systems: It's child's play." In J. S. Perkell and D. H. Klatt (Eds.), *Invariance and Variability of Speech Processes.* Hillsdale, NJ: Lawrence Erlbaum, 1986.

Ferguson, C. A., and C. B. Farwell, "Words and sounds in early language acquisition." *Language, 51* (1975): 419–439.

Ferguson, C. A., and O. K. Garnica, "Theories of phonological development." In E. H. Lenneberg and E. Lenneberg (Eds.), *Foundations of Language Development.* New York: Academic Press, 1975.

Ferguson, C. A., and M. A. Macken, "The role of play in phonological development." In K. E. Nelson (Ed.), *Children's Language*, Vol. 4. Hillsdale, NJ: Lawrence Erlbaum, 1983.

Ferguson, C. A., L. Menn, and C. Stoel-Gammon, *Phonological Development: Models, Research, Implications.* Parkton, MD: York Press, 1992.

Ferguson, C. A., D. B. Peizer, and T. A. Weeks, "Model-and-replica phonological grammar of a child's first words." *Lingua, 3* (1973): 35–65.

Fernald, A., and T. Simon, "Expanded intonation contours in mothers' speech to newborns." *Developmental Psychology, 20* (1984): 104–113.

Francescato, G., "On the role of the word in first language acquisition." *Lingua, 21* (1968): 144–153.

Fry, D. B., "The development of the phonological system in the normal and the deaf child." In F. Smith and G. Miller (Eds.), *The Genesis of Language: A Psycholinguistic Approach.* Cambridge, MA: M.I.T. Press, 1966.

Garnica, O. K., "The development of phonemic speech perception." In T. Moore (Ed.), *Cognitive Development and the Acquisition of Language.* New York: Academic Press, 1973.

Goldsmith, J. A., *Autosegmental and Metrical Phonology.* Oxford: Blackwell, 1990.

Greenlee, M., "Learning the phonetic cues to the voiced-voiceless distinction: An exploration of parallel processes in phonological change." Ph.D. thesis, University of California, Berkeley, 1978.

Grunwell, P., "The development of phonology." *First Language, 2* (1981): 161–191.

Hallé, P. A., B. de Boysson-Bardies, and M. M. Vihman, "Beginnings of prosodic organization: Intonation and duration patterns of disyllables produced by French and Japanese infants." *Language and Speech, 34* (1991): 299–318.

Householder, F. W., "Unreleased PTK in American English," In M. Halle (Ed.), *For Roman Jakobson.* The Hague: Mouton, 1956.

Ingram, D., *Phonological Disability in Children.* London: Edward Arnold, 1976.

Iverson, G., and D. Wheeler, "Hierarchical structures in child phonology." *Lingua, 73* (1987): 243–257.

Jakobson, R., *Child Language, Aphasia and Phonological Universals,* A. R. Keiler (Tr.). The Hague: Mouton, 1968. [Original title *Kindersprache, Aphasie und allgemeine Lautgesetze.* Uppsala: Almqvist and Wiksell, 1941.]

Jusczyk, P. W., and J. Bertoncini, "Viewing the development of speech perception as an innately guided learning process." *Language and Speech, 31* (1988): 217–238.

Jusczyk, P. W., J. Murray, and J. Bayly, "Perception of place of articulation in fricatives and stops by infants." Paper presented at Biennial Meeting of Society for Research in Child Development, San Francisco, 1979.

Karzon, R. B., "Discrimination of polysyllabic sequences by one-to- four-month-old infants." *Perception and Psychophysics, 39* (1985): 105–109.

Kent, R. D., "The biology of phonological development." In C. A. Ferguson, L. Menn, and C. Stoel-Gammon (Eds.), *Phonological Development: Models, Research, Implications.* Parkton, MD: York Press, 1992.

Kent, R. D., and H. R. Bauer, "Vocalizations of one-year-olds." *Journal of Child Language, 13* (1985): 491–526.

Kent, R. D., and A. D. Murray, "Acoustic features of infant vocalic utterances at 3, 6, and 9 months." *Journal of the Acoustical Society of America, 72* (1982): 353–365.

Kiparsky, P., and L. Menn, "On the acquisition of phonology." In J. Macnamara (Ed.), *Language Learning and Thought.* New York: Academic Press, 1977.

Kuhl, P. K., "Perception of speech and sound in early infancy." In P. Salapatek and L. Cohen (Eds.), *Handbook of Infant Perception*, Vol. 2. *From Perception to Cognition.* New York: Academic Press, 1987.

Leopold, W. F., *Speech Development of a Bilingual Child*, Vol. 2. *Sound-Learning in the First Two Years.* Evanston, IL: Northwestern University Press, 1947.

Lewis, M. M., *Infant Speech: A Study of the Beginnings of Language.* New York: Harcourt Brace, 1936.

Lieberman, P., "On the development of vowel production in young children." In G. Yeni-Komshian, J. Kavanagh, and C. A. Ferguson (Eds.), *Child Phonology*, Vol. 1, *Production.* New York: Academic Press, 1980.

Lindblom, B., "Phonological units as adaptive emergents of lexical development." In C. A. Ferguson, L. Menn, and C. Stoel-Gammon (Eds.), *Phonological Development: Models, Research, Implications.* Parkton, MD: York Press, 1992.

Lindner, G., *Aus dem Naturgarten der Kindersprache.* Leipzig: Th. Grieben's Verlag, 1898.

Lisker, L., "Rabid vs. rapid: A catalogue of acoustic features that may cue the distinction." Haskins Laboratories Status Report on Speech Research (SR-54). New Haven, CT, 1978.

Lisker, L., and A. S. Abramson, "A cross-language study of voicing in initial stops: Acoustical measurements." *Word, 20* (1964): 384–422.

Locke, J. L., *The Child's Path to Spoken Language.* Cambridge, MA: Harvard University Press, 1993.

Locke, J. L., "The child's processing of phonology." In W. A. Collins (Ed.), *Minnesota Symposium on Child Psychology*, Vol. 12. Hillsdale, NJ: Lawrence Erlbaum, 1979.

Locke, J. L., "The inference of speech perception in the phonologically disordered child. Part I: A rationale, some criteria, the conventional tests." *Journal of Speech and Hearing Disorders, 4* (1980a): 432–444.

Locke, J. L., "The inference of speech perception in the phonologically disordered child. Part II: Some clinically novel procedures, their use, some findings." *Journal of Speech and Hearing Disorders, 4* (1980b): 445–468.

Locke, J. L., *Phonological Acquisition and Change.* New York: Academic Press, 1983.

Locke, J. L., "Variation in human biology and child phonology: A response to Goad and Ingram." *Journal of Child Language, 15* (1988): 663–668.

Locke, J. L., "Structure and stimulation in the ontogeny of spoken language." *Developmental Psychobiology, 23* (1990): 621–643.

Locke, J. L., and D. Pearson, "Vocal learning and the emergence of phonological capacity: A neurobiological approach." In C. A. Ferguson, L. Menn, and C. Stoel-Gammon (Eds.), *Phonological Development: Models, Research, Implications.* Parkton, MD: York Press, 1992.

McCune, L., M. M. Vihman, L. Roug-Hellichius, D. B. Delery, and L. Gogate, "Grunt communication in human infants (*Homo sapiens*)," *Journal of Comparative Psychology, 110* (1996): 27–37.

MacKain, K. S., "Assessing the role of experience on infants' speech discrimination." *Journal of Child Language, 9* (1982): 527–542.

Macken, M. A., "Developmental reorganization of phonology: A hierarchy of basic units of acquisition." *Lingua, 49* (1979): 11–49.

Macken, M. A., "The child's lexical representation: The 'puzzle-puddle-pickle' evidence." *Journal of Linguistics, 16* (1980): 1–17.

Macken, M. A., and C. A. Ferguson, "Cognitive aspects of phonological development: Model, evidence and issues." In K. E. Nelson (Ed.), *Children's Language*, Vol. 4. Hillsdale, NJ: Lawrence Erlbaum, 1983.

MacNeilage, P. F., and B. F. Davis, "Acquisition of speech production: Frames, then content." In M. Jeannerod (Ed.), *Attention and Performance XIII: Motor Representation and Control.* Hillsdale, NJ: Lawrence Erlbaum, 1990.

Maxwell, E. M., "On determining underlying phonological representations of children: A critique of the current theories." In M. Elbert, D. A. Dinnsen, and G. Weismer (Eds.), *Phonological Theory and the Misarticulating Child.* ASHA Monographs, 22. Rockville, MD: ASHA, 1984.

Menn, L., "Pattern, control, and contrast in beginning speech: A case study in the development of word form and word function." Ph.D. thesis, University of Illinois, 1976. (Reprinted by the Indiana University Linguistics Club, 1978).

Menn, L., "Phonological units in beginning speech." In A. Bell and J. B. Hooper (Eds.), *Syllables and Segments.* Amsterdam: North-Holland, 1978.

Menn, L., "Theories of phonological development." In H. Winitz (Ed.), *Native Language and Foreign Language Acquisition.* New York: Academy of Sciences, 1981.

Menn, L., "Development of articulatory, phonetic, and phonological capabilities." In B. Butterworth (Ed.), *Language Production*, Vol. 2. London: Academic Press, 1983.

Menyuk, P., L. Menn, and R. Silber, "Early strategies for the perception and production of words and sounds." In P. Fletcher and M. Garman (Eds.), *Language Acquisition: Studies in First Language Development*, 2nd ed. Cambridge (UK): Cambridge University Press, 1986.

Mitchell, P. R., and R. D. Kent, "Phonetic variation in multisyllable babbling." *Journal of Child Language, 17* (1990): 247–265.

Moskowitz, A. I., "The acquisition of phonology and

syntax: A preliminary study." In K. J. J. Hintikka, J. M. E. Moravcsik, and P. Suppes (Eds.), *Approaches to Natural Language*. Dordrecht: Reidel, 1973.

Mowrer, O., *Learning Theory and Symbolic Processes*. New York: John Wiley, 1960.

Mulford, R., "First words of the blind child." In M. D. Smith and J. L. Locke (Eds.), *The Emergent Lexicon: The Child's Development of a Linguistic Vocabulary*. New York: Academic Press, 1988.

Nespor, M., and I. Vogel, *Prosodic Phonology*. Dordrecht: Foris Publications, 1986.

Oller, D. K., "The emergence of the sounds of speech in infancy." In G. Yeni-Komshian, J. Kavanagh, and C. A. Ferguson (Eds.), *Child Phonology*, Vol. 1, *Production*. New York: Academic Press, 1980.

Oller, D. K., and R. E. Eilers, "The role of audition in infant babbling." *Child Development, 59* (1988): 441–449.

Olmsted, D., *Out of the Mouth of Babes*. The Hague: Mouton, 1971.

Paradis, C., "On constraints and repair strategies." *The Linguistic Review, 6* (1988): 71–97.

Porges, S., "Autonomic regulation and attention." In B. A. Campbell, H. Hayne, and K. Richardson (Eds.), *Attention and Information Processing in Infants and Adults*. Hillsdale, NJ: Lawrence Erlbaum, 1992.

Priestly, T. M. S., "One idiosyncratic strategy in the acquisition of phonology." *Journal of Child Language, 4* (1977): 45–65.

Ramer, A. L. H., "Syntactic styles in emerging language." *Journal of Child Language, 3* (1976): 49–62.

Richards, J. E., and B. J. Casey, "Development of sustained visual attention in the human infant." In B. A. Campbell, H. Hayne, and R. Richardson (Eds.), *Attention and Information Processing in Infants and Adults*. Hillsdale, NJ: Erlbaum, 1992.

Robb, M. P., and J. H. Saxman, "Syllable durations of preword and early word vocalizations." *Journal of Speech and Hearing Research, 33* (1990): 583–593.

Roug, L., I. Landberg, and L. J. Lundberg, "Phonetic developoment in early infancy: A study of four

Swedish children during the first eighteen months of life." *Journal of Child Language, 16* (1989): 19–40.

Schwartz, R., and L. B. Leonard, "Do children pick and choose? An examination of phonological selection and avoidance in early lexical acquisition." *Journal of Child Language, 9* (1982): 319–336.

Shibamoto, J. S., and D. L. Olmsted, "Lexical and syllabic patterns in phonological acquisition." *Journal of Child Language, 5* (1978): 417–456.

Shvachkin, N. K. H., "The development of phonemic speech perception in early childhood." In C. A. Ferguson and D. I. Slobin (Eds.), *Studies of Child Language Development*. New York: Holt, Rinehart & Winston, 1973. [Original title "Razvitiye fonematicheskogo vospriyatiya rechi v rannem vozraste." *Izvestiya Akademii Pedagogicheskikh Nauk RSFSR, 13* (1948): 101–132.]

Skinner, B. F., *Verbal Behavior.* New York: Appleton–Century–Crofts, 1957.

Slobin, D. I., "Cognitive prerequisites for the development of grammar." In C. A. Ferguson and D. I. Slobin (Eds.), *Studies of Child Language Development*. New York: Holt, Rinehart & Winston, 1973.

Smit, A. B., and J. Bernthal, "Performance of articulation-disordered children on language and perception measures." *Journal of Speech and Hearing Research, 26* (1983): 124–136.

Smith, B. L., S. Brown-Sweeney, and C. Stoel-Gammon, "Reduplicated and variegated babbling." *First Language, 9* (1989): 175–189.

Smith, N. V., *The Acquisition of Phonology: A Case Study*. Cambridge (UK): Cambridge University Press, 1973.

Spencer, A., "Towards a theory of phonological development." *Lingua, 68* (1986): 3–38.

Stampe, D., "The acquisition of phonetic representation." Paper presented at the Fifth Regional Meeting of the Chicago Linguistic Society, Chicago, Illinois, 1969.

Stark, R. E., "Features of infant sounds: The emergence of cooing." *Journal of Child Language, 5* (1978): 379–390.

Stark, R. E., "Stages of speech development in the first year of life." In G. Yeni-Komshian, J. Kavanagh, and C. A. Ferguson (Eds.), *Child Phonology*, Vol. 1. *Production*. New York: Academic Press, 1980.

Stark, R. E., "The coupling of early social interaction and infant vocalization." Paper presented at Biennial Meeting of Society for Research in Child Development, New Orleans, 1993.

Stark, R. E., L. E. Bernstein, and M. E. Demorest, "Vocal communication in the first 18 months of life." *Journal of Speech and Hearing Research, 36* (1993): 548–558.

Stemberger, J., and C. Stoel-Gammon, "The underspecification of coronals: Evidence from language acquisition and performance errors." In C. Paradis and J. F. Prunet (Eds.), *Phonetics and Phonology*, Vol. 3. *The Special Status of Coronals*. New York: Academic Press, 1991.

Stoel-Gammon, C., and J. A. Cooper, "Patterns of early lexical and phonological development." *Journal of Child Language, 11* (1984): 247–271.

Stoel-Gammon, C., and K. Otomo. "Babbling development of hearing-impaired and normally hearing subjects." *Journal of Speech and Hearing Disorders, 51* (1986): 33–41.

Straight, H. S., "Auditory versus articulatory phonological processes and their development in children." In G. Yeni-Komshian, J. Kavanagh, and C. A. Ferguson (Eds.), *Child Phonology*, Vol. 1. *Production*. New York: Academic Press, 1980.

Strange, W., and P. A. Broen, "Perception and production of approximate consonants by 3-year-olds: A first study." In G. Yeni-Komshian, J. Kavanagh, and C. A. Ferguson (Eds.), *Child Phonology*, Vol. 2. *Perception*. New York: Academic Press, 1980.

Streeter, L. A., "Language perception of 2-month-old infants shows effects of both innate mechanisms and experience." *Nature, 259* (1976): 39–41.

Thevenin, D. M., R. E. Eilers, D. K. Oller, and L. La Voie, "Where's the drift in babbling drift? A cross-linguistic study." *Applied Psycholinguistics, 6* (1985): 3–15.

Trehub, S. E., "Auditory-linguistic sensitivity in infants." Ph.D. thesis, McGill University, Montreal, 1973.

Trehub, S. E., "The discrimination of foreign speech contrasts by infants and adults." *Child Development, 44* (1976): 466–472.

Trevarthan, C., and P. Hubley, "Secondary intersubjectivity: Confidence, confiding and acts of meaning in the first year." In A. Lock (Ed.), *Action, Gesture and Symbol: The Emergence of Language*. New York: Academic Press, 1978.

Tyler, A. A., and T. E. Langsdale, "Consonant-vowel interactions in early phonological development." *First Language, 16* (1996): 159–191.

Velleman, S. L., "The role of linguistic perception in later phonological development." *Applied Psycholinguistics, 9* (1988): 221–236.

Velleman, S. L., "A nonlinear model of early child phonology." Paper presented at Linguistic Society of America, Philadelphia, 1992.

Vihman, M. M., "Consonant harmony: Its scope and function in child language." In J. H. Greenberg (Ed.), *Universals of Human Language*, Vol. 2. *Phonology*. Stanford, CA: Stanford University Press, 1978.

Vihman, M. M., "A note on children's lexical representations." *Journal of Child Language, 9* (1982): 249–253.

Vihman, M. M., "Ontogeny of phonetic gestures: Speech production." In I. G. Mattingly and M. Studdert-Kennedy (Eds.), *Modularity and the Motor Theory of Speech Perception*. Hillsdale, NJ: Lawrence Erlbaum, 1991.

Vihman, M. M., "Early syllables and the construction of phonology." In C. A. Ferguson, L. Menn, and C. Stoel-Gammon (Eds.), *Phonological Development: Models, Research, Implications*. Parkton, MD: York Press, 1992.

Vihman, M. M. "Variable paths to early word production." *Journal of Phonetics, 21* (1993): 61–82.

Vihman, M. M. *Phonological Development: The Origins of Language in the Child*. Oxford: Blackwell, 1996.

Vihman, M. M., and B. de Boysson-Bardies, "The nature and origins of ambient language influence on infant vocal production and early words." *Phonetica, 51* (1994): 159–169.

Vihman, M. M., C. A. Ferguson, and M. Elbert, "Phonological development from babbling to speech: Common tendencies and individual differences." *Applied Psycholinguistics, 7* (1986): 3–40.

Vihman, M. M., and M. Greenlee, "Individual differences in phonological development: Ages one and three years." *Journal of Speech and Hearing Research, 30* (1987): 503–521.

Vihman, M. M., E. Kay, B. de Boysson-Bardies, C. Durand, and U. Sundberg, "External sources of individual differences: A cross-linguistic analysis of the phonetics of mother's speech to one-year-old children." *Developmental Psychology, 30* (1994): 652–663.

Vihman, M. M., M. A. Macken, R. Miller, H. Simmons, and J. Miller, "From babbling to speech: A reassessment of the continuity issue." *Language, 61* (1985): 395–443.

Vihman, M. M., and R. Miller, "Words and babble at the threshold of lexical acquisition." In M. D. Smith and J. L. Locke (Eds.), *The Emergent Lexicon: The Child's Development of a Linguistic Vocabulary.* New York: Academic Press, 1988.

Vihman, M.M., and S. Velleman, "Phonological reorganization: A case study." *Language and Speech, 32* (1989): 149–170.

Vihman, M. M., S. Velleman, and L. McCune, "How abstract is child phonology? Towards an integration of linguistic and psychological approaches." In M. Yavas (Ed.), *First and Second Language Phonology.* San Diego: Singular Publishing Group, 1994.

Vincent-Smith, L., D. Bricker, and W. Bricker, "Acquisition of receptive vocabulary in the toddler-age child." *Child Development, 45* (1974): 189–193.

Waterson, N., "Child phonology: A prosodic view." *Journal of Linguistics, 7* (1971): 179–211.

Waterson, N., "A tentative developmental model of phonological representation." In T. Myers, J. Laver, and J. Anderson (Eds.), *The Cognitive Representation of Speech.* Amsterdam: North-Holland, 1981.

Werker, J. F., "Ontogeny of speech perception." In I. G. Mattingly and M. Studdert-Kennedy (Eds.), *Modularity and the Motor Theory of Speech Perception.* Hillsdale, NJ: Lawrence Erlbaum, 1991.

Werker, J. F., J. H. V. Gilbert, K. Humphrey, and R. C. Tees, "Developmental aspects of cross-language speech perception." *Child Development, 52* (1981): 349–353.

Werker, J. F., and J. E. Pegg, "Infant speech perception and phonological acquisition," In C. A. Ferguson, L. Menn, and C. Stoel-Gammon (Eds.), *Phonological Development: Models, Research, Implications.* Parkton, MD: York Press, 1992.

Werker, J. F., and R. C. Tees, "Developmental changes across childhood in the perception of non-native speech sounds." *Canadian Journal of Psychology, 37* (1983): 278–286.

Werker, J. F., and R. C. Tees, "Cross-language speech perception: Evidence for perceptual reorganization during the first year of life." *Infant Behavior and Development, 7* (1984): 49–63.

Zlatin, M., "Explorative mapping of the vocal tract and primitive syllabification in infancy: The first six months." *Purdue University Contributed Papers, 5* (1975): 58–73.

Chapter *3*

Later Phonological Development

MARILYN MAY VIHMAN,
University of Wales–Bangor

The two different research strategies most commonly used in the study of later phonological development lead to somewhat different pictures of that process. In the **longitudinal** studies of individual children, extensive data are collected from different points in a particular child's development. This strategy, typically used by linguists, highlights the variability in any one child's productions at one point and over time, and across different children. Close analysis of individual differences can provide insight into the learning process. But such intensive data analyses are available for only a relatively small number of children, and therefore the validity of any generalizations about the time-course for acquisition of specific speech sounds is uncertain. Child development specialists and speech-language pathologists interested in the study of normal phonological development for the purpose of comparison with disordered speakers most often use a different strategy—a **cross-sectional** research design. In this approach, no single child is followed over time; rather, different children at different age levels are tested at a single point in time on their ability to produce speech sounds, and a composite profile is extrapolated from the data.

We will begin our discussion of later phonological development by reviewing some of the best-known large-scale studies. This will set the stage for a closer look at the particular paths followed by a smaller number of individual children. We will also consider issues relating to the perception of running speech by older children in comparison with adults. Finally, we will review ways in which phonetic and phonological variation and change continue beyond the early childhood years.

Establishing Group Norms: Large-Scale Studies

Long before the field of child language acquisition began to burgeon in the 1960s, there was considerable practical interest in determining the age at which most children are able to correctly produce each of the phonemes of their language; that is, there was a need to establish developmental norms. Such an enterprise, however, has inherent methodological and theoretical problems. In order to establish production norms, one must test large numbers of children, but fully adequate evaluation of any one child's ability to produce contrasts between speech sounds requires both time and patience. Use of imitation may yield different results than spontaneous speech, and speech sound production in single words may differ from that in running conversation, as it does in adults. Many intensive studies of small groups (e.g., Ingram, Christensen, Veach, and Webster, 1980) have confirmed what a careful reading of earlier diary data suggested: Individual differences across children are so great in some areas—in the acquisition of fricatives, for example—that it may be impossible to establish meaningful age norms. Nevertheless, the need for such normative information is undeniable. Furthermore, developmental norm studies are based on the testing of children covering a broad age range (2 to 10 years) and, thus, can provide a useful overview of development beyond the earliest period of lexical acquisition.

Table 3.1 lists salient characteristics of the major cross-sectional studies undertaken in the United States in this century. These large-sample studies generally follow the same model, which may be described as follows.

Subject Selection

First of all, an effort is made to ensure that the sample reflects the socioeconomic distribution of the population as a whole; Templin (1957), who reported the parameters of her study in full, weighted her sample toward the lower end of the scale (70 percent of the children, based on father's occupation) and included only urban children. Second, audiometric screening and parental report are typically used to exclude children with hearing losses or delayed language development.

TABLE 3.1   Major Cross-Sectional Production Studies in the United States (I = initial, M = medial, F = final; Sp = spontaneous, Im = imitated)

Date	Author(s)	No.ss	Age Range	Word Position	SP/IM	Criterion
1931	Wellman et al.	204	2;0–4;0	I, M, F	Sp, Im	75%
1934	Poole	140	2;5–8;5	I, M, F	Sp	100%
1957	Templin	480	3;0–8;0	I, M, F	Sp, Im	75%
1963	Snow	438	6;5–8;7	I, M, F		
1967	Bricker	90	3;0–5;0	I	Im	
1971	Olmsted	100	1;3–4;6	I, M, F	Sp	
1972	Sax	535	5;0–10;0	I, M, F	Sp	93%
1975	Prather et al.	147	2;0–4;0	I, F	Sp, Im	75%
1976	Arlt and Goodban	240	3;0–5;6	I, M, F	Im	75%
1990	Smit et al.	997	3;0–9;0	I, F	Sp, Im	75%

Obtaining the Sample

Children are asked to name a picture representing a target word, usually only once; if the child does not produce the word spontaneously, an imitation is elicited. Consonants and clusters are tested in initial, medial, and final position, or a subset of those; vowels and diphthongs are also tested in some studies.

Analysis

A criterion is set to determine "age of acquisition" *for the group as a whole.* For Templin, this criterion was correct production in each of three word positions by 75 percent of the children. For Prather, Hedrick, and Kern (1975), it was correct production in two positions, again by 75 percent of the children, and scores were averaged over the two positions. Vowels and diphthongs were generally found to be acquired by age three, and will not be further considered here.

In these studies, only group data are used. No results are given regarding individual responses, so there is no information regarding either individual differences between children of the same age or actual errors made for a given sound. The basic goal is to establish the age at which parents, teachers, and clinicians may reasonably expect a child's production of a given sound to match the adult standard.

Sander (1972) pointed out that the widely quoted ages of acquisition for speech sounds, based on the earlier studies cited in Table 3.1, are misleading if taken to reflect "average" performance, given the strict criteria used. Instead, they must be understood to represent upper age limits for acquisition. In an effort to derive a more representative profile, Sander reanalyzed the Wellman, Case, Mengert and Bradbury (1931) data and the Templin data. He established a range between "customary production" (correct production in two out of three word positions by 50 percent of the children) and "mastery" (correct production in all three word positions by 90 percent of the children). Prather et al. (1975) also utilized this strategy; they presented their normative data in a similar manner, and then compared it with Sander's reanalysis (see Chapter 7, Figure 7.1).

Figure 7.1 vividly illustrates the difference between customary production and mastery, given data based on group behavior. Acquisition of /k/, for example, ranges from customary production (i.e., use by half the children sampled) at age 2 to correct production by virtually all the children at nearly age 4. The data regarding correct production of /t/ are strikingly discrepant in the two studies. Whereas Prather and colleagues report a range from under 24 months to 32 months, Sander's reanalysis of the data from Wellman and colleagues and from Templin shows a range from 24 months to over 48 months. However, Sander points out that the late age of acquisition cited for /t/ in Templin (age 6) is entirely due to the younger children's failure to produce a voiceless [t] in medial position. In fact, in American English /t/ is normally produced as a (voiced) flap in medial position following a stressed vowel (as in *skating*). The coding of an error here reflects an unrealistic, idealized standard based on British rather than American usage, since the British do use a true medial [t].

Relatively small differences in methodology may greatly affect the age of acquisition reported. Smit (1986) analyzed the differences between Templin's study, which appears to be the one most frequently consulted by clinicians, and the more recent studies by Prather et al. (1975) and Arlt and Goodban (1976). The latter studies reported younger ages of acquisition for most sounds, as is evident for Prather and colleagues. Arlt and Goodban suggested that children were learning speech sounds at younger ages at the time of their study than 20 years earlier. Use of this more recent standard, then, would entail concern about children at an earlier age if their production of some sounds (most likely fricatives or liquids) failed to meet expectations based on the reported data.

Smit noted several methodological reasons for the discrepancy, particularly differences in analysis, like the decision to use two positions instead of three and to *average* scores across word-positions rather than require that 75 percent of the children produce a sound correctly in *each* position. Furthermore, Templin reported data only for children who attempted all sounds, whereas Prather and colleagues reported *partial* data, especially at the younger ages. Since missing data likely reflect an unwillingness to make errors in producing a difficult sound, this difference alone can have a significant effect on the results.

Given their cursory sampling (one production per segment in each word-position) and the differences in methods of analysis of these large-scale studies, it would clearly be a mistake to place a great deal of faith in an exact age at which a given phoneme can be expected to be produced correctly. Nevertheless, the results of the studies do agree sufficiently to provide a general picture of the order of acquisition of English consonants up to the point of mastery of the system as a whole. Nasals, stops, and glides are acquired relatively early; fricatives and affricates are mastered relatively late. Consonant clusters are also acquired late, with two-consonant clusters (for example, /kl/ and /st/) preceding the three-consonant clusters (for example, /str/ and /spl/). Most single consonants and consonant clusters are apparently mastered by age 7 or 8. As Locke (1983) has pointed out, the consonants acquired early are, generally speaking, those which occur most frequently in the languages of the world.

Three other large-scale studies carried out in the United States provided more qualitative data than those described so far. Snow (1963) tested 438 first-grade children, using two test words per consonant for each of three word-positions. Unlike Templin, Snow reported in some detail the particular errors made on each sound. Bricker (1967) tested imitation of word-initial consonants in nonsense syllables by 90 children aged 3 to 5, and reported substitutions for the 10 consonants which elicited the most errors. Finally, Olmsted (1971) collected spontaneous speech samples of varying lengths from 100 children aged 1;3 to 4;6. He, too, reported substitutions for the 10 consonants most "prone to error."

Noting that these three studies are "more sophisticated in methodology and interpretation" than the earlier large-scale studies, Ferguson (1975) provided a thorough review and comparison of their data on fricatives, which account for the largest proportion of errors in all three. Despite differences in testing procedure, analysis, and the reporting of results, Ferguson found that the order of acquisition of the eight English fricatives across all three studies could be summarized in terms of three (internally unordered) groups: first /f, s, ʃ/, then /v, z/, and finally /θ, ð, ʒ/—an ordering which is largely consistent with the predictions of Jakobson (1941/68). On the other hand, the specific substitutions reported for these fricatives are not typically stops, as Jakobson predicted, except for /v/ (> /b/) and sometimes /ð/ (> /d/). Instead, /s/ substitutes for several other fricatives, /f/ substitutes for /θ/, and the affricate /dʒ/ is the most common substitute for /ʒ/, which has marginal status in English and is often replaced by /dʒ/ word-finally, even by adults. Linguists have yet to provide a plausible or widely accepted explanation for the occurring pattern of fricative to stop and fricative to fricative substitutions, whether based on the physiology of the speech tract, the nature of mental processes, the structure of English phonology, or the phonological usage of different members of society in the English-speaking world.

Smit, Hand, Freilinger, Bernthal, and Bird (1990) reported on a study conducted in Iowa and Nebraska which was larger in scale than anything undertaken previously. The study excluded data from 2-year-olds because of the large number who either failed to complete the test or refused to produce some of the test words. For the remaining children, Smit et al. reported a significant gender difference for children at ages 4;0, 4;6, and 6;0. Comparing their overall results with Templin's, they reported a plateau in the *boys'* developmental speech sound curve, between ages 3;6 and 4;0 or 4;6. a comparable plateau appears in the Templin data for boys beginning six months later. Close analysis of the various speech sounds tested reveals that the gender difference can be traced back to consonant cluster development, with either a plateau or a drop in performance for most clusters for boys, beginning at age 3;6. No explanation for this developmental difference is apparent at this time.

Summary

Despite methodological difficulties, investigators have attempted to establish age norms based on the testing of large numbers of children at different age levels. Several cross-sectional studies of 100 or more English-speaking children have been conducted. Most reports group data in terms of a set criterion, such as the age at which three quarters of the children correctly produce each consonant in three word-positions. It is important to bear in mind that there is often a long temporal gap between average age of customary production of a sound (correct use by 51 percent of the children in two out of three positions), and mastery of the sound (correct use in all positions by 90 percent of the children). Analysis in terms of customary production yields lower ages of acquisition. Other methodological variables—such as inclusion versus exclusion of data from subjects who fail to attempt some of the target sounds—also strongly affect the resultant chronology.

Large-scale studies do agree on certain general points. Nasals, stops, and glides are acquired early; fricatives, affricates, and consonant clusters are acquired later. Reporting of qualitative results (e.g., specification of the errors made for each sound) greatly enhances the value of a cross-sectional study. Developmental norm studies are designed to provide information about a large number of children and thus afford an overview of phonological development. Their limitation in principle is their inability to reveal the particular course of development of any one child. In providing a broad range of data, such studies can serve as a useful complement to the more narrowly based diaries, and longitudinal studies of small groups of children.

Phonological Processes: Systematicity in Production Errors

One fact about phonological development on which linguists of virtually all theoretical persuasions can agree is the **systematic** nature of the child's simplifications and restructuring of adult words (Macken and Ferguson, 1981). As Oller (1975) explicitly puts it, "the sorts of substitutions, deletions and additions which occur in child language are not merely random errors on the child's part, but are rather the result of a set of systematic tendencies" (299). It is the systematic relationship between the adult target and the child's reproduction of that target that is expressed by the linguist's "rewrite" or "realization rule":

$$X \rightarrow Y/Z$$

or "X 'goes to' [is substituted by or realized as] Y in the environment Z." For example, when a 3-year-old produces a series of words like [tænt] for *can't*, [tɔz] for *'cause*, [taᵘ] for *cow*, and [oᵘˈteⁱ] for *okay*, the linguist formulates a rule to express the observed regularity: [k] → [t]; in this case no "conditioning environment" or context is given since the substitution appears to occur in a wide range of contexts. In fact, when we notice that the child also says [dɛt] for *get*, [doᵘ] for *go*, [ˈdoᵘfɚs] for *gophers*, and [diːn] for *green*, we can express the rule more generally as "a velar stop is realized as a dental (or alveolar) stop."

Phonological substitutions typically show great regularity in the language of children past the earliest stage of lexical acquisition. Linguists express that regularity by using phonological rules, or what have come to be known in the child language literature as "phonological processes." The theoretical status—and the psychological reality—of these processes remains highly controversial. If perception of phonological contrasts continues to develop over the preschool years, the phonological processes that the child appears to operate with may not be strictly production rules; rather, they may be perception or "interpretation" rules, meaning that the error underlying the mismatch between child form and adult form is actually present in the child's internal representation of the target word. Most likely, distortions of different kinds occur in both perception and production and may be due to a variety of factors including such idiosyncrasies as affective peculiarities of certain words and interrelationships between lexical items which the child associates. In any case, our understanding of phonological development has undoubtedly benefited from the extensive cataloging of common processes used by different children learning different languages. At our present stage of knowledge regarding the child's actual processing of language, references to phonological processes are generally a description convenience rather than an attempt to directly reflect the child's mental activity.

Let us now take a closer look at the most common phonological processes that children have been found to apply to adult words. In general, these processes appear to be used regardless of the particular language the child is learning, although the structure of the adult language may affect the frequency with which a given process is used (Ingram, 1986; Vihman, 1978, 1980). The processes are used to some extent by virtually all children in the earlier stages of word acquisition, but a given child will quickly master certain difficulties (e.g., the production of velars or fricatives or closed syllables, depending on his or her phonetic preferences and the words he or she has been attempting) and thereby obviate the need for the corresponding processes (velar fronting, stopping, final consonant deletion) while continuing to make use of other processes. Finally, more than one process may be implicated in a child's production of a single word (e.g., cluster simplification as well as velar fronting must be posited to account for the realization of *green* as [diːn], cited above).

Phonological processes may be grouped into two functionally distinct categories: **whole-word processes**, which simplify word or syllable structure and segmental contrast within a word (generally through reduction or assimilation), and **segment change processes**, which involve (context-free) changes in specific segments or segment types, regardless of syllable- or word-position. We will briefly characterize a few of the most common processes representing each of these types; further discussion, using examples taken from the extensive literature on normal phonological acquisition, follows. For a fuller list of common phonological processes, see Chapter 7.

Whole-Word Processes

Unstressed syllable deletion: omission of an unstressed syllable of the target word

>*Ramon* → [mən]   (Si: Macken, 1979)

Final consonant deletion: omission of a final consonant of the target word

>*because* → [pi'kʌ]
>*thought* → [fɔ]   (Vihman and Greenlee, 1987)

Reduplication: production of two identical syllables, based on one or more of the syllables of the target word

>*Sesame Street* → [si:si]   (Deborah: Vihman et al., 1986)
>*hello* → [jojo]   (Hildegard: Leopold, 1947)

Consonant harmony: one of the contrasting consonants of the target word takes on features of another consonant in the same word

>*duck* → [gʌk]
>*tub* → [bʌb]   (Daniel: Menn, 1971)

Consonant cluster simplification: a consonant cluster is simplified in some manner

>*cracker* → [kæk]   (Molly: Vihman et al., 1986)

Assimilatory processes (like consonant harmony) take the whole word as their domain, whereas reduction processes (involving consonant or syllable deletion) alter the phonotactic or syntagmatic structure of the adult model, reducing the number of syllables or simplifying the shape of syllables. The two types of reduction processes are often treated together and have variously been referred to as "phonotactic rules" (Ingram, 1974), "syllable structure processes" (Ingram, 1986: see also Ch. 7), "structural simplifying processes" (Grunwell, 1981), "syntagmatic processes" (Nettelbladt, 1983), or "processes affecting sequential structure" (Magnusson, 1983). Following the order of processes given above, we will first consider two of the most common reduction processes, syllable deletion and consonant deletion, and then two assimilatory processes, reduplication and consonant harmony;

finally, we will illustrate consonant cluster simplification, which is closely related to the segment change processes.

Reduction Processes

Vihman (1980) examined "long word reduction" in 11 children (aged 1;0 to 2;9) acquiring five languages. She restricted analysis to words of three syllables or more in the adult model. She found a strict language-based order for the proportion of long words attempted: Frequencies ranged from about 25 percent for two Spanish-speaking children to about 3 percent for three English-speaking children. Use of syllable deletion to handle the long words varied independently of the particular language spoken, and ranged from 90 percent for Hildegard Leopold (German- and English-speaking) to 26 percent for Jiri, a Czech-speaking child.

   Syllable deletion most often affects an unstressed syllable. Even a stressed syllable may be omitted, especially if it is the first of three or more syllables. There is a strong tendency for children to preserve a final syllable, whether it is stressed or not, presumably because final position is perceptually salient. Klein (1981) provides a great many examples of syllable deletion. The following instances were produced by Jason, a child who made moderate use of the process of deletion.

   alligator → ['ægejʌ]
   banana → ['nænæ]
   butterfly → ['bʌfaɪ]
   watermelon → ['mõmĩn]   (omitting the stressed initial syllable)

One of the 3-year-olds included in the study reported in Vihman and Greenlee (1987) was continuing to apply syllable deletion to many words:

   animals → ['æml̩z]
   ambulance → ['æmʌns]
   dessert → [ʒɹ̩t]

   Consonant deletion most often affects final consonants, though initial and medial consonants may also be omitted. Berman (1977) reported that her daughter Shelli (age 18 to 23 months, acquiring both Hebrew and English) frequently used consonant deletion, particularly to avoid producing word-forms with both initial and final consonants. Difficulty with individual segments appears to have dictated the choice of segment to omit: Stops and nasals were retained, with preference for stops; fricatives and liquids were omitted. The chief mark of phonological advance in the period under study was the production of formerly omitted consonants and the admission of new CVC words without reduction. Some examples of consonant deletion (from Berman, 1977):

   1. Word-initial

   /'ruti/ → ['uti] "Ruthie" (mother's name)
   /ʃa'lom/ → ['alom] "hello"
   /xam/ → [am] "hot"

2. Word-final

peach → [pi]

spoon → [pu]

/tov/ → [to] "good"

Deletion of a medial consonant is cited for one 3-year-old in Vihman and Greenlee (1987):

mommy → [mãi]

Assimilatory Processes

Although some writers view use of **reduplication** as the mark of a developmental stage that all children pass through (Moskowitz, 1973; Fee and Ingram, 1982), others maintain that reduplication, like other phonological processes, represents an individual strategy characterizing the speech of some but not all children at the same developmental point (Schwartz, Leonard, Wilcox, and Folger, 1980; cf. also Schwartz and Leonard, 1983). The function of reduplication is also a subject of controversy. It may serve as a strategy for producing multisyllabic adult words—retaining the syllable count while reducing the number of contrasting elements, or as a way to avoid final consonant production.

Schwartz and colleagues collected spontaneous speech data from 12 (English-speaking) children aged 1;3 to 2;0, half of whom proved to be "reduplicators," using full or partial reduplication in 20 percent or more of their recorded lexicon. Fee and Ingram drew on 24 heterogeneous data sets (mostly parental diaries) for children aged 1;1 to 2;6. Some examples of reduplication provided by Schwartz and colleagues (1980):

Christmas → [dzɪdzɪ]

kitten → [kɪkɪ]

water → [wɔwɔ]

Whereas Schwartz and colleagues found no correlation between age or linguistic stage and relative use of reduplication for their narrower age range, Fee and Ingram found that the reduplicators in their sample were younger than the non-reduplicators (they did not assess stage of linguistic development). Both studies found that reduplication is primarily used to reduce the complexity of multisyllabic words. (Application of the process to monosyllables—e.g., *ball* → [bʌbə]—proved rare.) The relation between reduplication and final consonants remains unclear. Moreover, the suggestion that heavy use of reduplication may characterize slower learners (Ferguson, Peizer, and Weeks, 1973) has yet to be tested on a large scale.

Ferguson (1983) pointed out that reduplication has also been found to serve a "play" or "practice" function, not only in babbling but also in the sound-play of 2- to 5-year-olds (cf. Ferguson and Macken, 1983). Furthermore, reduplication may help the child to identify and learn to produce phonologically distinctive syllables and segments; production of a reduplicative pattern reflecting the shape of one of the syllables of the adult model seems to provide the child with a well-controlled way to move from a whole-word to a segment-based phonology (cf. Macken, 1978; Lleó, 1990).

Consonant harmony, or the assimilation of non-contiguous consonants, is essentially the same as "partial reduplication" (vowel harmony is a parallel process but is less frequently noted in child language data). Unfortunately, neither Schwartz et al. nor Fee and Ingram specified the proportion of full versus partial reduplication (i.e., assimilation) in their data. In a study of relatively large data sets from 13 children (aged 1;0 to 2;9) acquiring six languages, Vihman (1978) found a range from 1 percent to 32 percent in the use of consonant harmony (for words containing different consonants in the adult model); mean use was 14 percent. Differences in frequency of harmony use did not appear to be tied to differences in target language.

Smith suggested that consonant harmony is "part of a universal template which the child has to escape from in order to learn his language" (1973; 206). In some children, however, it is rare, and when it is used, it often enters the child's lexicon as a simplification of words produced earlier in a form closer to the adult model. The use of consonant harmony can be taken to reflect the child's effort to systematize his or her word production. More specifically, consonant harmony often provides a way of avoiding difficult segments (such as liquids and fricatives) or of allowing the child to produce new segments or longer words by reducing overall complexity. For a recent study of patterns of consonant harmony in a large sample of children acquiring English, see Stoel-Gammon and Stemberger, 1994.

Consonant harmony may also be described as "full" or "partial," depending on the resultant child form. In full harmony, the consonants of a word, which contrasted in the adult model, are identical in the child form; in partial harmony, the consonants of the child form are more similar than in the adult model but are not identical. Some examples (from Vihman, 1978):

1. Full

   | Amahl Smith | *tiger* → [gaigə] |
   | Virve Vihman | *tuppa* → [pup:a] "into the room" |

2. Partial

   | Virve Vihman | *suppi* → [fup:i] "some soup" |

Notice that the differences reflected here between adult and child forms could all be described in terms of a single distinctive feature: alveolar to velar (plus automatic word-initial voicing) for *tiger*, alveolar to labial or labiodental for *tuppa* and *suppi*. Full versus partial harmony describes only the resultant form, not the extent of the difference between adult and child form.

Grunwell's chronology (1981) showed that neither reduplication nor consonant harmony is normally used by age 3. Full reduplication did not occur in the 3-year-old samples in Vihman and Greenlee (1987), and consonant harmony occurred only sporadically (a few instances in a three-hour sample) and only for a few of the children.

1. Full

   yellow → [ˈlɛlou]

   mailboxes → [ˈmeɪlmaksɪz]

2. Partial

slimy → [ˈsnaɪmi]

Consonant Cluster Simplification

Like the reduction processes, cluster simplification alters syllable structure, but it is also closely related to the segment change processes in that the specific consonants omitted or changed are typically those difficult to produce as singleton consonants. Cluster simplification is virtually always present in the first year of language use, and it is one of the longest lasting processes. At age 3, cluster simplification still accounted for a substantial proportion of the phonological errors made by the 10 children followed in Vihman and Greenlee (1987), and it still accounts for over 10 percent of the errors of 5-year-olds responding to standardized test items (Haelsig and Madison, 1986; Roberts, Burchinal, and Footo, 1990).

Among the 11 younger subjects of Vihman (1980), cluster simplification affected from 52 percent to 100 percent (mean 80 percent) of all target words with clusters (which themselves made up nearly a third of the children's words, on average; the three children learning Slavic languages averaged 38 percent words with clusters). Several general relationships emerged in this study. In clusters made up of liquid plus another consonant, the liquid was typically omitted, and when stop and fricative were combined, the stop was the more likely to be preserved. Nasal plus stop clusters were more likely to be maintained as clusters, but when such a cluster was reduced, the nasal was likely to be retained before a voiced stop and omitted before a voiceless stop. Perceptual rather than articulatory factors may be at work here (Braine, 1976) since nasals, like vowels, are longer before voiced obstruents and, thus, may be more easily perceived in that context.

In a study of the acquisition of stop-plus-liquid clusters Greenlee (1974) found the course of development to be very similar in all six of the languages investigated. She identified three stages: (1) omission of the liquid, (2) substitution for the liquid (usually by a glide), and (3) correct production. Some examples (from Greenlee, 1974):

Amahl Smith: *bread* → [bɛd], [blɛd]

Edmond Grégoire (a Belgian child acquiring French):

bras → [bwa] "arm"
croute → [tut] "crust"
grillé → [dije] "toasted"
tram → [kam], [tʃam] "streetcar"

From English-speaking 3-year-olds (Vihman and Greenlee, 1987):

flower → [ˈfawr]
monster → [ˈmãtr]
stinker → [ˈsɪʃkr]
thread → [sɛd]

Segment Change Processes

Velar fronting: a velar is replaced by an alveolar or a dental

/kikeriki:/ → [titi:]   (Virve: Vihman, 1976)

Stopping: a fricative is replaced by a stop

    sea → [ti:]
    say → [tʰei]   (Amahl: Smith, 1973)

Gliding: a liquid is replaced by a glide

    lie → [jaɪ]   (Hildegard: Leopold, 1947)

Of the commonly found changes, **velar fronting** is the only one to affect stops, and it is, no doubt, the first common change process to be outgrown (Preisser, Hodson, and Paden, 1988). A case study by Berg (1995) provides an unusually detailed account of the loss of velar fronting—or, more accurately, the acquisition of velar stops (both as singletons and in clusters)—as his daughter acquired her first language, German, between the ages of 3 and 4 years. The study , based on daily recording, begins with the first successful production of a word-initial velar and ends with virtual mastery of velar production; the process took a full 15 months. Of the ten 3-year-olds described in Vihman and Greenlee, only one exhibited consistent velar fronting. Regular use of velar fronting contributed significantly to the relative unintelligibility of the speech of that child, who was very advanced syntactically and thus often produced long, complex sentences. For example:

    called → [tald]
    cow → [taʊ]
    gophers → [ˈdoufɚs]

The process of **gliding**, which also plays a role in the acquisition of stop + liquid clusters, persists considerably longer. Examples can be found in many languages, but Ingram (1986) claimed that this process does not appear in French acquisition data. Examples of gliding from English-speaking 3-year-olds (Vihman and Greenlee, 1987):

    love → [jʌv]
    red → [wɛd]

Mastering Fricatives

The most common process affecting fricatives is **stopping**, but replacement by a stop is not the only error type found. In particular, the interdentals—the most difficult segments for English-speaking children to acquire (comparable to r-trills in languages which have them)—are frequently substituted by other fricatives (/f/ or /s/ for /θ/, somewhat less commonly /v/, /z/, or even /l/ for /ð/). As mentioned earlier, perceptual difficulties have been implicated in production errors involving both fricatives and liquids, although the low incidence of fricatives in babbling suggests that these sounds present articulatory problems for many children. Some examples of stopping from English-speaking 3-year-olds (Vihman and Greenlee, 1987):

> *move* → [mu:b]
> *shoes* → [ʃu:t]
> *some* → [tʌm]

Perhaps the most important lesson to be learned from the rather extensive literature on the acquisition of fricatives (e.g., Moskowitz, 1975; Edwards, 1979; Ingram, Christensen, Veach, and Webster, 1980) is that each fricative is acquired by its own individual path of development. There is no rapid spread of a feature of "frication" or "continuancy" to relevant segments (Ferguson, 1975). Other points of particular interest raised by Ferguson include the following: (1) Fricatives may be acquired in postvocalic, final position or intervocalically before initial position, and may precede the acquisition of stops in these word-positions, and (2) language-specific constraints on the frequency and freedom of occurrence of particular fricatives may affect the order of acquisition (e.g., English /ʒ/ is rare and largely limited to word-medial position, and it consequently tends to be a late acquisition).

The Acquisition of Voicing

Ingram (1986) noted that the voicing of prevocalic consonants has been reported primarily for English. This raises a question as to whether English-speaking transcribers may be mishearing **lack of aspiration** as "voicing." Acoustic studies of voice onset time in children's productions suggest that both aspiration, or "long lag," and pre-voicing, or "voicing lead," are relatively difficult for children to master (Gilbert, 1977; Barton and Macken, 1980; Macken and Barton, 1980; Clumeck, Barton, Macken, and Huntington, 1981; Eilers, Oller, and Benito-Garcia, 1984; Allen, 1985). Children first produce only voiceless unaspirated stops (regardless of the language being learned); any contrasting stop classes will be acquired later (Macken, 1980).

Smit and Bernthal (1983) found that their 11 normally developing (English-speaking) 4-year-old subjects tended to use fewer fully voiced stops in initial position than adults. But these children did maintain a phonological voicing contrast in initial position: They used disproportionately long voice onset times (or heavy aspiration) in producing (word-) initial voiceless stops (all productions were embedded in a carrier phrase, "the ___ away").

In a study of consonantal devoicing in **final position** in English, Smith (1979) found that both 2- and 4-year-old subjects used substantially fewer voiced stops in all contexts than adults. He reported as much as 50 percent (partial) devoicing in final position by adults, but over 90 percent partial devoicing by both 2- and 4-year-olds. Smith attributed these results to the difficulty children have in controlling the physiological mechanisms needed to sustain voicing during stop closure.

The evidence from acoustic analyses suggests that the observed contrast between early word-initial voicing of stops and word-final "devoicing" is derived from adult (mis)interpretation of a single child phonetic type—voiceless unaspirated stop. Because final stops are not necessarily aspirated (or even released) in English, the voiceless unaspirated phone (used to realize final voiced as well as voiceless stops in target words) is perceived by observers as devoicing, whereas in initial position, where aspiration is an important cue to the English phonemic voicing contrast, the same child phone (again used to realize voiced as well as voiceless stop targets) is heard as voicing. For illustration of the unusual strategies children may resort to in the effort to produce an acceptable voiced stop word-finally, see Fey and Gandour (1982) and Clark and Bowerman (1986).

Summary

The regularity found in phonological substitutions after the earliest stage of lexical acquisition can be conveniently formulated in terms of phonological rules or processes. Two types of processes are usually distinguished on functional grounds. Whole-word processes simplify word or syllable structure and segmental contrast within a word, and segment change processes account for errors involving difficulty with specific segments. Whole-word processes are generally typical of the earlier stages of phonological development. They include assimilatory processes (reduplication and consonant harmony) and consonant cluster simplification. The most common segment changes are velar fronting, gliding, and various substitutions affecting fricatives. Only voiceless unaspirated stops are used in the earliest stage of phonological development, regardless of the language being learned; later, any contrasting classes of stops found in the adult language will gradually be added.

Profiling the Preschool Child: Individual Differences Revisited

We have reviewed both the findings of large-scale studies aimed at establishing norms for the acquisition of particular phonemes of the adult language and the phonological processes found to apply most often in intensive studies of small groups of children (or even just one child). In both cases, the analyses involved may be termed *relational*; that is, they are concerned with the relationship between the child's productions and the adult forms (Stoel-Gammon and Dunn, 1985). "Independent" analyses, on the other hand, describe the sounds and syllable structures of the child's productions in their own right, without reference to the adult forms. In order to form an idea of the kind of phonological production that we can expect to characterize a normally developing 2- or 3-year-old child, we will consider the results of two studies reporting phonological analyses of data drawn from naturally occurring conversation. The first is a study of 2-year-olds and makes use of both relational and independent analyses; the second is an intensive examination of the kinds of errors made by a smaller group of 3-year-olds. In addition, we will consider the results of two longitudinal studies, one comparing the phonological status at age 3 of the two 1-year-old girls profiled in Chapter 2, the other comparing phonological process use in two boys at ages 2, 3, and 6.

Phonetic Tendencies of Two-Year-Olds

Stoel-Gammon (1987) characterized the "phonological skills" of thirty-three 2-year-old children acquiring English. Subjects were recruited through a mailing to parents of newborn children in the Seattle area and observed from the age of 9 to 24 months on a trimonthly basis (cf. also Stoel-Gammon, 1985). The data were derived from two half-hour play sessions involving conversational interaction between child and observer rather than from attempts to elicit pre-selected target words. Stoel-Gammon pointed out that the "large-scale" studies of Wellman et al. (1931), Sander (1972), and Prather et al. (1975) were, in fact, based on a rather small number of 2-year-old subjects (no more than 10 or 20), since a large number of children failed to produce many of the target words. She argued that a better assessment of a 2-year-old's phonological skills can be attained through the recording of naturally occurring conversational data.

Stoel-Gammon established the use of at least 10 different adult-based words in the course of one hour of recording as a base criterion for including a speech sample in the 2-year-old analyses. She then developed a corpus of up to 50 words for each subject, taken from the first fully or partially intelligible utterances in each sample. No one word *type* was represented by more than two variable *tokens* or productions of the same word (e.g., [su] and [du] for *shoe*). The number of words analyzed ranged from 20 to 50 per child (mean 36). Three different analyses were carried out.

Word and Syllable Shapes, Based on the Co-Occurrence of Consonants and Vowels

All the children produced at least two different open monosyllables (CV), and only one child failed to produce two different closed monosyllables (CVC). Disyllabic word shapes (CVCV[C]) occurred in over half the samples, as did word-initial clusters. Word-final clusters were produced by 48 percent of the children and medial clusters by only 30 percent.

Phonetic Inventories

Word-initial consonant inventories typically included stops at all three places of articulation ([t, k, b, d, g] occurred in at least 50 percent of the samples). In addition, nasals ([m, n]), fricatives ([f, s, h]), and a glide ([w]) typically occurred in initial position. In final position, three voiceless stops, one nasal ([n]), one fricative ([s]), and one liquid ([r]) were typically used. There was a strong tendency for children with large inventories in initial position to have a large inventory in final position as well. No one cluster (such as [sp-, pl-]) was used by more than half the children in either initial or final position.

Accuracy of Consonant Production

The mean percentage of correct consonants, based on a procedure developed by Shriberg and Kwiatkowski (1982), was 70 percent (range 43 percent to 91 percent). There was a tendency for the children with larger inventories to achieve greater accuracy with respect to the adult form than those with smaller inventories. Stoel-Gammon pointed out that the difference in inventory size between adult English and the "typical" 2-year-old in her study is considerable, and thus, the 70 percent accuracy level achieved by the children suggests that 2-year-olds attempt mainly words with consonants that fall within their productive range. The relationship between the number of different consonants produced and the use of consonant phones that match adult segments further suggests that phonetic and phonological abilities are developing parallel to one another.

Phonological Process Use at Age Three

After age 3, the majority of simplifying phonological processes no longer apply regularly in most cases. The data we will describe were derived from three hours of recorded natural interaction between each of ten 36-month-old children and the child's mother (30 minutes), a familiar peer (30 minutes) and the observer (including phonological, grammatical, and cognitive probes: Vihman and Greenlee, 1987). The children were drawn from a middle-class population in California and were the same children observed weekly for seven months in the period of transition to speech (Vihman et al., 1985). Despite the socioeconomic homogeneity of the sample, wide differences were found in intelligibility, specific processes used, and phonological organization.

Intelligibility

All of the children could be clearly understood more than half the time; on average, 73 percent of their utterances were judged intelligible by three raters unfamiliar with the children, but the range was broad: 54 percent to 80 percent. As might be expected, the children judged most intelligible were generally those who made the fewest phonetic or phonological errors. Yet misarticulation and phonological process use were not the only factors contributing to unintelligible speech at this age. The children who used the highest proportion of complex sentences tended to be relatively difficult to understand. Some examples of complex sentences produced by these children:

> It's sort of necklace, but it's a string where you put beads on.
>
> It hurts when I crash into something.
>
> I can buckle 'em when people say that's alright, and then when they say that's not alright, I don't do it.

Most of the 3-year-olds were apparently unable to produce complex sentences and still speak clearly enough to be easily understood by unfamiliar adults.

Only the substitution of interdental fricatives by other consonants (stops or other fricatives) was regularly used by all subjects. Two other processes—gliding and palatal fronting—were regularly used by over half the subjects. The remaining processes were used by no more than one to three subjects. Of the processes affecting sequential structure, cluster simplification was regularly used by three subjects, but the prosodic processes typical of 1-year-olds were each regularly used by only one or (in the case of consonant and syllable deletion) two of these 3-year-old subjects.

Phonological Organization: Profile of Two Three-Year-Old Girls

Earlier, we described two talkative firstborn girls, Deborah and Molly. Both had developed large vocabularies by the time they were 16 months old, but they showed different phonetic preferences and differences in phonological organization; we characterized Deborah's style as exploratory and Molly's as systematic. To what extent were the differences between the two girls present at age 3?

Both the girls were still quite talkative. Molly ranked first and Deborah fourth in average length of conversational turn at age 3 (based on interaction with their mothers). Both were also still lexically advanced, with Deborah ranking first and Molly second on a scale of lexical diversity (reflecting the number of different words used in the course of interaction with their mothers). And, with respect to phonology, they continued to diverge. Deborah was judged the most intelligible of the 10 children in the study and was found to make the next-to-least use of phonological processes (i.e., had the next-to-fewest phonological errors). Molly was third from last of the 10 children on both the intelligibility ranking and the phonological error score.

Deborah and Molly continued to differ in their respective error patterns. Deborah's errors were fairly evenly balanced between whole-word and segment change processes. She was the only 3-year-old who made relatively high use of **metathesis**, the reordering of segments. She made regular use of the segment change processes typical of the majority of the 3-year-olds (**palatal fronting**, **interdental fricative substitution**), and she was one of four children who did not replace liquids with glides. All of Molly's whole-word errors were sporadic or rare, as was true of the group as a whole, but she had a great many more cluster and segment errors than Deborah had. She was one of the three children who often, although inconsistently, reduced Cl-clusters.

What kind of comparison can be made with the specific phonetic preferences exhibited by these children at age 1 (see Chapter 2)? Several of the phonetic preferences seen at age 1 are no longer present at age 3. For example, place of articulation errors were rare at this age and were not made by Deborah or Molly. At age 1, Deborah made unusually extensive use of fricatives, yet at age 3, it was Molly, not Deborah, who showed relatively high accuracy in fricative use. On the other hand, Molly was exceptional at age 1 in her high use of final consonants, yet it was Deborah, not Molly, who showed no tendency to delete final consonants at age 3. In general, the specific phonetic tendencies found at age 1 seemed to be unrelated to the phonological errors made at age 3 (Vihman and Greenlee, 1987).

Turning to the question of phonological organization, the chief difference between Deborah and Molly at age 3 was Deborah's willingness to abbreviate words and to slur or scramble segments (e.g., ['dalfoz]~[du'ralfoz] for *Ruldolfo's*), despite her relatively accurate production of individual consonants. Molly made relatively few errors affecting the structure of the word as a whole, yet she was unintelligible some of the time because of her difficulty with a number of individual consonants (especially /l/, /r/, and /ʃ/). Recall that Molly's systematic approach to phonological learning was expressed in (1) her highly constrained choice of words—rarely attempting fricatives, in particular (whereas Deborah attempted a wider range of sound patterns), and (2) the unusually low degree of variability across different tokens of the same word. In general, the children who, like Molly, were relatively more constrained in their word selection patterns at age 1 were very likely to make little use of whole-word processes at age 3; and those who, like Deborah, explored a wide range of sounds at age 1 were also more likely to delete consonants and syllables, assimilate consonants, and change the order of segments in a word at age 3. Furthermore, there was a tendency for children whose word shapes were more variable at age 1 to make more *inconsistent* use of phonological processes at age 3 (Vihman and Greenlee, 1987). In summary, Deborah's phonological style at both ages was typical of more *exploratory* children, those with a high "tolerance for variability" (Kamhi, Catts, and Davis, 1984), and Molly's was typical of children with a lower tolerance for variability and hence, a more systematic approach.

Profile of Two Boys Recorded at Ages Two, Three, and Six Years

Klein (1985) reported the results of a longitudinal study of phonological process usage of two boys, Jason and Joshua. The boys were first recorded at ages 1;8 and 2;0, during a four-hour naturalistic play session with the investigator (see also Klein, 1981). Analyses focused on a comparison of monosyllabic versus polysyllabic productions. The boys proved similar in many ways, each attempting polysyllabic words in a little over half of their single-word productions (Jason 60 percent, Joshua 51 percent), and each matching the syllable count of the adult model in the majority of their productions. However, they differed in their more specific production strategies. Joshua tended to use consonant harmony and reduplication, while Jason typically replaced the consonants in unstressed syllables with either glottals or glides. In addition, Jason made greater use of syllable deletion than Joshua, and was thus more variable in his approach to the production of polysyllabic words. These are some examples of words produced by both boys in the course of the first recording:

Adult model	Joshua	Jason
bunny	[babi]	[bʌɪ]
tiger	[tada]	[daɪja]
pocketbook	[bababuk]	[paʔəwu]
motorcycle	[mumulalak]	[modaɪʔu]

At ages 3 and 6 the boys were recorded for about one hour each, including both **continuous speech**, produced during play with the same materials provided at age 2, and **single words**, produced in response to the *Photo Articulation Test* (Pendergast, Dickey, Selmar, and Soder, 1969). Analysis of these data focused on comparison of phonological process use (instances of use relative to opportunities for use in the child's productions) in single-word versus continuous speech. A "whole word accuracy" score was derived by comparing the number of error-free words with the total number of intelligible productions. Based on norms reported by Schmitt, Howard, and Schmitt (1983), Joshua was found to fall one standard deviation above the mean for his age at both ages 3 and 6, while Jason fell slightly more than one standard deviation below the mean for his age. At both ages the boys made many more errors in continuous speech than on single-word productions; in fact, at age 6 Joshua failed to make any errors on the articulation test, while Jason evidenced only **stopping** and **deaffrication**. In continuous speech both children sometimes deleted final consonants, stopped /ð/, and simplified consonant clusters.

The relationship between use of supraglottal consonants at age 2 and relative accuracy in phonological production at ages 3 and 6 is striking. Klein (1985) suggested that an **articulatory timing factor** may explain Jason's difficulty with the production of both affricates (or consonant clusters which pattern as **segmental units** in English) and consonant clusters in general, particularly in the flow of running speech (see Gilbert and Purves, 1977, discussed below). As Klein pointed out, the same difficulty with articulatory timing may account for Jason's earlier overuse of glottals and glides, which require less precise articulatory control than other consonants. Interestingly, Vihman and Greenlee (1987) found low use of "true consonants" (or overuse of glottals and glides) to be the best phonetic indicator at age 1 of slower phonological advance at age 3.

Summary

Analysis of the naturally occurring conversation of 2-year-old English-speaking children revealed that open monosyllables were still the dominant production shape at this time, followed by closed monosyllables, and open or closed disyllables. Word-initial consonant clusters were used frequently as well. Stops and nasals continued to be the most common consonants; word-initial inventories were richer than word-final inventories in every consonant category except liquids. The children were more accurate in consonant production than might be expected, given their relatively incomplete inventories.

Analysis of ten 3-year-old English-speaking children engaged in natural conversation revealed that over half their speech was intelligible to outsiders. Both specific phonological errors and high use of complex sentences appeared to contribute to unintelligibility. All the children made errors involving interdental fricatives; gliding and palatal fronting were also common.

Comparison of the phonological error patterns of two 3-year-old children whose phonological development at age 1 was described earlier showed that the specific phonetic strengths they had exhibited at age 1 bore no relationship to the errors made at age 3. On the other hand, their differing approaches to phonological learning—systematic versus exploratory—manifested themselves at both ages.

Comparison of two boys across three time points, ages 2, 3, and 6 years, suggested that difficulty with articulatory timing may underlie relatively slow phonological development, and may be identifiable as early as age 1 or 2 years in the relatively high use of glottals and glides, or relatively slow mastery of supraglottal articulation.

Development of Perception Beyond Early Childhood: Understanding Running Speech

Perceptual issues relevant to the time when the child must construct both a repertoire of lexical forms and a store of knowledge about the sound system of the language were discussed previously. As the child becomes a more fluent speaker and enters the world of discourse with unfamiliar adults as well as peers, one challenge is to master the complex task of understanding continuous or running speech. What factors enter into that task? Do children process spoken language differently than adults?

Under ordinary circumstances, listeners do not identify isolated words but rather retrieve a message from the flow of speech. Recently, investigators have begun to study the factors affecting the perception of continuous speech, by children as well as adults. A variety of research methods have been designed to investigate the complex process by which listeners interpret speech "on-line," without taking the time to make sure of what was heard, consult a lexicon of possible words, and compare the plausibility of one word or interpretation against another.

Studies addressing the comprehension of natural, continuous speech have exploited one of two research methods: (1) **fast reaction time** tasks, in which the listener is required to shadow the input speech (Marslen-Wilson, 1985) or to monitor the speech for occurrences of particular words (identical monitoring) or word categories (Tyler and Marslen-Wilson,

1981), or of mispronunciations deliberately included in ongoing sentences or stories (Cole, 1981), and (2) the **gating** task, developed by Grosjean (1980), in which the listener is presented with successively longer fragments of a word (either isolated or in sentential context), and required to respond at each new increment with a guess as to what word they are hearing.

Recognizing spoken words is thought to involve integrating two different sources of information (Tyler and Frauenfelder, 1987): (1) **sensory input**, or "bottom-up" (phonetic) information, deriving from the speech signal itself; and (2) **contextual constraints**, or "top-down" information, deriving from the speaker's knowledge of what has already been said, what might plausibly follow, what semantic and syntactic structures the language allows, and what words the language makes available, given the unfolding message.

Experimental evidence suggests that words are typically (though not always) identified *before* sufficient acoustic-phonetic information has become available to allow all words but one to be eliminated on the basis of the sound pattern alone (Marslen-Wilson, 1987). Such "early selection" means that word recognition is based on informed guessing as well as perception. That is, the listener is continually engaged in constructing an interpretation of the incoming message, so that the more predictable a particular word is, given the conversation up to that point, the preceding sentence, or the phrase in which the word is located, the more rapidly a listener can guess or "recognize" it from a brief phonetic clue—such as the first sound or the first syllable.

In addition to the important role of context in word recognition, word frequency must also be taken into account: Experimental manipulations have shown that high-frequency words are recognized more rapidly than low-frequency words, when both provide equally good matches to the initial phonetic shape of the input and each are plausible in context.

To what extent do children resemble adults in the recognition of words in running speech? Each of the factors that enter into adult word recognition—ongoing analysis of the acoustic-phonetic signal, expectations based on the semantic, syntactic, and pragmatic context, and relative lexical familiarity—may potentially reflect a long period of development. Both increasing *experience with language* and possible changes in *processing abilities* may affect the child's capacity to carry out the complex task of interpreting running speech.

Adult–Child Differences in Word Recognition

Analysis of the Phonetic Signal

Elliott, Hammer, and Evan (1987) used a **forward gating procedure** to test children, teenagers, and adults aged 70 to 85 on their recognition of highly familiar spoken monosyllabic nouns under conditions of **limited acoustic information**. The subjects were required to make a response (i.e., to guess, if the word had not yet been recognized) to each successive stimulus. The teenagers performed more successfully on this task than either the children or adults. They recognized more words and did so more rapidly. Their guesses were usually real words which were phonetically compatible with the sounds heard, whereas the children's responses sometimes failed to match the phonetic stimuli. These results are consistent with the hypothesis, advanced by Walley (1984), that children require more acoustic information to identify stimuli than do teenagers or adults.

Cole and his colleagues (Cole and Jakimik, 1980; Cole and Perfetti, 1980) used a mispronunciation task to compare the processing of continuous speech by children and adults.

The subjects' reaction times are assumed to reflect the time it takes to (1) identify the intended or target word (e.g., *pajamas*), and (2) note the acoustic mismatch (e.g., /pədaməz/ or "padamas"). By manipulating both the words and their sentence context, Cole has tested several hypotheses about the process of word recognition in context. Cole's work supports three major theoretical assumptions regarding the process of decoding or recognizing words in running speech.

1. Words are recognized through the *interaction* of sound perception and linguistic and pragmatic knowledge.

2. Words are typically recognized *in order*. As each word is recognized, it allows the listener to establish word boundaries. In addition, each decoded word imposes syntactic and semantic constraints on the following words, which enables the listener to progressively narrow the field of possible interpretations.

For example, after decoding the word *picnic*, the listener is well prepared for a word like *basket*. When the phonetic pattern [pʰæskət] is heard instead, a mispronunciation is quickly identified. When [pʰæskət] follows a word with which *basket* is less likely to be combined—such as *plastic*—the mispronunciation is detected less rapidly.

3. Words are decoded sequentially, using earlier-occurring sounds to narrow the range of possible candidates. Adults have been found to detect errors in second syllables more rapidly than in first syllables, presumably because the target word has already been identified when the mispronounced second-syllable error is heard. Similarly, mispronunciations in the second syllable of words beginning with relatively unusual first syllables (e.g., *sham-*) are recognized more rapidly than those in words with common first syllables (*com-*), presumably because the set of possible lexical matches can more quickly be narrowed to one. On the other hand, mispronounced word-final consonants are less likely to be detected than mispronounced word-initial consonants. This likely reflects the limited attention paid to the end of a word, even under the special circumstances of a mispronunciation-detecting task.

In three experiments with 4- and 5-year-old children and adults, Cole (1981) investigated the effects of word-position, consonant substituted, and phonotactic structure, or permissible versus impermissible consonant clusters, on the detection of mispronunciations in running speech. The children were tested on familiar songs and nursery rhymes. The main results were:

1. The children averaged about 50 percent detection in word-initial position; in medial position, detection fell to 25 percent, and in final position, to 12 percent. Adult detection frequencies were 95 percent, 86 percent, and 71 percent, respectively, in the three word-positions. Thus, the children, like the adults, paid most attention to initial position and least to final position.

2. In word-initial position, children were most sensitive to changes in place of articulation of stops and to changes of stop to nasal and of voiced to voiceless stop. Interchanges among nasals, fricatives, or liquids were less often detected. Most easily detected were common articulatory substitutions of a stop for a fricative. In a follow-up study, Bernthal, Greenlee, Eblen, and Marking (1987) also found that **developmental substitutions** were more easily detected than nondevelopmental substitutions by normally developing and misarticulating 4- to 6-year-old children as well as by adults.

Cole and Perfetti (1980) reported one important difference between children and adults. Though the children, like adults, detected errors more readily in words predictable from the context (an advantage of about 14 percent, across all ages), they failed to identify second-syllable errors more readily than first-syllable errors. This difference may mean that, unlike adults, children put off deciding which word was intended until they have heard several syllables. Such a strategy seems reasonable for listeners who, to some extent, lack confidence in their ability to recognize words. In other words, if a great many words in adult conversation are still unfamiliar, it is easy to see why children would be slower to settle on a lexical interpretation.

Contextual Effects

Tyler and Marslen-Wilson (1981) investigated the role of discourse and of syntactic context alone on the comprehension of running speech of children aged 5, 7, and 10 years. Children were tested on two tasks, **identical monitoring**, in which the occurrence of a particular word is to be noted as soon as it is spoken, and **category monitoring**, in which a word belonging to a particular category (body part, fruit, furniture) is to be identified when heard. The target words fell toward the end of the second of a pair of sentences of one of three kinds: normal prose, in which the first sentence provides a normal discourse context for the second; syntactic prose, in which the sentences are anomalous in meaning but syntactically correct; and random word order, which violates both semantic and syntactic structure and thus provides no contextual support for word recognition. Examples (with the target word in boldface):

> John had to go back home. He had fallen out of the swing and had hurt his **hand** on the ground. (normal)

> John had to sit on the shop. He had lived out of the kitchen and had enjoyed his **hand** in the mud. (syntactic)

> The on sit shop to had John. He lived had and kitchen the out his of had enjoyed **hand** mud in the. (random)

The results suggested that children as young as age 5 are able to make good use of discourse and even of syntactic context: Mean reaction times decreased significantly with age, but all three groups showed a marked facilitatory effect from the normal discourse, and a lesser effect from normal syntax only. The category monitoring task was considerably more difficult for the children than the identical monitoring task. The normal discourse context again aided recognition, but the semantically anomalous "syntactic" sentence sequences gave no significant advantage in this case.

Another study suggested that children's ability to make use of **semantic knowledge** continues to improve up to as late as age 15. Elliott (1979) tested 24 children at each of four age levels (11, 13, 15, and 17 years) on their understanding of sentences against a background of multitalker babble. The test sentences were designed to fall into two groups: **high predictability** and **low predictability**—a function of the presence or absence of two or three semantically related "pointer" words that could help cue the listener as to the identity of the final (target) word, always a monosyllabic noun. The test consisted of 25 sentences of each type; none was longer than 8 syllables. The subject's task was to repeat back the last word of the sentence.

Under just one set of conditions, when the target sentence was presented at the same intensity as the noise, a significant age trend was found, with the 11- and 13-year-olds performing less well on high-predictability sentences than the 15- and 17-year-olds, who did about as well as young adults tested earlier with written responses. No age differences were found in quiet or in comprehension of the low-predictability sentences. A later test of 9-year-old children showed significantly poorer performance than that of the 11-year-olds. The age-related differences are not a direct auditory effect since only the high-predictability sentences proved easier for older subjects. Rather, the difference appears to reflect the extent to which children of different ages were able to use the semantic information in the pointer syllables to guess at the final, difficult-to-hear, target noun.

Lexical Familiarity

Cole and Perfetti (1980) reported a significant difference between children and adults in the detection of mispronunciations in a simple, clearly articulated story: On average, preschool children (ages 4 to 5) detected about 50 percent of the mispronounced words, children kindergarten through fifth grade about 60 percent, and adults 95 percent. Cole and Perfetti suggested that children probably treat mispronunciations as unfamiliar words: "It seems likely that children learn to tolerate (or actively ignore) unfamiliar words, so that each occurrence of an unfamiliar word does not result in a breakdown of the comprehension process" (313).

It is important to note that the children detected mispronunciations in isolated words (95 percent) far more readily than in fluent speech. The high detection rate for isolated words is due in part to their slower articulation, and also to the cues provided by pictures that accompanied the test words. This procedure is commonly used in clinical tests of phonetic discrimination, and therefore, the tests may overestimate children's ability to perceive phonetic differences in the course of conversational speech (Cole, 1981).

The issue of **word familiarity** itself has also received attention. Walley and Metsala (1990) used mispronunciation tasks to test children aged 5 and 8. Subjective age-of-acquisition ratings were used to categorize test words as "early," "current," and "late." The familiarity factor proved to be important: Young children were more likely to detect mispronunciations in early and current words. Furthermore, the children were biased toward identifying late (or for age 5, both late and current) words as mispronounced—including words which were correctly pronounced ("intact" words). Thus, whereas the subjects in Cole and Perfetti (1980) were found to treat mispronounced words as unfamiliar, Walley and Metsala showed through analysis of "false alarms" that their subjects were reluctant to treat unfamiliar words as intact, and preferred to label them mispronounced. These results call to mind the biasing role of familiarity in early tests of linguistic perception, mentioned in Chapter 2 (Barton, 1976; Clumeck, 1982). They are reminiscent also of several anecdotes reported in Vihman (1981: 248), in which preschool children misperceived unfamiliar words as relatively more familiar ones, disregarding the fact that their interpretation was at odds with the ongoing discourse context.

Summary

Word recognition is a complex process, involving the integration of the sensory input (acoustic-phonetic signal), contextual information (including both pragmatic and general knowledge-based inferences regarding the gist of the incoming message) and specific structural effects relating to the phonotactic, syntactic, and semantic restrictions characteristic of the language code. The listener's lexical expectations are also influenced by word frequency.

On the whole, school-age children process continuous speech in an adult-like way, making use of context to aid in the interpretation of the acoustic signal. Also, developmental mispronunciations are more salient than other consonant substitutions to children as young as age 4 as well as to adults. In several respects children are different from adults, however. They appear to need more acoustic information before they commit themselves to a decision as to word identity, perhaps because so many words continue to be unfamiliar, at least up to the teens. Furthermore, their use of semantic knowledge as a clue to the unfolding message is not fully developed until the teen years. Finally, school-age children, like younger children, perceive familiar words more accurately than unfamiliar words, and take a cautious approach to apparent mispronunciations in running speech.

Production in the School-Age Child: Continuing Change

In characterizing the phonological production of 3-year-olds, we noted that the majority of simplifying phonological processes no longer apply at that age although consonant clusters are still frequently reduced and certain segment types (especially fricatives and liquids) continue to be substituted by other segments. According to the normative articulation data presented in Figure 7.1, half of the children tested had succeeded in using all of the relevant sounds correctly by age 4. However, fricatives and liquids correct production by 90 percent of the children was achieved only later. Hodson and Paden (1981) reported that articulation by the 60 normally developing 4-year-old children they tested closely resembled that of adults.

It is reasonable, then, to ask whether phonetic and phonological acquisition can be said to be complete for most normally developing children by the time they reach school age. With respect to basic articulatory mastery and intelligibility outside the family, the answer is probably yes. It is important to note, however, that both phonetic and phonological variation and change continue in a number of respects, not only beyond early childhood but also throughout a person's life span. We will illustrate this point by briefly discussing three areas of continuing change: (1) temporal coordination of speech production, (2) phonological reorganization under the influence of literacy, and (3) phonetic and phonological influence from the peer group.

Temporal Coordination of Speech Production

Smith (1978) inferred from durational measurements that segment and word production by 2- and 4-year-old children was consistently slower than adult productions of the same forms. However, the proportional relationships between segments were much like those of adults: For example, final syllables and stressed syllables tended to be longer than non-final and unstressed syllables; voiceless stops were longer than voiced stops while vowels were shorter before the (longer) voiceless stops. Smith concluded that children possess quite sophisticated timing-control systems, despite their still immature neuromuscular control capacities (as reported for other aspects of motor performance, such as reaction time in general, maximum rate of syllable repetition, and maximum finger-tapping rate).

A gradual increase in rate of articulation with age was reported by Hulme, Thomson, Muir, and Lawrence (1984). They tested children aged 3 to 4, 7 to 8, and 10 to 11 as well as adults on their maximum rate of repetition of one-, two-, and three- or four-syllable words. They found an increase in speech rate with age, as well as a tendency for subjects to repeat short words more quickly than long ones, but with less difference in rate for different word lengths in the younger subjects. Hulme and colleagues were not primarily interested in speech rate per se, however, but in the possible relationship between speech rate—and, hence, maximum potential rate for verbal *rehearsal*—and short-term memory. Their results showed a close connection between increases in verbal short-term memory and speech rate. They viewed this finding as strong support for the hypothesis that verbal short-term memory "is a time-based system limited by the amount of speech which it can store" (251): see Baddeley, Thomson, and Buchanan (1975); Baddeley (1986).

A number of studies of children's speech production have addressed the question of the timing of individual segments embedded in clusters, syllables, and words. There is evidence that word-initial clusters may first be represented as single consonants combining features of both the consonants in the cluster (cf., e.g., Menyuk, 1972). Only later is the cluster "unpacked" into its separate component segments. Gilbert and Purves (1977) pointed out that the level at which the child represents the cluster as a single segment—in perception, in the production plan, or only in the execution of the plan—is not clear. If, for example, the child perceives the cluster but cannot produce the segments sequentially, the problem could be purely articulatory (difficulty with the timing and/or motor control of the separate articulatory gestures), or it could reflect difficulty in applying the appropriate "segmentalization rules," that is, in sorting out the overlapping articulatory gestures (at the planning level) to achieve the proper sequential output. It has been hypothesized that the child may be constrained at first by a **timing-dominant system**, in which a rigid time schedule governs the execution of articulatory gestures (cf. Ohala, 1970; Hawkins, 1973). As the timing-dominant system is gradually replaced by an **articulation-dominant** system, the limited time constraints are relaxed, leading to slower but more accurate speech production.

Results from detailed analyses of children's productions tend to support such a developmental sequence. Hawkins (1973) measured consonant durations based on production by seven children aged 4 to 7. Comparing her findings with results reported for adults, Hawkins found that in clusters, /l/ tended to be longer in the children's speech. There was, however, no apparent age trend in her data. Hawkins suggested that once the child is able to produce "acceptable but not necessarily mature forms" of particular sounds or sequences of sounds, speech production may remain essentially unchanged for several years (perhaps until puberty) (204).

Gilbert and Purves (1977) tested four groups of five children, one group each at age 5, 7, 9, and 11, and five adults on the production of closed monosyllables, beginning with /s/, /f/, /l/, /w/, /sl/, /fl/, and /sw/, to determine the relative duration of the fricatives, liquids, and glides as singletons and as part of a cluster. They found greater variation in duration values in the younger children's productions. Like Hawkins (1973), they also found that the only significant timing differences across age groups involved clusters with /l/. In adult production, consonants are shorter when combined in a cluster. Five-year-olds failed to shorten /l/ appropriately; they produced a longer /l/ after fricatives. For the remaining age groups, there was a progressive decrease in the duration of /l/ in clusters, as compared with singleton /l/, up to age 11, when the relative durations were about the same as those for adults. The positional differences in duration, however, were not significant.

In the view of Gilbert and Purves, these results reflected a late stage in the acquisition of consonant clusters. At first, /l/ is likely to be omitted. Later, some children "split" the cluster, producing *blue* (/blu/) as [bəlu]. This may reflect the child's attempt to circumvent the constraints of a timing-dominant system: Since the child lacks the articulatory control needed to produce the cluster within a single syllabic unit, an additional syllable is produced. Gilbert and Purves's data suggest that the elongation of the /l/ may represent a further stage in the splitting process. As the child's timing control improves, the lengthening of /l/ is no longer needed.

In another study involving timing, Gilbert and Johnson (1978) tested eleven 6-year-old children on the (imitative) production of 73 polysyllabic words containing the syllable C/jul/ (as in *ambulance, ridiculous*). Since most of the words were unfamiliar to the children, they could be considered the equivalent of nonsense words.

Correct production of the C/jul/ segment (in *folliculous*, for example) characterized only 14 percent of the tokens. The remaining tokens generally displayed one of four (cumulative) error patterns: (1) unrounding (sometimes with reduction) of the vowel, to [ɪ] or [ə] (13 percent), (2) with glide deletion ([kɪ], [kəɪ]: 24 percent), (3) with methathesis ([klɪ]: 23 percent), and (4) with vowel deletion ([kl]: 7 percent). In adult production, the duration of the first two syllables is slightly less than that of the last two (43 percent : 57 percent of total duration). This ratio typically was maintained in the children's productions as well, despite a tendency toward greater shortening of the last two syllables with each cumulative error type. In the case of the last error type, the ratio is reversed (54 percent : 46 percent).

Although all of the subjects tested could produce the component segments of the C/jul/ sequence in isolation, production of these segments within the sequence and time constraints posed by a long word proved difficult. Gilbert and Johnson contend that it is the relation between syllable durations that must be modified as the child learns the articulatory program for a new polysyllabic word.

In summary, studies of timing problems posed by the production of consonants in clusters and in long words have shown that school-age children, although able to produce acceptably adult-like speech, are continuing to develop fluency in the planning and production of complex sequences of sounds.

Phonological Reorganization: The Influence of Literacy

Linguistic theory in this century has strongly emphasized the primacy of oral as opposed to written language. As a corollary, it is typically assumed that the unconscious systemic knowledge which underlies productive language use derives solely from the learning of oral language in early childhood. Yet in a literate society, individuals spend many of their formative years learning to read, to write, to spell, and to alphabetize. Indeed, as Ferguson (1968) has pointed out, spoken language changes in subtle ways as a society becomes literate, as indicated, for example, by the sporadic occurrence of spelling pronunciations (such as /ˈfɔrˋhɛd/ in lieu of /ˈfɔrɪd/ for *forehead*; /ˈɔftən/ in lieu of /ˈɔfən/ for *often*). It is likely that what children are taught in school "reshapes the psychological structures . . . built up previously, so that what is psychologically real for literate speakers includes at least some of what they have been taught about their language" (Jaeger, 1984; 22). Three types of studies have investigated the role of literacy in forcing a restructuring of phonological knowledge. These studies have focused on (1) knowledge of the vowel alternations partially reflected in the English spelling system, (2) the influence of spelling on perception and production, and (3) differences in lexical organization between children and adults.

Knowledge of Vowel Alternations

In their highly influential work *The Sound Pattern of English*, Chomsky and Halle (1968) posited a set of phonological rules to capture the systematic relationship between different vowels that is reflected in such word-pairs as *divine–divinity* (/ai:ɪ/), *serene–serenity* (/i:ɛ/), *profane–profanity* (/ey:æ/), *cone–conical* (/ow:a/), *lose–lost* (/u:ɔ,a/), *profound–profundity* (/aw:ʌ/). These and other phonological rules in Chomsky and Halle's account have been said to reflect psychologically real patterns of alternation; that is, it is assumed that speakers will unconsciously apply these rules to new words fitting into the same pattern. But this particular set of rules, which reflects a historical sound change known as the Great English Vowel Shift (fourteenth to seventeenth century), is no longer productive or transparent in present-day English, since many words entered the lexicon *after* the shift took place and now participate in other alternations (e.g., *retain–retention* (/e:ɛ/), *genteel–gentility* (/i:ɪ/). Jaeger (1984) reviewed a series of psycholinguistic tests carried out on adults and children in an effort to probe the psychological reality of the vowel shift rule for English speakers.

Moskowitz (1973) obtained positive results on a concept formation task used in testing children aged 9 to 12 on knowledge of the vowel shift alternations. She concluded, however, that these results were based on the children's knowledge of *spelling rules* rather than of the phonological rules underlying derived words that were still largely unfamiliar to them. Jaeger (1984) followed up on Moskowitz's suggestion with a concept formation task carefully designed to distinguish between responses based on the vowel shift alternations and responses based on spelling rules. The crucial patterns involved the pair /aw/–/ʌ/, in which the alternations are not spelled with the same letter, and /u/–/ʌ/, in which the alternations are spelled with *u* (as in *reduce–reduction*) but are not part of the vowel shift rule. Jaeger trained 15 adults to respond positively to English words reflecting the vowel shift alternations and negatively to other derivationally related word-pairs exhibiting other phonological relationships, such as tense–lax (*retain–retention*, *peace–pacify*), or the same vowel (*promise–promissory*). She then tested subjects with new word-pairs exhibiting these two types of relationships as well as pairs belonging to the two critical categories (/aw/–/ʌ/ or /u/–/ʌ/). The results were clear. Pairs containing the critical spelling-based pair /u/–/ʌ/ were generally accepted, while pairs containing the irregular vowel shift pair /aw/–/ʌ/ were generally rejected. Later interviews with the subjects further confirmed a tendency to rely on the spelling rule, as when the training category was described by one subject as "a long and a short version of the same vowel." Jaeger concluded that "certain entities can be psychologically real either because they have been brought to speakers' conscious attention as part of their education or because they have been intuited from the orthographic system of their language" (34).

Influence of Spelling on Perception and Production

Ehri (1984) reviewed the various ways in which learning to read and spell have been found to affect children's competence in the production and perception of speech. In Ehri's view, "the full representational system offered by printed language is acquired and stored in memory during acquisition" (123), including both the whole-word ("lexical") gestalt and the segmental ("phonetic") letter-sound correspondences that characterize each word. Specifically, Ehri maintains that in the course of learning to read, the "alphabetic" or "orthographic" image of a word is *added* to the store of information associated with each item in the mental lexicon. The orthographic image is integrated with other information about a word as printed words are read and understood in context. Gradually, orthographic representations come to stand for a word's meaning as well as its form and to be as intimately associated with the word as are the phonological, semantic, and syntactic aspects of its identity. (For words acquired later, through reading, the orthographic image may even be established *before* the actual oral pronunciation is known.)

Ehri's experimental investigations on the effect of orthography on perception and production have led to a number of interesting results. She found that knowledge of spelling helps children to detect and accurately segment out the sounds embedded in words. For example, through spelling children become aware of extra syllabic segments (e.g., in words like *different*, *comfortable*, *decimal*). On the other hand, knowledge of spelling may also misleadingly influence perception, as in the case of the English alveolar flap /D/ (as in *latter* or *ladder*), which children typically hear as /d/ until they learn that many words containing the flap are spelled with *t*. Surprisingly, knowledge of related words in which the flap is realized as /t/ or /d/ (*sit–sitting*, *ride–riding*) was not found to affect perception.

In a series of studies of older children, Templeton (1979, 1983; Templeton and Scarborough-Franks, 1985) established that knowledge of the complex phonological alternations between derivationally related English words, such as those investigated by Moskowitz and Jaeger, continues to increase at least through grade 10 and is typically acquired through *prior* learning of the more transparent orthographic relationship between these words. Templeton and Scarborough-Franks pointed out that it is easier to relate complex derived English words through spelling than through verbal production for two reasons: The derivational stem is more stable in orthography than in surface phonetics, and the processes which must be applied to relate the base and derived forms of the word are also less complex (compare the spelling and pronunciation shifts needed to relate *incline* and *inclination*, for example). These authors concluded that the subjects in their study (both "good" and "poor" spellers, in grades 6 and 10) had abstracted the orthographic patterns associated with such words by the end of elementary school, but in grade 10 they were still in the process of abstracting the patterns in pronunciation (so that they could be automatically applied to the production of novel forms, for example: see also Jaeger, 1986).

Differences in Lexical Organization

The study of malapropisms (e.g., *ornaments* or *monuments* in lieu of *condiments*), or the mistaken production of one word in lieu of another, can shed light on the organization of the mental lexicon. Aitchison and Straf (1981) analyzed 680 malapropisms, almost a third of which were produced by children (aged 12 or under). Separate analysis of the adult and child malapropisms in comparison with their target words was carried out with respect to number of syllables, stress pattern, initial and final consonant, and identity of the stressed vowel. The results for adults and children were then compared. The child malapropisms were found to be as close to the targets as those produced by adults. For both adults and children, the number of syllables, initial consonant, and stressed vowel all were likely to match the target. Where all three were not retained, adults were most likely to produce the same initial consonant (e.g., *acapulco* in place of *acupuncture:* 77 percent), whereas children were more likely to retain the number of syllables (e.g., *naughty story* in place of *multistory* [*carpark*]: 84 percent, vs. 68 percent for adults) and least likely to retain the initial consonant (57 percent). Stress pattern largely correlated with number of syllables for both adults and children. Although final consonants were retained more or less equally often by adults (e.g., *jungle* for *conjugal:* 72 percent) and children (e.g., *faint* for *fête:* 68 percent), the initial consonant was more often retained than the final consonant in the adult data; children retained the final consonant (marginally) more often than the initial consonant. In longer words, the final consonant was especially likely to be preserved by both children and adults, perhaps because of the derivational suffixes in which target and malapropism often matched (especially in the adult data where about 50 percent of the malapropisms included a suffix: Recall the errors for *condiments*).

Aitchison and Straf (1981) suggested five interacting factors to account for the differences between adult and child lexical retrieval and storage:

1. Children may pay more attention to perceptually salient aspects of words, such as rhythm (i.e., *giggle* for *wriggle, fascination* for *vaccination*).
2. Children appear to pay more attention to word endings (cf. Slobin, 1973) and, perhaps consequently, less attention to initial consonants.
3. Consonant harmony, a preference for open syllables, and a tendency to alter unstressed syllables appear to affect older children's memory for unfamiliar words, just as they affect word production in younger children and perhaps for the same reasons (cf. Aitchison and Chiat, 1981, who implicate "faulty perception," or incomplete representation, together with memory overload to account for the role of phonological processes in both younger and older children).
4. Literacy and experience with dictionaries may enhance the importance of initial consonants for adults.
5. Growth in importance of word beginnings may accompany growth in vocabulary since the high frequency of derivational affixes in more sophisticated English vocabulary renders attention to word endings relatively inefficient as a way of differentiating between words.

In summary, the analysis of adult and child malapropisms reveals some of the salient features that must characterize words in the mental lexicon since these features influence word retrieval. Rhythmic structure and word endings are salient from early childhood (cf. Vihman, 1981); with schooling, experience with dictionary and library work, and the growth of a more abstract, derived lexicon, the importance of the initial consonant increases. An experimental study of ninety 5- to 9-year-olds showed that, at those ages, the consonants of the stressed syllable were still more likely to be recalled than the initial consonant (Aitchison and Chiat, 1981). It is not clear at what age the shift to a preferential reliance on initial consonants begins to affect lexical retrieval.

Influence from the Peer Group

In the introduction to Chapter 2 we mentioned that by the time children are speaking clearly enough to be understood outside the family, their speech patterns will have been stamped with the phonetically distinguishing features of the language of their home community. Yet phonetic and phonological development do not come to an end at this point. An extensive sociolinguistic study by Payne (1975, 1980) demonstrated the influence of the peer group on both the phonetic and the phonological levels after the period of early childhood.

In order to investigate ongoing linguistic change, Payne designed a study to observe the speech patterns of a large number of children who had moved from one dialect area to another. By noting the age at which the children moved to the new community as well as their length of stay there, she was able to roughly distinguish between parental and peer influence.

Payne carried out her investigation in King of Prussia, a small middle-class community on the outskirts of Philadelphia that had become a thriving industrial center attracting a large number of recent arrivals. She interviewed some 200 families, making contact through children playing on the block and through church leaders, and finally, extended her investigation to the school where some 50 groups of children were interviewed, including 10 of the children originally approached in the family context. Payne (1975) presented in detail the acquisition of the Philadelphia dialect by one family of four children that had moved to the area from New York five years earlier; the children were aged 8, 10, 11, and 13 at the time of the study.

Payne concentrated her analysis on seven specific vowel patterns that characterize the "stable, central core" of the Philadelphia dialect. These patterns include three phonological differences from other dialects of English (splitting or merger of classes of phonemically distinct vowels; for example, the stressed vowels of *merry–Murray* and *ferry–furry* are merged) and four phonetic differences, in which the phonemic structure is not affected (e.g., the nucleus of /oy/ is raised to [u]).

Payne found that the phonetic variables had all been acquired by all of the children, whereas the phonological variables were only incompletely acquired. Furthermore, she found a correlation for the three older children between degree of acquisition of the Philadelphia dialect and number of years spent under the influence of the King of Prussia peer group. The youngest child, Mike, aged 3 on arrival in the new area, showed about the same degree of influence as the oldest child, Richard (aged 8 on arrival). Liz (aged 6 on arrival) showed more influence and Dan (aged 5 on arrival) showed full acquisition of the phonological and phonetic variables. Payne explained this pattern of dialect change in terms of the proportion of a child's peer-influence years (from about 4 to 14) spent in the new dialect area (see Figure 3.1). Liz and Dan had spent a larger proportion of their peer-influence years in King of Prussia than had Richard, and they showed it by sounding more like Philadelphians; Mike was presumably too young to be influenced by peers for two of the five years he had spent in the area at the time of the study.

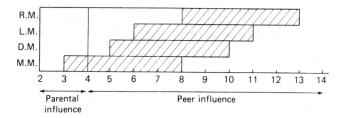

FIGURE 3.1 Peer group influence. Number of years the Morgan children have spent under King of Prussia peer-group influence versus New York City and parental influence.

From A. Payne, "The Reorganization of Linguistic Rules: A Preliminary Report." *Pennsylvania Working Papers on Linguistic Change and Variation, 2,* 1975. Used with permission.

Although Payne (1975) reported results for only a single family, she noted that observation of the community as a whole supports the generality and consistency of the pattern of findings reported. Payne's study suggests that the dialect a child learns from his or her parents can change almost completely in later years under the influence of peers (but see Deser, 1991).

Summary

Phonetic and phonological variation and change continue at least into the school-age years. Difficulties with the precise timing of sequential articulatory gestures continue to be smoothed out over a period of several years. The learning of a written language supplies a visual-spatial model for speech that is internalized as a representational system in memory (Ehri, 1984). Once children begin learning to read and spell, they acquire an important added dimension of language that subtly affects many aspects of language processing and use. Lexical organization, as revealed by lexical selection errors, is also influenced by literacy skills and by the growth, associated with advancing education, of the derived-word vocabulary. Finally, language in the school-age years comes under strong peer influence. Where parental and peer dialects differ in this period the peer norm is likely to triumph.

References

Note: References cited in both Chapter 2 and Chapter 3 are listed only in Chapter 2.

Aitchison, J., and S. Chiat, "Natural phonology or natural memory? The interaction between phonological processes and recall mechanisms." *Language and Speech, 24* (1981): 311–326.

Aitchison, J., and M. Straf, "Lexical storage and retrieval: A developing skill?" In A. Cutler (Ed.), *Slips of the Tongue and Language Production.* Amsterdam: Mouton, 1981.

Allen, G. D., "How the young French child avoids the pre-voicing problem for word-initial voiced stops." *Journal of Child Language, 12* (1985): 37–46.

Arlt, P. B., and M. J. Goodban, "A comparative study

of articulation acquisition as based on a study of 240 normals, aged three to six." *Language, Speech, and Hearing Services in Schools, 7* (1976): 173–180.

Baddeley, A., *Working Memory*. Oxford: Clarendon Press, 1986.

Baddeley, A. D., N. Thomson, and M. Buchanan, "Word length and the structure of short-term memory." *Journal of Verbal Learning and Verbal Behavior, 14* (1975): 575–589.

Barton, D., and M. A. Macken, "An instrumental analysis of the voicing contrast in word-initial stops in the speech of four-year-old English-speaking children." *Language and Speech, 23* (1980): 159–169.

Berg, T., "Sound change in child language: A study of inter-word variation." *Language and Speech, 38* (1995): 331–363.

Berman, R. A., "Natural phonological processes at the one-word stage." *Lingua, 43* (1977): 1–21.

Bernthal, J. E., M. Greenlee, R. Eblen, and K. Marking, "Detection of mispronunciations: A comparison of adults, normal speaking children and children with articulation errors." *Applied Psycholinguistics, 8* (1987): 209–222.

Bricker, W. A., "Errors in the echoic behavior of preschool children." *Journal of Speech and Hearing Research, 10* (1967): 67–76.

Chomsky, N., and M. Halle, *The Sound Pattern of English*. New York: Harper & Row, 1968.

Clark, E. V., and M. Bowerman, "On the acquisition of final voiced stops." In J. A. Fishman, A. Tabouret-Keller, M. Clyne, Bh. Krishnamurti, and M. Abdulaziz (Eds.), *The Fergusonian Impact*, Vol 1. *From Phonology to Society*. Berlin: Mouton de Gruyter, 1986.

Clumeck, H., D. Barton, M. A. Macken, and D. A. Huntington, "The aspiration contrast in Cantonese word-initial stops: Data from children and adults." *Journal of Chinese Linguistics, 9* (1981): 210–224.

Cole, R. A., "Perception of fluent speech by children and adults." In H. B. Winitz (Ed.), *Native Language and Foreign Language Acquisition*. New York: New York Academy of Sciences, 1981.

Cole, R. A., and J. Jakimik, "A model of speech perception." In R. A. Cole (Ed.), *Perception and Pro-*

duction of Fluent Speech. Hillsdale, N. J.: Lawrence Erlbaum, 1980.

Cole, R. A., and C. A. Perfetti, "Listening for mispronunciations in a children's story: The use of context by children and adults." *Journal of Verbal Learning and Verbal Behavior, 19* (1980): 297–315.

Deser, T., "Dialect transmission and variation: An acoustic analysis of vowels in six urban Detroit families." Ph.D. thesis, Boston University, 1990. (Reprinted by the Indiana University Linguistics Club, 1991).

Edwards, M. L., "Patterns and processes in fricative acquisition: Longitudinal evidence from six English-learning children." Ph.D. thesis, Stanford University, 1979.

Ehri, L. C., "How orthography alters spoken language competencies in children learning to read and spell." In J. Downing and R. Valtin (Eds.), *Language Awareness and Learning to Read*. New York: Springer-Verlag, 1984.

Eilers, R. E., D. K. Oller, and C. R. Benito-Garcia, "The acquisition of voicing contrasts in Spanish and English learning infants and children: A longitudinal study." *Journal of Child Language, 11* (1984): 313–336.

Elliott, L. L., "Performance of children aged 9–17 years on a test of speech intelligibility in noise using sentence material with controlled word predictability." *Journal of the Acoustic Society of America, 66* (1979): 651–653.

Elliott, L. L., M. A. Hammer, and K. E. Evan, "Perception of gated, highly familiar spoken monosyllabic nouns by children, teenagers, and older adults." *Perception and Psychophysics, 42* (1987): 150–157.

Fee, J., and D. Ingram, "Reduplication as a strategy of phonological development." *Journal of Child Language, 9* (1982): 41–54.

Ferguson, C. A., "Language development." In J. A. Fishman, J. Das Gupta, and C. A. Ferguson (Eds.), *Language Problems of Developing Nations*. New York: John Wiley, 1968.

Ferguson, C. A., "Fricatives in child language acquisition." In L. Hellman (Ed.), *Proceedings of the Eleventh International Congress of Linguists*. Bologna: Mulino, 1975. (Also in V. Honsa and

M. H. Hardman-Bautista (Eds.), *Papers on Linguistics and Child Language*. The Hague: Mouton, 1978.)

Ferguson, C. A., "Reduplication in child phonology." *Journal of Child Language, 10* (1983): 239–243.

Fey, M. E., and J. Gandour, "The pig dialogue: Phonological systems in transition." *Journal of Child Language, 9* (1982): 517–519.

Gilbert, J. H. V., "A voice onset time analysis of apical stop production in 3-year-olds." *Journal of Child Language, 4* (1977): 103–110.

Gilbert, J. H. V., and C. E. Johnson, "Temporal and sequential constraints on six-year-olds' phonological productions: Some observations on the 'ambliance' phenomenon." *Journal of Child Language, 5* (1978): 101–112.

Gilbert, J. H. V., and B. A. Purves, "Temporal constraints on consonant clusters in child speech production." *Journal of Child Language, 4* (1977): 417–432.

Greenlee, M., "Interacting processes in the child's acquisition of stop-liquid clusters." *Papers and Reports on Child Language Development, 7* (1974): 85–100.

Grosjean, F., "Spoken word recognition and the gating paradigm." *Perception and Psychophysics, 28* (1980): 267–284.

Haelsig, P. C., and C. L. Madison, "A study of phonological processes exhibited by 3-, 4-, and 5-year-old children." *Language, Speech, and Hearing Services in Schools, 17* (1986): 107–114.

Hawkins, S., "Temporal coordination of consonants in the speech of children: Preliminary data." *Journal of Phonetics, 1* (1973): 181–217.

Hodson, B. W., and E. P. Paden, "Phonological processes which characterize unintelligible and intelligible speech in early childhood." *Journal of Speech and Hearing Disorders, 46* (1981): 369–373.

Hulme, C., N. Thomson, C. Muir, and A. Lawrence, "Speech rate and the development of short-term memory span." *Journal of Experimental Child Psychology, 38* (1984): 241–253.

Ingram, D., "Phonological rules in young children." *Journal of Child Language, 1* (1974): 49–64.

Ingram, D., "Phonological development: Production." In P. Fletcher and M. Garman (Eds.), *Language Acquisition: Studies in First Language Development*, 2nd ed. Cambridge (U.K.): Cambridge University Press, 1986.

Ingram, D., L. Christensen, S. Veach, and B. Webster, "The acquisition of word-initial fricatives and affricates in English by children between 2 and 6 years." In G. Yeni-Komshian, J. Kavanagh, and C. A. Ferguson (Eds.), *Child Phonology*, Vol. 1, *Production*. New York: Academic Press, 1980.

Jaeger, J. J., "Assessing the psychological status of the vowel shift rule." *Journal of Psycholinguistic Research, 13* (1984): 13–36.

Jaeger, J. J., "On the acquisition of abstract representations for English vowels." *Phonology Yearbook, 3* (1986): 71–97.

Kamhi, A. G., H. W. Catts, and M. K. Davis, "Management of sentence production demands." *Journal of Speech and Hearing Research, 27* (1984): 329–338.

Klein, H., "Productive strategies for the pronunciation of early polysyllabic lexical items." *Journal of Speech and Hearing Research, 24* (1981): 389–405.

Klein, H., "Relationship between early pronunciation processes and later pronunciation skill." *Journal of Speech and Hearing Disorders, 50* (1985): 156–165.

Lleó, C., "Homonymy and reduplication: On the extended availability of two strategies in phonological acquisition." *Journal of Child Language, 17* (1990): 267–278.

Macken, M. A., "Permitted complexity in phonological development: One child's acquisition of Spanish consonants." *Lingua, 44* (1978): 219–253.

Macken, M. A., "Aspects of the acquisition of stop systems: A cross-linguistic perspective." In G. Yeni-Komshian, J. Kavanagh, and C. A. Ferguson (Eds.), *Child Phonology*, Vol. 1. *Production*. New York: Academic Press, 1980.

Macken, M. A., and D. Barton, "The acquisition of the voicing contrast in English: A study of voice onset time in word-initial stop consonants." *Journal of Child Language, 7* (1980): 41–74.

Macken, M. A., and C. A. Ferguson, "Phonological universals of language acquisition." In H. B. Winitz (Ed.), *Native Language and Foreign Language*

Acquisition. New York: New York Academy of Sciences, 1981.

Magnusson, E., *The Phonology of Language Disordered Children: Production, Perception, and Awareness*. Travaux de l'Institut de Linguistique de Lund, 17. Lund: CWK Gleerup, 1983.

Marslen-Wilson, W. D., "Speech shadowing and speech comprehension." *Speech Communication, 4* (1985): 55–73.

Marslen-Wilson, W. D., "Functional parallelism in spoken word-recognition." In U. H. Frauenfelder and L. K. Tyler (Eds.), *Spoken Word Recognition*. Amsterdam: Elsevier-Science Publishers, 1987.

Menn, L., "Phonotactic rules in beginning speech." *Lingua, 26* (1971): 225–251.

Menyuk, P., "Clusters as single underlying consonants: Evidence from children's production." *Proceedings of the Seventh International Congress of Phonetic Science, Montreal, 1971*. The Hague: Mouton, 1972.

Moskowitz, A. I., "The acquisition of fricatives: A study in phonetics and phonology." *Journal of Phonetics, 3* (1975): 141–150.

Nettelbladt, U., *Development Studies of Dysphonology in Children*. Travaux de l'Institut de Linguistique de Lund, 19. Lund: CWK Gleerup, 1983.

Ohala, J. J., "Aspects of the control and production of speech." *U.C.L.A. Working Papers in Phonetics, 15* (1970).

Oller, D. K., "Simplification as the goal of phonological processes in child speech." *Language Learning, 24* (1975): 299–303.

Payne, A., "The reorganization of linguistic rules: A preliminary report." *Pennsylvania Working Papers on Linguistic Change and Variation, 2* (1975).

Payne, A. C., "Factors controlling the acquisition of the Philadelphia dialect by out-of-state children." In W. Labov (Ed.), *Locating Language in Time and Space*. New York: Academic Press, 1980.

Pendergast, K., S. Dickey, J. Selmar, and A. L. Soder, *Photo Articulation Test*. Danville, Ill.: Interstate, 1969.

Poole, E., "Genetic development of articulation of consonant sounds in speech." *Elementary English Review, 11* (1934): 159–161.

Prather, E., D. Hedrick, and C. Kern, "Articulation development in children aged two to four years." *Journal of Speech and Hearing Disorders, 40* (1975): 179–191.

Preisser, D. A., B. W. Hodson, and E. P. Paden, "Developmental phonology: 18–29 months." *Journal of Speech and Hearing Disorders, 53* (1988): 125–130.

Roberts, J. E., M. Burchinal, and M. M. Footo, "Phonological process decline from $2\frac{1}{2}$ to 8 years." *Journal of Communication Disorders, 23* (1990): 205–217.

Sander, E., "When are speech sounds learned?" *Journal of Speech and Hearing Disorders, 37* (1972): 55–63.

Sax, M., "A longitudinal study of articulation change." *Language, Speech, and Hearing Services in Schools, 3* (1972): 41–48.

Schmitt, L. S., B. H. Howard, and J. F. Schmitt, "Conversational speech sampling in the assessment of articulatory proficiency." *Language, Speech, and Hearing Services in Schools, 14* (1983): 210–222.

Schwartz, R., and L. B. Leonard, "Some further comments on reduplication in child phonology." *Journal of Child Language, 10* (1983): 441–448.

Schwartz, R., L. B. Leonard, M. J. Wilcox, and K. Folger, "Again and again: Reduplication in child phonology." *Journal of Child Language, 7* (1980): 75–88.

Shriberg, L., and Kwiatkowski, J., "Phonological disorders III: A procedure for assessing severity of involvement." *Journal of Speech and Hearing Disorders, 47* (1982): 256–270.

Smit, A. B., "Ages of speech sound acquisition: Comparisons of several normative studies." *Language, Speech, and Hearing Services in Schools, 17* (1986): 175–186.

Smit, A. B., and J. Bernthal, "Voicing contrasts and their phonological implications in the speech of articulation-disordered children." *Journal of Speech and Hearing Research, 26* (1983): 486–500.

Smit, A. B., L. Hand, J. J. Freilinger, J. E. Bernthal, and A. Bird, "The Iowa articulation norms project and its Nebraska replication." *Journal of Speech and Hearing Disorders, 55* (1990): 779–798.

Smith, B. L., "Temporal aspects of English speech production: A developmental perspective." *Journal of Phonetics, 6* (1978): 37–67.

Smith, B. L., "A phonetic analysis of consonantal devoicing in children's speech." *Journal of Child Language, 6* (1979): 19–28.

Snow, K., "A detailed analysis of articulation responses of 'normal' first grade children." *Journal of Speech and Hearing Research, 6* (1963): 277–290.

Stoel-Gammon, C., "Phonetic inventories, 15–24 months: A longitudinal study." *Journal of Speech and Hearing Research, 28* (1985): 505–512.

Stoel-Gammon, C., "The phonological skills of two-year-olds." *Language, Speech, and Hearing Services in Schools, 18* (1987): 323–329.

Stoel-Gammon, C., and C. Dunn, *Normal and Disordered Phonology in Children.* Baltimore: University Park Press, 1985.

Stoel-Gammon, C., and J. P. Stemberger, "Consonant harmony and phonological underspecification in child speech." In M. Yavas (Ed.), *First and Second Language Phonology.* San Diego: Singular Publishing Group, 1994.

Templeton, S., "Spelling first, sound later: The relationship between orthography and higher order phonological knowledge in older students." *Research in the Teaching of English, 13* (1979): 255–264.

Templeton, S., "The spelling-meaning connection and the development of word knowledge in older students." *Journal of Reading, 27* (1983): 8–14.

Templeton, S., and L. Scarborough-Franks, "The spelling's the thing: Knowledge of derivational morphology in orthography and phonology among older students." *Applied Psycholinguistics, 6* (1985): 371–390.

Templin, M. C., *Certain Language Skills in Children.* Minneapolis: University of Minnesota Press, 1957.

Tyler, L. K., and U. H. Frauenfelder, "The process of spoken word recognition: An introduction." In U. H. Frauenfelder and L. K. Tyler (Eds.), *Spoken Word Recognition.* Amsterdam: Elsevier-Science Publishers, 1987.

Tyler, L. K., and W. D. Marslen-Wilson, "Children's processing of spoken language." *Journal of Verbal Learning and Verbal Behavior, 20* (1981): 400–416.

Vihman, M. M., "From pre-speech to speech: On early phonology." *Papers and Reports on Child Language Development, 3* (1976): 51–94.

Vihman, M. M., "Sound change and child language." In E. C. Traugott, R. Labrum, and S. Shepherd (Eds.), *Papers from the Fourth International Conference on Historical Linguistics.* Amsterdam: John Benjamins B.V., 1980.

Vihman, M. M., "Phonology and the development of the lexicon: Evidence from children's errors." *Journal of Child Language, 8* (1981): 239–264.

Walley, A. C., "Developmental differences in spoken word identification." Ph.D. thesis, Indiana University, 1984.

Walley, A. C., and J. L. Metsala, "The growth of lexical constraints on spoken word recognition." *Perception and Psychophysics, 47* (1990): 267–280.

Wellman, B. L., I. M. Case, E. G. Mengert, and D. E. Bradbury, *Speech Sounds of Young Children.* University of Iowa Studies in Child Welfare, 5. Iowa City: University of Iowa Press, 1931.

Chapter *4*

Language and
Dialectal
Variations

AQUILES IGLESIAS,
Temple University

BRIAN GOLDSTEIN,
St. Louis University

Introduction

The speech patterns of a child's community are an important consideration in assessing a child's phonological status. For example, if members of a child's speech community consist of individuals who are bilingual (e.g., Spanish and English) and the variety of English spoken in the child's community is African American Vernacular English (AAVE), the child will most likely speak a variety of English that has been influenced by both AAVE and Spanish. It follows then, that phonological assessment of such a child must take into account the influence AAVE and Spanish may have on the child's phonological patterns.

Information on the characteristics of particular languages and dialects, together with data on normal phonological development, can be extremely useful in conducting least-biased phonological assessments and in differentiating children with dialectal differences from those with phonological disorders. Speech-language pathologists must develop intervention programs for children that reflect the social situations in which they interact and the linguistic characteristics of their speech communities. Sensitivity and knowledge of the linguistic influences on a child's speech, as well as the social characteristics of the child's community, are required for clinicians who serve children with phonological disorders from culturally diverse backgrounds. A similar sensitivity is required for clinicians who serve clients who elect to modify their cultural dialects.

Language Varieties

Several varieties of American English are spoken in the United States, some of which depend on context and interlocutors (**register**), while others are related to social, ethnic, and geographical characteristics of the speakers (**dialect**). **Registral varieties** are dependent on participants, settings, and topics. For example, we would usually use one register when talking to friends about an enjoyable weekend and another when speaking to a policeman about a speeding violation. **Dialects** are mutually intelligible forms of a language associated with a particular region, social class, or ethnicity. Southern White Standard, Appalachian English, Caribbean English, AAVE, General American English (GAE), Mexican American Spanish, Puerto Rican Spanish, and Cuban Spanish are but a few of the dialects spoken in the United States.

Thoughts can be expressed using any dialect of any language; thus, no dialect of any language is superior to another. This is not to say, however, that all varieties of a language are viewed as equal. Some, specifically those used by the dominant groups in any socially stratified society, will be considered to have higher prestige (Wolfram, 1986), a phenomenon promulgated both within the educational system (Adler, 1984) and the private sector (Shuy, 1972; Terrell and Terrell, 1983).

The promulgation of GAE, the prestige dialect in the United States, within the educational system has partially reduced dialectal diversity (**dialect leveling**). Contact through broadcast media among members of different regional dialects has decreased differences between dialects. At the same time, isolation of some groups, especially those of lower socioeconomic status, has resulted in a communicative seclusion that has had nearly the opposite effect. Moreover, the increased immigration and ethnic isolation that has occurred among some subgroups has further increased the number of ethnic dialects. Indeed, with regard to dialects, the "melting pot" hypothesis appears to be a myth for certain segments of our society.

The courts have acknowledged the rights of linguistic minority populations, which has resulted in greater acceptance of dialects other than GAE. In addition, there has been a realization that although English is the most common and dominant language spoken in the United States, other languages have a right to exist in our linguistically plural society.

Historically, the general trend for most immigrants to the United States was to adopt English as their native tongue. Some immigrant groups, however, maintained the use of their first language from generation to generation with reinforcement from new immigrants and travel to their countries of origin. A notable example of this phenomenon is evidenced by the Latino population in the United States, over 20 percent of which do not speak English "well or at all" (U.S. Department of Commerce, 1995).

Simply put, English is spoken in numerous distinctive ways, often described under the rubrics of pidgins, creoles, and dialects. In addition, there are many non-English languages spoken in the United States. In the following sections, we will examine phonological characteristics in each of these areas.

Pidgins and Creoles

Language is always changing. This change is represented in all areas of language—phonology, syntax, semantics, lexicon, and pragmatics—and may occur as a result of a number of factors, including geography, social prestige, and the introduction of new vocabulary (Crystal, 1987). Pidgins and creoles are two important examples of language change.

A **pidgin language** is a communication system used by groups of people who wish and need to communicate with each other but have different languages. They use a limited vocabulary and "simplified" syntactic structure compared with their respective native languages (Crystal, 1987). Pidgins, however, do not simply degrade natural languages but develop their own language rules over time. Crystal notes, however, that a pidgin often has a short life span (perhaps a few years) and disappears when the need for a common communication system ceases to exist. Alternately, he suggests that a pidgin may develop into a creole.

A **creole** is "a pidgin language which has become the mother tongue of a community— a definition which emphasizes that pidgins and creoles are two stages in a single process of linguistic development" (Crystal, 1987, p. 336). In essence, a creole is a pidgin which serves as primary input to the next generation of speakers. That is, a pidgin becomes a creole when it is passed on to child speakers. Compared with pidgins, creoles show increased complexity in syntax, phonology, lexicon, semantics, and pragmatics (Muyksen and Smith, 1995). Creoles tend to show rules that were not exhibited by their pidgin ancestor (Holm, 1988).

Common Creoles in the U.S.

There are three main creoles spoken in the United States: Gullah, Hawaiian Creole, and Louisiana French (Nichols, 1981). Speech-language pathologists may periodically encounter a fourth, somewhat less prevalent variety—Haitian Creole. In this section, important characteristics of these creoles are briefly outlined. (See Table 4.1.)

Gullah (or "Geechee" or "Sea Island Creole," as it is sometimes called) is spoken by approximately 250,000–300,000 individuals, most of whom reside on the barrier islands off the coasts of South Carolina and Georgia (Holm, 1989). This English Creole is closely related to other creoles such as Sierra Leone Krio, Cameroon Creole, Jamaican Creole, the Creole of British Guiana, and the Creoles of Surinam (Cunningham, 1992). Its origin is debated. Some believe that Gullah arrived in the American colonies from the West coast of Africa as a fully developed creole (Nichols, 1981). Others link its development to a complex interaction of white British settlers, Africans, and Caribbeans (Holm, 1989). Notable phonological features of Gullah (compared with GAE) include the use of [a] for /æ/, [t] for /θ/, [d] for /ð/, [dʒ] for /z/, and deletion of postvocalic /r/.

Hawaiian Creole arose in the nineteenth century and culminates from the influence of many sources such as Polynesian, European, Asian, and pidgin languages (Holm, 1989). Distinctive phonological features of Hawaiian Creole (compared with GAE) include [t] for /θ/, [d] for /ð/, backing in the environment of [r] (/θr/ → [tʃr]; /tr/ → [tʃr]; /str/ → [ʃr]), deletion of postvocalic /r/, and deletion of the second member of word-final abutting consonants, for example, /nɛst/ → [nɛs] (Bleile, 1996).

Louisiana French Creole evolved as the native language of descendants of West African slaves brought to southern Louisiana by French colonists (Nichols, 1981). The creole has also been influenced by features of Cajun, a variety of regional French brought from Canada (Holm, 1989). There are an estimated 60,000–80,000 speakers of this creole. The vowel system consists of four front vowels, /i, e, ɛ, a/, four back vowels, /u, o, ɔ, a/, schwa /ə/, and

TABLE 4.1   Characteristics of Common Creoles in the United States

Rule	Example
Gullah	
Low vowel backing	
/æ/ → [a]	/bæt/ → [bat]
Stopping	
/θ/ → [t]	/θæŋk/ → [tæŋk]
/ð/ → [d]	/ðe/ → [de]
/z/ → [dʒ]	/bʌz/ → [bʌdʒ]
Deletion of postvocalic /r/	
/ɚ/ → [Ø]	/pepɚ/ → [pep]
Hawaiian Creole	
Stopping	
/θ/ → [t]	/θæŋk/ → [tæŋk]
/ð/ → [d]	/ðe/ → [de]
Backing in the environment of [r]	
/θr/ → [tʃr]	/θri/ → [tʃri]
/tr/ → [tʃr]	/tre/ → [tʃre]
/str/ → [ʃr]	/stret/ → [ʃret]
Deletion of postvocalic /r/	
/ɚ/ → [Ø]	/pepɚ/ → [pep]
Deletion of word-final abutting consonants	
/st/ → [s]	/nɛst/ → [nɛs]
Louisiana French Creole	
Voicing assimilation (across word boundaries)	
$C_{[-vc]}$ # $C_{[+vc]}$ → $C_{[-vc]}$ # $C_{[+vc]}$	/pæsði/ → [pæzði]
Deletion of word-final consonants	
C # → Ø	/wak/ → [wa]
Deletion of word-final unstressed syllables	
Syllable$_{[-str]}$ # → Ø	/mʌðɚ/ → [mʌð]
Vowel raising	
/ɛ/ → [i]	/pɛn/ → [pin]

three nasalized vowels /ɛ̃, ɔ̃, ã/ (Morgan, 1959; Nichols, 1981). The consonant system contains six oral stops /b, d, g, p, t, k/, three nasal stops /m, n, ñ/, seven fricatives /f, s, ʃ, v, z, ʒ, h/, two liquids /l, r/, and one glide /j/. Nichols (1981) noted two common phonological patterns manifested in French Creole. First, abutting consonants across word boundaries are often assimilated to the voicing of the second member of the consonant pair. Second, word-final consonants may be deleted. Third, word-final unstressed syllables are often weakened or deleted. Finally, vowel raising may take place such that [i] is substituted for /ɛ/.

Haitian Creole, spoken in Haiti, has almost 6 million speakers (Muyksen and Veenstra, 1995). There are three dialects of Haitian Creole: northern, central (including the capital

Port-au-Prince), and southern. The Haitian Creole vowel system contains seven segments, /i, u, e, o, a/ and two front rounded vowels /ø/ and /o̯e/. This creole also contains 17 consonants, six stops /b, d, g, p, t, k/, six fricatives /f, s, ʃ, v, z, ʒ/, three nasals /m, n, ɲ/, and two liquids /l/ and /r/.

Dialectal Variations

Dialects of English

Although it is possible that speech-language pathologists will encounter speakers of one of the creoles listed above, it is more likely that they will serve individuals who speak a dialectal variety of English. As mentioned earlier, a number of dialects of English are spoken in the United States; three of the most prevalent will be discussed in this section: AAVE, Appalachian English, and Ozark English.

Characteristics of AAVE

AAVE is spoken by many, but not all, African Americans. One of the most widely accepted theories explaining the origin of AAVE places its roots in West Africa. When Europeans traveled to the African continent for trade and exploration, *lingua francas*, or trade languages, developed between various European and African speakers as they attempted to communicate verbally regarding business matters. As the slave trade evolved and Africans were brought from Africa to the Caribbean and the American colonies in the southeastern United States, an African-European language combination developed from a *lingua franca* to a pidgin. As the African and European languages (especially English) became more blended, the pidgin evolved into a creole.

The exodus of African Americans from the southeast to the northeast and other parts of the United States in the early 1900s brought AAVE to the urban areas of the north (Stewart, 1971). In many cases, individuals from a particular state tended to migrate to particular cities (e.g., South Carolinians moving to Philadelphia). The restricted social environments in which many African Americans lived, in addition to the continued contact with their southern families and communities, reinforced the use of AAVE.

AAVE is generally considered a dialect of American English. Like all American-English dialects, AAVE is systematic, complete with rule-governed phonological, semantic, syntactic, pragmatic, and proxemic systems. Wolfram (1994), however, indicates that AAVE may be a descendent of a creole. Wolfram notes that Plantation Creole was commonly used by African Americans on plantations in the South, but was not spoken by European Americans at the time. AAVE, then, may be related more to this creole than to European English and may be seen undergoing a *decreolization* process showing few links to its creole past. Wolfram points out, however, that not all aspects of AAVE can be traced to a creole relative; some features of AAVE phonology, such as stopping of interdental fricatives, cannot be related to a creole.

A number of linguistic features distinguish AAVE from GAE, the most notable of which are listed in Table 4.2. These features are always optional, are not used in each possible phonetic context, and are not used by all AAVE speakers. For example, the simplification of word-final clusters tends to occur when one of the consonants is an alveolar and the other

TABLE 4.2 Major Phonological Features that Distinguish African-American Vernacular English (AAVE) and General American English (GAE)

1. Word-final consonant cluster reduction, particularly when one of the two consonants is an alveolar (e.g., "test" /tɛst/ → [tɛs]).
2. Stopping of word-initial interdentals (e.g., "they" /ðe/ → [de], "thought" /θat/ → [tat]).
3. Substitution of f/γ and v/ð in intervocalic position (e.g., "nothing" /nʌθiŋ/ → [nʌfiŋ], "bathing" /beðiŋ/ → [beviŋ]).
4. Substitution of f/θ in word-final position (e.g., "south" /sauθ/ → [sauf]).
5. Deletion of /r/ (e.g., "sister" /sɪstɚ/ → [sɪstə], "Carol" /kærəl/ → [kæəl], "professor" /prʌfɛsɚ/ → [pʌfɛsə]).
6. Deletion of /l/ in word-final abutting consonants (e.g., "help" /hɛlp/ → [hɛp]).
7. Substitution of [ɪ] for /ɛ/ before nasals (e.g., "pin" /pɪn/ and "pen" /pɛn/ pronounced as pɪn).
8. Deletion of nasal consonant in word-final position with nasalization of preceding vowel (e.g., "moon" /mun/ → [mũ]).

(i.e., the deleted consonant) is a morphological marker. Hence, some AAVE speakers may not differentiate between the present and past tense of the same verb (e.g., both *miss* and *missed* are pronounced as /mɪs/), but would retain the cluster in a word such as *mist*.

The extent to which particular individuals use features of the dialect often depends on socioeconomic status. For example, middle-class African Americans use AAVE features to a lesser extent than working-class African Americans, especially in formal situations (Wolfram, 1986). Wolfram refers to this sociolinguistic phenomenon as *social diagnosticity*, a term applied to the observation that linguistic features sometime exhibit dissimilar patterns of usage across socioeconomic levels.

Wolfram observed the frequency of occurrence of selected AAVE features among the speech of individuals representing four socioeconomic groups: upper middle class, lower middle class, upper working class, and lower working class. His research revealed that certain AAVE linguistic features showed **gradient stratification** across the four groups. That is, there was a progressive decrease in the usage of a particular linguistic feature from lower to higher class groups. The lack of realization of postvocalic *r* (e.g., /sɪstɚ/ → [sɪstə]) is a particularly good example of this pattern, as this phonological feature is used by all four socioeconomic groups, albeit with different levels of frequency. On the other hand, certain AAVE features show a pattern of usage referred to as **sharp stratification**. This term applies to linguistic features that, based on frequency of usage, more clearly differentiates socioeconomic groups. One example of this type of stratification is the substitution of [f] for /θ/. The use of this feature contrasts middle-class with working-class groups, with working-class groups using the feature much more frequently than middle-class speakers. According to Wolfram, features revealing sharp stratification are of greater social diagnosticity than those showing gradient stratification.

Phonological Development in AAVE

Little information exists on the development of AAVE phonology. Seymour and Seymour (1981) compared the performance on a standard articulation test of 4- and 5-year-old African-American children to that of a group of white children. They reported that both groups evidenced phonological variations characteristic of AAVE (e.g., f/θ in medial and final positions; d/ð in initial and medial positions; b/v in initial and medial positions); however, the AAVE features occurred more frequently in the productions of the African-American children. Thus, both groups produced the same types of substitutions, but with different frequencies. These results suggest that for the population studied, the contrast between AAVE and GAE was *qualitatively* undifferentiated at this age level. The same qualitative differences have been demonstrated with similar populations in their use of phonological processes (Haynes and Moran, 1989).

Seymour and Seymour (1981) also reported considerable intersubject variability among the African-American subjects, all of whom were AAVE speakers. Although the prevalence of AAVE phonological features was higher among African-American subjects than white subjects, not all of the target features were present in each African-American speaker nor were the features equally distributed. These researchers inferred that African-American children from AAVE-speaking communities would likely show developmental variations similar to existing normative data.

Bleile and Wallach (1992) compared the articulation of nonspeech-delayed and speech-delayed African-American children ranging in age from 3;6 to 5;5. Head Start teachers of African-American descent differentiated the two groups of children; data analysis was based on non-AAVE phonological patterns exhibited by the children in a picture-identification, single-word test. The delayed and nondelayed groups reflected differences in the type and quantity of their speech errors. Speech-delayed children showed more (1) stop errors (especially velars), (2) fricative errors in all positions (especially fricatives other than /θ/), and (3) affricate errors in all positions. Nonspeech-delayed subjects evidenced greater devoicing of final /d/, sonorant errors, and errors related to /r/. Both groups produced a large number of consonant cluster errors, with the speech-delayed children exhibiting a larger number of cluster errors. Bleile and Wallach concluded that, as is the case with non-African-American populations, a combination of characteristics, rather than a single indicator, appears to be the most reliable index of speech delay in African-American speakers.

The acquisition of AAVE features by English-speaking Puerto Rican children has also been the subject of study. Wolfram (1974) studied the speech characteristics of Puerto Rican teenagers living in East Harlem, New York. His findings suggest that the degree of contact his subjects had with AAVE speakers greatly influenced the number of AAVE features in their speech (individuals with the greatest contact showed the largest number of features). Poplack (1978) examined AAVE, Puerto Rican Spanish, and Philadelphia English variants in the speech of sixth-grade Puerto Rican boys and girls. She concluded that the specific variants used by the children were more related to "covert prestige" than to their linguistic environment, with the boys assigning more prestige to AAVE speakers and the girls assigning more prestige to Philadelphia English. Though they utilized speakers of different age groups, locale, and ethnic background, both studies support the assertion that speech patterns are greatly affected by peer interaction.

Appalachian English and Ozark English
In addition to AAVE, Appalachian English (AE) and Ozark English (OE) are among the dialects frequently observed in the United States. Christian, Wolfram, and Nube (1988) indicate that AE and OE are related linguistically, and share many similar features. Given the

TABLE 4.3   Characteristics of Appalachian English (AE) and Ozark English (OE)

Rule	Example (IPA)	Example (Orthography)
Epenthesis following clusters CCC# → CC C#	/gosts/ → [gost s]	"ghosts" → "ghostes"
Intrusive *t* (more common in AE) /s/# → [st] /f/# → [ft]	/wʌns/ → [wʌnst] /klɪf/ → /klɪft/	"once" → "oncet" "cliff" → "clifft"
Stopping of fricatives /θ/ → [t] /ð/ → [d]	/θat/ → [tat] /ðe/ → [de]	"thought" → "tought" "they" → "dey"
Initial *w* reduction /w/ → Ø	/wɪl/ → [ɪl]	"will" → "'ll"
Initial unstressed syllables (IUS) ISU → Ø	/əlaud/ → [laud]	"allowed" → "'llowed"
h retention Ø → [h]	/ɪt/ → [hɪt]	"it" → "hit"
Retroflex *r* /r/ → Ø postconsonantal /r/ → Ø intervocalic	/θro/ → /θo/ /kæri/ → [kæi]	"throw" → "thow" "carry" → "ca'y"
Lateral *l* /l/ → Ø before labials	/wʌlf/ → [wʌf]	"wolf" → "wof"

phonological similarities of these two dialects, they will be discussed together. AE is spoken chiefly in areas of Kentucky, Tennessee, Virginia, North Carolina, and West Virginia (parts of Georgia and Alabama may also be included). OE is most prevalent in an area encompassing northern Arkansas, southern Missouri, and northwestern Oklahoma.

Christian and colleagues (1988, pp. 153–159) have outlined the following characteristics of AE and OE. (See Table 4.3. Only the most common features are outlined here; see Christian et al., 1988, for more details.)

As with AAVE as spoken by African-American speakers, not all features of AE/OE are utilized by every speaker, in every situation, in every context. For example, the rule termed *intrusive t*, in which [t] may be added to words ending in /s/ or /f/, is usually limited to a small set, most commonly the words *once* and *twice*. Interestingly, the number of words exhibiting this rule seems to be more extensive in AE than in OE.

Phonological Development in Speakers of Languages Other than English

If current birthrates and immigration trends continue in the United States, a marked increase in the size of culturally and linguistically diverse populations will occur. It is estimated that by the end of the twentieth century the population of Latinos will increase by 21 percent, the Asian population by 22 percent, the African-American population by 12 percent, and the white population by slightly greater than 2 percent (Battle, 1993). These increases, coupled with the more than 200 Native American languages currently spoken in the United States (Harris, 1993), suggest that speech-language pathologists will likely encounter speakers of languages other than English. To conduct appropriate phonological assessments that guide the treatment process, speech-language pathologists need to gather segmental, syllabic, and developmental information about the languages of their clients. In this section, the characteristics of Spanish, Asian languages, and Native American languages, as well as information about phonological acquisition and development in speakers of those language groups, will be described.

The Influence of the Home Language on English

When there is contact between speakers representing two languages, there is a tendency for each to influence the other. For example, English phonology may influence the production of Spanish (e.g., "Como se llama su niño?" [komo se dzama su niño]→[ko̞umo̞ʊ se̞ ɪ dʒama su niɲo̞ʊ] "What is your child's name?"); alternately, Spanish phonology can influence the production of English (e.g., "Let me try to explain the theme." [le mi trai tu eʰple di tim]). In the first case, the speaker substitutes English vowels, while in the second case the speaker primarily substitutes Spanish vowels and deletes all final consonants.

Simply stated, sounding like a native speaker entails not only producing the correct phones—although this helps considerably—but also knowing when to apply phonological rules. For example, application of the English rule of regressive assimilation of voicing in final clusters does not increase intelligibility as much as it increases one's ability to sound like a native English speaker.

Several factors influence the extent to which one phonological system influences another. The influence may be due to the absence of phonemes or allophones in a language (e.g., [pʰ, tʰ, and kʰ, ʃ, v, dʒ] do not occur in Spanish); differences in the distribution of sounds (e.g., in Spanish, the only word-final consonants are /s, n, ɾ, l, d/); or differences in place of articulation for consonants (Spanish /d/ and English /d/). Other important influential factors are how and when pronunciation is acquired. For example, for some individuals learning English as a second language, first exposure to English may be the written form. As English lacks one-to-one correspondence between grapheme and phoneme (e.g., the grapheme "s" in English is produced as [s] in *basin* and as [ʒ] in measure), acquisition may be adversely affected.

Spanish

Characteristics of Spanish

Spanish has become the second most common language spoken in the United States, with more than 11 million speakers, or 5 percent of the population. According to Dalbor (1980), there are six major dialects of American Spanish: Mexican and Southwestern United States; Central American; Caribbean; Highlandian; Chilean; and Southern Paraguayan, Uruguayan, and Argentinean. The principal differences among these dialects are lexical and phonological. Although all are spoken in the mainland United States, the two most common are Southwestern United States and Caribbean. Their prevalence is attributable to the large number of Mexican immigrants, the prolific migration of Puerto Ricans, and the immigration of political refugees from Cuba, El Salvador, and Nicaragua.

The English dialect spoken in the geographical community of a Spanish speaker will influence that person's Spanish and English dialects alike. Other important influential factors include the degree of contact with Spanish and English speakers; whether the speaker is learning both languages simultaneously or sequentially; and the prestige attached to the various dialects with which the individual comes in contact. These factors interact in highly complex ways, resulting in multiple variations and considerable linguistic diversity within the population. Thus, it is important to have a working knowledge of the salient characteristics of Spanish to understand how English and Spanish dialects interact.

Spanish Phonology

A brief overview of the Spanish consonant and vowel system is presented here (for a more complete analysis, see Goldstein, 1995). There are five primary vowels in Spanish. The two front vowels are /i/ and /e/, and the three back vowels are /u/, /o/, and /a/. There are 18 phonemes in "standard" Spanish: the voiceless unaspirated stops, /p/, /t/, and /k/; the voiced stops, /b/, /d/, and /g/; the voiceless fricatives, /f/, /χ/, and /s/; the affricate, /tʃ/; the glides, /w/ and /j/; the lateral, /l/; the tap /ɾ/ and trill /r/; and the nasals, /m/, /n/, and /ŋ/.

Differences between Spanish dialects further complicate the process of characterizing phonological patterns in Spanish-speaking children. Unlike English, in which dialectal variations are generally defined by variations in vowels, Spanish dialectal differences primarily affect consonant sound classes rather than vowels or a few specific phonemes. The dialect differences affect certain sound classes more so than others. Fricatives and liquids (in particular /s/, /ɾ/, and /r/) tend to show more variation than stops, glides, or the affricate. These differences make it paramount that speech-language pathologists identify the dialects their clients are speaking; otherwise, the likelihood of misdiagnosis dramatically increases.

Phonological Development in Normally Developing Spanish-Speaking Children

Normative data (summarized in detail in Goldstein, 1995) show that normally developing Spanish-speaking infants will tend to produce CV syllables containing oral and nasal stops with front vowels (e.g., Oller and Eilers, 1982). It is likely that, by the time normally developing Spanish-speaking children reach 3 years of age, they will use the dialectal features of the community and will have mastered the vowel system and most of the consonant system (Anderson and Smith, 1987; Pandolfi and Herrera, 1990). By completion of preschool, normally developing children will exhibit some difficulty with consonant clusters and a few phones, specifically, [ð], [χ], [s], [ŋ], [tʃ], [ɾ], [r], and [l] (Acevedo, 1991; Jimenez, 1987). To some degree, these children will still occasionally exhibit specific phonological processes—cluster reduction, unstressed syllable deletion, stridency deletion, and tap/trill /r/ deviation—but will likely have suppressed velar and palatal fronting, prevocalic singleton omission, stopping, and assimilation (Goldstein and Iglesias, 1996a; Stepanof, 1990). For some Spanish-speaking children, phonetic mastery will continue into the early elementary school years, when they continue to show some, although infrequent, errors on the fricatives [χ] and [s], the affricate [tʃ], the liquids [r, ɾ, l], and consonant clusters (Bailey, 1982; De la Fuente, 1985).

Children's acquisition and development of vowels have received increased attention recently (e.g., Clement and Wijnen, 1994; Pollock and Keiser, 1990), although few studies have examined the production of vowels in Spanish-speaking children. Oller and Eilers (1982) found that the mean proportion occurrence of vowel-like productions in 12- to 14-month-old English- and Spanish-speaking children was remarkably similar. They noted that, in general, the children were likely to produce more anterior-like than posterior-like vowels. The rank order of the first ten vowels in Spanish-speaking infants was: (1) [ɛ]; (2) [æ]; (3) [e]; (4) [i]; (5) [a]; (6) [ʌ]; (7) [ʊ]; (8) [u]; (9) [ɪ]; (10) [o] (p. 573). Maez (1981) indicated that by 18 months the three subjects in the study had mastered (i.e., produced correctly at least 90 percent of the time) the five basic Spanish vowels, [i], [e], [u], [o], and [a]. Maez's study, however, focused on consonant development and did not indicate if vowel errors occurred.

Goldstein and Pollock (1995) examined vowel productions in 23 Spanish-speaking children (10 3-year-olds and 13 4-year-olds) with phonological disorders. Fourteen of the 23 children (10 girls and 4 boys) in the study exhibited vowel errors. Only one child exhibited more than one vowel error (5 errors); the other 13 each exhibited only one vowel error. Across all subjects, the results indicated that there were only 18 total vowel errors, almost half (8 of 18 errors) of which were on the vowel /o/. There were four errors each exhibited on /e/ and /a/, and one each on /i/ and /u/.

Phonological Development in Spanish-Speaking Children with Phonological Disorders

Although a number of studies have described phonological patterns in normally developing children, the data remain scarce for Spanish-speaking children with phonological disorders. Data indicate that the percentage of Spanish-speaking children with phonological disorders who exhibit specific processes is similar across studies (e.g., Bichotte, Dunn, Gonzalez, Orpi, and Nye, 1993; Goldstein and Iglesias, 1996b; Maez, 1983). Phonological processes exhibited by a large percentage of children (in excess of 40 percent) include cluster reduction, unstressed syllable deletion, stopping, liquid simplification, and assimilation.

Asian Languages

There are three main families of languages spoken in Asia (Crystal, 1987). The first consists of the more than 100 Austro-Asiatic languages, which represent most of the languages spoken in Southeast Asia (the countries between China and Indonesia), including Khmer, Hmong, and Vietnamese. The second is the Tai family, centered on Thailand and extending into Laos, North Vietnam, and parts of China. The third branch is Sino-Tibetan, comprising the languages of China, Tibet, and Burma, including Mandarin and Cantonese. Together, these families contain in excess of 440 languages spoken by more than 1 billion people. Two other families, Austronesian (containing languages such as Chamorro, Hawaiian, Ilocano, Samoan and Tagalog, and Papuan (to which belongs New Guinean) comprise languages spoken in the Pacific Islands (Cheng, 1993).

There are a number of features of Asian languages that speech-language pathologists need to recognize. With this in mind, the following topics will be discussed here: tone, acquisition of tone, segmental inventory, syllable structure and stress, dialect differences, and phonological development in children speaking Asian languages. For more detail on these subjects, see Cheng (1987, 1993).

Tone

Many, but not all, Asian languages are tone languages; for example, Cantonese is a tone language but Japanese is not. In **tone languages**, differences in word meaning are signified by differences in pitch. Tone languages are generally composed of *register tones* (typically two or three in a language) and *contour tones* (also usually two or three per language) (O'Grady, Dobrovolsky, and Aranoff, 1993). Register tones are level tones, usually signaled by high, mid, and low tones; contour tones are a combination of register tones over a single syllable. An example from Mandarin Chinese is provided in Table 4.4.

Acquisition of Tone

There have been very few studies of tone acquisition in Asian languages. Some studies have examined this phenomenon in specific dialects such as Mandarin (Chao, 1973), while others have analyzed tone spectrographically in adults (Wang and Li, 1967). Two studies, Li and Thompson (1977) and Tse (1978), examined tone acquisition in Chinese speakers and

TABLE 4.4 Examples of Tone in Mandarin Chinese

H ↓ [ma]	'mother'	high tone
LH ↓ [ma]	'hemp'	low rise
MLH ↓ [ma]	'horse'	fall rise
HL ↓ [ma]	'scold'	high fall

Adapted from O'Grady, Dobrovolsky, and Aranoff (1993).

obtained similar results. These studies illustrate well the developmental process of tone. Li and Thompson (1977) examined the acquisition of lexical tone in 17 Mandarin-speaking children ranging in age from 1;6 to 3;0 in Taipei. They found that (1) these children acquired the correct tone system relatively quickly, (2) mastery of tone occurred before segmental mastery, (3) high and falling tones were acquired earlier and more easily than rising and contour tones, and (4) substitution errors often exist for rising and contour tones during the two- and three-word stages. Tse (1978) completed a longitudinal study on the acquisition of tone in a single Cantonese-speaking child from the age of 2;8 to 4;10. Tse found that (1) perceptual discrimination of tone began as early as 10 months, (2) the tonal system was acquired in about 8 months (from 1;2 to 1;9), (3) the tone system was acquired before the segmental system, and (4) the falling tone was acquired before the rising tone.

Segmental Inventory

In general, there are few syllable-final segments and few consonant clusters in Asian languages. For example, (1) the only syllable final consonants in Mandarin Chinese are /n/ and /ŋ/, (2) there are no labiodental, interdental, or palatal fricatives in Korean, and (3) Hawaiian contains only five vowels and eight consonants. There are, however, segmental systems in Asian languages which are relatively complex. For example, Hmong (the language spoken by dwellers in mountainous areas of Indochina) contains 56 initial consonants, 13 or 14 vowels (depending on dialect), seven tones, and one final consonant /ŋ/ (Cheng, 1993). Given these differences between Asian languages and English, Cheng (1987) notes possible phonetic "interference" by speakers of Asian languages learning English. (For segmental information on specific languages and dialects, it is suggested that the reader consult Cheng, 1987, 1993; Tipton, 1975; and Wang, 1989. These sources contain segmental information on Cantonese/Mandarin, Vietnamese, Hmong, Khmer, Pilipino, Korean, Japanese, and Chamorro.)

Syllable Structure and Stress

Syllable structure varies greatly in Asian languages. For example, while Laotian contains but three syllable types (CVC, CVVC, and CVV), Khmer exhibits eight (CVC, CCVC, CCCVC, CVVC, CCVVC, CCCVVC, CVV, CCVV) yet contains few polysyllabic words (Cheng, 1987). Many Asian languages also show restrictions on the types of segments that may appear in certain syllable positions: Vietnamese has a limited number of final consonants (voiceless stops and nasals); the only final consonant in Hmong is /ŋ/; Korean contains no fricatives or affricates in word-final position.

The use of stress in Asian languages often contrasts sharply with English. For example, there is no tonic word stress in Korean, so native speakers of Korean may sound somewhat monotonous to native English speakers when they speak English (Cheng, 1993).

Dialectal Differences

Like English, Asian languages contain a number of dialectal variations (Wang, 1990). For example, two main dialects of Chinese are spoken in the United States (Mandarin and Cantonese), each of which contains several subdialects. Conversely, though, Japanese has relatively few dialects, unlike Khmer's four dialects, and they are mutually unintelligible.

Phonological Development in Speakers of Asian Languages

Few studies have investigated phonological development in children who speak Asian languages. Those that have been conducted have examined chiefly phonological development in specific language/dialect groups.

So and Dodd (1994) investigated phonological development in Cantonese-speaking children with phonological disorders and also provided data on development in normally developing Cantonese-speaking children. In the latter group they noted phoneme acquisition similar to English but at a more rapid rate. In general, anterior consonants were acquired before posterior consonants, and oral and nasal stops and glides were acquired before fricatives and affricates. They also noted the exhibition of phonological processes and found that by age 4;0 no process was exhibited more than 15 percent of the time. Between the ages of 2;0 and 4;0, these children showed processes similar in quantity (greater than 15 percent) and kind to English-speaking children: assimilation, cluster reduction, stopping, fronting, affrication, and final consonant deletion.

So and Dodd (1994, pp. 238–240) also outlined and defined four subgroups of children with phonological disorders: articulation disorder ("consistent distortion of a phoneme"), delayed phonological development ("rules or processes used by more than 10 percent of children acquiring phonology normally"), consistent use of one or more unusual rules ("rules not used by more than 10 percent of children acquiring phonology normally"), and inconsistent errors ("production of specific words or particular phonological segments"). These researchers applied these categories to 17 Cantonese-speaking children with phonological disorders aged 3;6–6;4. Their results revealed that 8 of 17 subjects (47 percent) displayed a phonological delay, 5 of 17 (30 percent) were categorized as consistent users of one or more unusual rules, 2 of 17 (12 percent) were articulation disordered, and 2 of 17 (12 percent) were defined as using inconsistent errors.

They provided increased detail on the phonological patterns exhibited by the 13 subjects labeled either "phonological delayed" or "consistently disordered," noting that delayed children tended to exhibit assimilation, cluster reduction, stopping, fronting, deaspiration, affrication, and final consonant deletion. Disordered children tended to exhibit final consonant deletion, final glide deletion, initial consonant deletion, aspiration, gliding, vowel rule, and backing.

Native American Languages

It is estimated that more than 200 Native American languages, including Eskimo and Amerindian languages, are currently spoken in North America. Combined, these languages are spoken by in excess of 760,000 individuals (Leap, 1981; U.S. Census, 1995). By the mid-1970s, approximately 150–200 North American Indian languages were spoken, only about 50 of which were spoken by more than 1,000 individuals (Crystal, 1987). Several languages teeter even more closely to extinction; Eyak (spoken in Alaska), for example, now has but two speakers (Krauss, 1992).

Native American languages in North America have been classified into six general families (Crystal, 1987). The following classification contains each family's general geographic area along with a limited number of member languages:

1. *Eskimo-Aleut* (Alaska, part of Canada, Greenland): Yupik, Inuit
2. *Na-Dané* (Alaska, northwest Canada, southwest U.S.): Apache, Navajo
3. *Algonquin* (central and eastern Canada, central and southern U.S.): Arapaho, Blackfoot, Cree, Ojibwa
4. *Penutian* (bridge between North and South America, southwest Canada, western U.S.): Maya, Quiché
5. *Macro-Siouan* (Canada through central U.S.): Cherokee, Dakota, Crow
6. *Aztec-Tanoan* (central, southern U.S.): Shoshone, Hopi

Segmental Inventory

Native American languages include sounds in their segmental inventories that do not appear in English (Ladefoged, 1993). First, many contain *ejectives*, sounds made with a glottalic egressive airstream. These phonemes include /p′, t′, k′, ts′/; for example, [p′o] ("foggy") in Lakhota. Second, they may show voiceless stops in combination with the velar fricative, /pˣ, tˣ, kˣ/; for example, [pˣa] ("bitter" in Lakhota). Third, *implosives*—stops made with an ingressive glottalic airstream—may be part of the segmental inventories of these languages. Fourth, ejective and nonejective stops and ejective affricates may be produced with a lateral release, /tl′/, /tl/, and /ts′/, respectively. Three examples from Navajo include [tl′èè?] ("night"), [tlàh] ("oil"), and [ts′áal] ("cradle"). Finally, these languages may contain nasalized vowels (Welker, 1995).

Phonological Development in Speakers of Native American Languages

Although there is some information on how Native Americans learn English, little developmental data exist on phonological acquisition and development in Native American children. Bayles and Harris (1982) performed a screening on 583 children on the Papago Indian Reservation (the total population in the reservation's two elementary schools). Only the results of the articulation testing will be presented here. The children's phonological skills were assessed in English using the *Goldman-Fristoe Test of Articulation* (Goldman and Fristoe, 1969). It is difficult to evaluate the results of this aspect of the study because 68 percent of the children indicated that English was the dominant language spoken at home; 12 percent said that Papago was the dominant home language; while 20 percent noted that both languages were spoken equally at home.

The authors noted that dialectal features such as diminished aspiration and deemphasis of final consonants were taken into account and not counted as errors. Twenty-nine of the 583 children (5 percent) were diagnosed with an articulation disorder. They noted that most misarticulations involved the phonemes /s/ and /z/ and /s/-blends.

Assessment

In assessing the speech and language skills of children from culturally and linguistically diverse populations, the same types of information are gathered as for all children: case histories are taken, oral-peripheral examinations and hearing screenings are conducted, language (e.g., syntax, semantics, etc.), voice, fluency, and phonological patterns are assessed. A detailed phonological assessment might include both formal measures (of which few are available for non-English-speaking children) and informal measures.

Considerations for Children from Culturally and Linguistically Diverse Populations

The assessment of phonological patterns in children from culturally and linguistically diverse populations requires determination of whether children's phonological systems are within the norm of acceptable speech for their linguistic communities. Thus, the assessment must be approached with an understanding of the social, cultural, and linguistic characteristics of the community from which a given child comes. It is vital that such information be obtained to guard against cultural stereotyping (Taylor, Payne, and Anderson, 1987). For example, it is inappropriate to assume that all African Americans speak AAVE. Members of the same race need not share the same speech community or culture. While one African American's production of f/θ in the word *mouth* may be regarded as a dialectal feature of AAVE, it would be inappropriate to make the same clinical judgment for another African American who also produced f/θ without further investigation. While the first speaker may be an AAVE speaker, the second speaker may not and therefore his or her production would be considered a phonological error.

Several issues must be considered in assessing an individual whose language or dialect differs from that of the examiner. Examiners must be aware of their own dialects and their effect on the assessment process. Indeed, Seymour and Seymour (1977) noted that the client's perception of the formality of the situation affects linguistic phonological usage. Casual speaking settings may encourage the use of AAVE, while formal settings may inhibit and stigmatize speech forms other than GAE. A similar issue may be encountered when a clinician uses Castillian Spanish (i.e., the standard dialect of Spanish spoken in Spain and taught in most educational systems in the U.S.) in conversing with a speaker of any of the other major Spanish dialects. This is not to say that one should force oneself to use the client's dialect. One must recognize, however, the potential effect one's own dialect may have on a client.

ASHA's position paper on social dialects officially acknowledges the distinction between a speech-language difference and a speech-language disorder (ASHA, 1983). A few investigators have attempted to determine if scoring dialectal features as "errors" would penalize the child for a pattern that is, in effect, a dialectal feature, thus artificially inflating the child's severity rating. Three studies, all of which used African-American children as subjects, have specifically examined the effect of dialect on the diagnosis of phonological disorders in children. In their examination of 10 children aged 5;11–6;11, Cole and Taylor (1990) found that not taking dialect into account resulted in the misdiagnosis of phonological disorders for half the subjects.

Two other studies, while advocating that dialect should be accounted for in phonological assessment, did not report results at the same level of significance as did Cole and Taylor. Fleming and Hartman (1989) examined 72 4-year-olds using the *Computer Assessment of Phonological Processes* (CAPP) (Hodson, 1985). They determined that while some test items were influenced by "Black English (BE) phonological rules," the assessment, as a whole, was not invalidated (p. 28). Moreover, they indicated that no normally developing child was labeled as having a disorder based solely on dialectal factors. Washington and Craig (1992) examined 28 preschool children aged 4;6–5;3. Their results indicated that dialect scoring changes did "not seem to penalize the BE-speaking preschooler to a degree that is clinically significant" (p. 203). These researchers ascribed the differences in their results as compared to those of Cole and Taylor (1990) to geographic location (the subjects in Cole and Taylor's study were from Mississippi, while the children in Washington and Craig's study resided in Detroit).

While the results of these studies suggest somewhat different conclusions about whether scoring dialectal features as "errors" affected severity ratings, the researchers all agreed that accounting for dialectal features is a prime consideration in the assessment of children from culturally and linguistically diverse populations. There are, of course, a number of dialectal differences among varieties of any language. Analysis of phonological information must be made that takes children's dialects into account. "Errors" can only be counted as such when they conflict with children's dialects. For example, in the Puerto Rican dialect of Spanish, the production of /dos/ as [do:] would not be scored as an error because syllable-final /s/ is often deleted. The production of /floɾ/ as [flo] would be scored as an error because syllable-final deletion of /ɾ/ is not considered a typical feature of the dialect. In short, not accounting for dialectal features may result in misdiagnosis.

In summary, all analyses should factor in the features of dialects, with extra care taken not to score dialectal features as errors. To account for dialect features in any particular linguistic group, the speech-language pathologist might (a) sample the adult speakers in the child's linguistic community, (b) obtain information from interpreters/support personnel, and (c) consult reliable background literature.

The assessment of speakers of languages other than English presents a challenge to the speech-language pathologist. Ideally, the assessment tools used should be designed specifically to assess phonological patterns in the child's native language. However, not only are such tools often unavailable, but the normative data necessary is often also unavailable. In such cases, it is recommended that speech-language pathologists familiarize themselves with the phonological rules of the language and develop, in cooperation with native speakers of the language, informal assessments that provide the examiner with a measure of the child's ability to produce the phonemes of the client's native language. In cases where non-English tests are available, primarily Spanish, dialectal features of the speaker must be taken into consideration. Assuming a given individual speaks both English and a language other than English, the clinician should assess, whenever possible, both languages, being conscious of possible interference errors and dialectal variations.

Intervention for Phonological Disorders in Children from Culturally and Linguistically Diverse Populations

Once the results of an assessment are gathered, speech-language pathologists must decide the next course of action. ASHA's 1983 position paper on social dialects provides guidelines to be followed if the client is a speaker of a dialect other than GAE. As reflected in this paper, the traditional role of a speech-language pathologist is to provide clinical services for communication disorders but not to treat dialectal differences. The paper (ASHA, 1983) does identify, however, the following expanded role for speech-language pathologists:

> Aside from the traditionally recognized role, the speech-language pathologist may also be available to provide *elective* clinical services to nonstandard English speakers who do not present a disorder. The role of the speech-language pathologist for these individuals is to prepare the desired competency in Standard English without jeopardizing the integrity of the individual's first dialect. The approach must be functional and based on context-specific appropriateness of the given dialect. (p. 24)

If elective services are to be provided, it is important that clinicians keep in mind that elective therapy does not necessarily mean that clients want to eliminate their first dialect (D_1). More often, the clients prefer to be bidialectal. Taylor (1986) proposed a series of steps to be followed in order to maintain both dialects. First, a positive attitude toward D_1 should be established. Second, clients learn to contrast the features of the first and second dialect (D_2). Finally, clients should practice D_2 in controlled, structured, and eventually spontaneous situations.

The speech-language pathologist must also recognize how dialectal variation and phonological disorders interact (Wolfram, 1994). Wolfram suggested the following guiding principles. He classifies impairments into three types. **Type I** impairments are judged to be atypical patterns regardless of speakers' dialects. For example, this would include patterns such as initial consonant deletion (e.g., [it] for /mit/) or velar fronting (e.g., [dot] for /got/). **Type II** impairments show cross-dialectal differences in normative (or underlying) forms. For example, the normative form for the word *bathing* would be [beðiɹ] for speakers of GAE but [beviŋ] for AAVE speakers, even though speakers from both dialect groups might misarticulate that word as [beziŋ]. **Type III** impairments affect forms that are shared across dialects but applied with different frequencies. For example, syllable-final cluster reduction is exhibited in many dialects, but is observed more frequently in AAVE than in other dialects. Wolfram (1994) noted that treating a Type I impairment would not necessitate gathering different norms across dialect groups. The treatment of Types II and III impairments, however, would involve taking into account both qualitative and quantitative differences between dialect groups.

Intervention in Non-English Speakers

Little information is available to direct treatment in non-English-speaking children with phonological disorders. There is no reason to suspect that the principles that guide intervention choices for English-speaking children would differ from those of culturally and linguistically diverse populations; still the conspicuous absence of data warrants attention. There are, however, a number of guidelines that speech-language pathologists might follow. First, the clinical management process should begin with an appropriate and least-biased assessment. The speech-language pathologist should:

1. Take the client's cultural values and learning styles into account.
2. Ask for help from colleagues, parents, teachers, and others if necessary.
3. Possess knowledge of phonological and dialectal features of the clients' languages.
4. Use nondiscriminatory assessment tools.
5. Complete phonological analyses in both L_1 (native language) and L_2 (English), if possible.
6. Compare clients' performances against reliable referents collected from both normally developing and phonologically disordered non-English-speaking children.

In addition, the speech-language pathologist should neither use normative phonological data gathered from English-speaking children to assess non-English speaking children, nor generalize developmental phonological data from one dialect group to another. Second, speech-language pathologists should apply sensitive treatment techniques. That is, remediation approaches may need to be varied depending on a number of factors, including the children's ages, language status (monolingual L_1, limited English proficiency, bilingual, etc.), length of exposure to L_1/L_2, and dialect (Perez, 1994). Third, the clinician must decide in which language (or languages) to treat the phonological disorder—often a difficult decision. There are little data to indicate when treatment for phonological disorders should be conducted in L_1 versus L_2. Much of our knowledge in this area comes from information on treating language disorders in children from culturally and linguistically diverse populations.

Speech-language pathologists should consider a number of factors when deciding in which language to conduct treatment (Beaumont, 1992). These include: length of residency, motivation, age, length of exposure to L_1 and L_2, families' goals, and language of the children's peers. For language disorders, Beaumont indicated that treatment in L_1 is warranted if it is the "dominant" language, is used for several aspects of communication, a majority of concepts and past experiences are coded in L_1, and L_1 reflects the cultural environment of the client. Given that these suggestions are designed to guide treatment for language impairments, they must be interpreted cautiously in their application to the management of children with phonological disorders.

Adapting Treatment Approaches to Individuals from Culturally and Linguistically Diverse Populations

Although there is scant specific information to guide the treatment of phonological disorders in speakers of languages other than English, specific treatment approaches developed for English-speaking children can be adapted for use with culturally and linguistically diverse populations. A number of different methods for remediating speech sound errors have been categorized into two main types: motoric and cognitive-linguistic (Bernthal and Bankson, 1993). Motoric approaches, such as the "traditional approach" (Van Riper,

1972) and the "multiple phoneme approach" (Bradley, 1985), and "cognitive-linguistic approaches," such as the "cycles approach" (Hodson and Paden, 1991) and "language-based approaches" (Hoffman, Norris, and Monjure, 1990), are examples of adaptable remediation techniques. Each of the two major types has its advantages and disadvantages.

Utilizing a motoric approach poses several difficulties unless the speech-language pathologist is a speaker of the clients' native/home languages. First, the speech-language pathologist must be able to carry out the perceptual training phase of this approach, which necessitates the ability to produce an auditory model. Second, the clinician must know the segments that comprise a given client's native language and repertoire, the order of acquisition and ease of production of sounds, the frequency of occurrence of each phone in the language, and phonetic contexts that may facilitate production of the target sound (Bernthal and Bankson, 1993).

A cognitive-linguistic approach also raises several issues for the speech-language pathologist. First, instructional methodology would have to be adapted to the clients' specific languages and dialects. Second, since this type of approach is based on patterns rather than individual sound segments, the clinician would need to be able to relate seemingly unrelated errors into one or more specific phonological rules (Bernthal and Bankson, 1993). Third, to apply this type of approach, the speech-language pathologist should be able to identify errors most affecting intelligibility, errors that cut across sound classes, and errors that typically disappear at the earliest age (Stoel-Gammon and Dunn, 1985). Finally, the order of treatment advocated by this approach might need to be altered for speakers of languages other than English. For example, Hodson and Paden (1991), in their "cycles approach," suggest treating syllabicity early in the remediation process. That is, if a child does not use two-syllable words, then increasing his or her production of multisyllabic words might be warranted. In a language such as Khmer, for example, which has complex syllable types but few polysyllabic words, this might not be the initial treatment target of choice.

A number of cognitive-linguistic approaches advocate the use of contrastive word pairs (i.e., minimal opposition pairs, *so–toe*, or maximal opposition pairs, *beet–seat*). Approaches using contrastive word pairs include the paired stimuli approach (Weston and Irwin, 1985), minimal phonemic contrast approach (Cooper, 1985), minimal "triads" (Nelson, 1995), metaphon (Howell and Dean, 1991), and maximal opposition (Gierut, 1989). Contrastive word pairs, however, may be difficult to adapt to speakers of languages other than English. English, unlike other languages, is replete with minimal pair words. The lack of a significant number of contrastive word pairs makes it more difficult to apply this methodology to languages other than English.

Summary

To provide adequate and appropriate speech and language services to linguistically diverse individuals, speech-language pathologists should be knowledgeable about the dialects of their clients. Furthermore, clinicians must be aware that not all speakers of a particular dialect will show or use its every characteristic. It is commonly accepted that the next 15 to 20 years will bring an increasing number of immigrants to the United States; many will speak English with either limited or non-English proficiency. These immigrants will join the large number of individuals for whom English is not a first language. Members of this population will include individuals speaking a variety of languages and dialects. Regardless of whether services are provided in the speakers' first or second languages, clinicians must know the phonological rules of the first language and its dialectal variations.

References

Acevedo, M., "Spanish consonants among two groups of Head Start children." Paper presented at the convention of the American Speech-Language-Hearing Association. Atlanta, Georgia, November 1991.

Adler, S., *Cultural Language Differences: Their Educational and Clinical-Professional Implications.* Springfield, Ill.: Charles C. Thomas, 1984.

American Speech-Language-Hearing Association, "Social dialects: A position paper." Rockville, Md.: American Speech-Language-Hearing Association, 1983.

Anderson, R., and B. Smith, "Phonological development of two-year-old monolingual Puerto Rican Spanish-speaking children." *Journal of Child Language, 14* (1987): 57–78.

Bailey, S., "Normative data for Spanish articulatory skills of Mexican children between the ages of six and seven." Master's thesis, San Diego State University, 1982.

Battle, D., "Introduction." In D. Battle (Ed.), *Communication Disorders in Multicultural Populations* (xv–xxiv). Boston, Mass.: Andover Medical Publishers, 1993.

Bayles, K., and G. Harris, "Evaluating speech-language skills in Papago Indian children." *Journal of American Indian Education, 21*(2) (1982): 11–20.

Beaumont, C., "Service delivery issues." In H. Langdon (Ed.), *Hispanic Children and Adults with Communication Disorders: Assessment and Intervention* (pp. 343–372). Gaithersburg, Md.: Aspen Publishers, 1992.

Bernthal, J., and N. Bankson, *Articulation and Phonological Disorders* (3rd ed.). Englewood Cliffs, N.J.: Prentice Hall, 1993.

Bichotte, M., B. Dunn, L. Gonzalez, J. Orpi, and C. Nye, "Assessing phonological performance of bilingual school-age Puerto Rican children." Paper presented at the convention of the American Speech-Language-Hearing Association. Anaheim, Calif., November 1993.

Bleile, K., *Articulation and Phonological Disorders: A Book of Exercises* (2nd ed.). San Diego, Calif.: Singular Publishing Group, 1996.

Bleile, K., and H. Wallach, "A sociolinguistic investigation of the speech of African-American preschoolers." *American Journal of Speech-Language Pathology, 1* (1992): 54–62.

Bradley, D., "A systematic multiple-phoneme approach to articulation treatment." In P. Newman, N. Creaghead, and W. Secord (Eds.), *Assessment and Remediation of Articulatory and Phonological Disorders* (pp. 315–335). Columbus, Ohio: Merrill, 1985.

Chao, Y., "The Cantian idiolect: An analysis of Chinese spoken by a twenty-eight-month-old child." In C. Ferguson and D. Slobin (Eds.), *Studies of Child Language Development* (pp. 13–33). New York: Holt, Rinehart and Winston, 1973.

Cheng, L. R. L., *Assessing Asian Language Performance: Guidelines for Evaluating Limited-English-Proficient Students.* Rockville, Md.: Aspen Publishers, 1987.

Cheng, L. R. L., "Asian-American cultures." In D. Battle (Ed.), *Communication Disorders in Multicultural Populations* (pp. 38–77). Boston, Mass.: Andover Medical Publishers, 1993.

Christian, D., W. Wolfram, and N. Nube, *Variation and Change in Geographically Isolated Communities: Appalachian English and Ozark English.* Tuscaloosa, Ala.: University of Alabama Press, 1988.

Clement, C., and F. Wijnen, "Acquisition of vowel contrasts in Dutch." *Journal of Speech and Hearing Research, 37* (1994): 83–89.

Cole, P., and O. Taylor, "Performance of working class African-American children on three tests of articulation." *Language, Speech, and Hearing Services in Schools*, *21* (1990): 171–176.

Cooper, R., "The method of meaningful minimal contrasts." In P. Newman, N. Creaghead, and W. Secord (Eds.), *Assessment and Remediation of Articulatory and Phonological Disorders* (pp. 369–382). Columbus, Ohio: Merrill, 1985.

Crystal, D., *The Cambridge Encyclopedia of Language.* Cambridge: Cambridge University Press, 1987.

Cunningham, I., *A Syntactic Analysis of Sea Island Creole.* Tuscaloosa, Ala.: University of Alabama Press, 1992.

Dalbor, J., *Spanish Pronunciation: Theory and Practice* (2nd ed.). New York: Holt, Rinehart and Winston, 1980.

De la Fuente, M. T., "The order of acquisition of Spanish consonant phonemes by monolingual Spanish-speaking children between the ages of 2.0 and 6.5." Unpublished doctoral dissertation, Georgetown University, 1985.

Fleming, K., and J. Hartman, "Establishing cultural validity of the computer analysis of phonological processes." *Florida Educational Research Council Bulletin*, *22* (1989): 8–32.

Gierut, J., "Maximal opposition approach to phonological treatment." *Journal of Speech and Hearing Disorders*, *54* (1989): 9–19.

Goldman, R., and M. Fristoe, *Goldman-Fristoe Test of Articulation.* Circle Pines, Minn.: American Guidance Service, 1969.

Goldstein, B., "Spanish phonological development." In H. Kayser (Ed.), *Bilingual Speech-Language Pathology: An Hispanic Focus* (pp. 17–38). San Diego, Calif.: Singular Publishing Group, 1995.

Goldstein, B., and A. Iglesias, "Phonological patterns in normally developing Spanish-speaking 3- and 4-year olds of Puerto Rican descent." *Language, Speech, and Hearing Services in Schools*, *27*(1) (1996a): 82–90.

Goldstein, B., and A. Iglesias, "Phonological patterns in Puerto Rican Spanish-speaking children with phonological disorders." *Journal of Communication Disorders*, *29* (1996b): 367–387.

Goldstein, B., and K. Pollock, "Vowel production in Spanish-speaking children with phonological dis-

orders." Paper presented at the 1995 Child Phonology Meeting, Memphis, Tenn., May 1995.

Harris, G., "American Indian cultures: A lesson in diversity." In D. Battle (Ed.), *Communication Disorders in Multicultural Populations* (pp. 78–113). Boston, Mass.: Andover Medical Publishers, 1993.

Haynes, W., and M. Moran, "A cross-sectional developmental study of final consonant production in Southern Black children from preschool through third grade." *Language, Speech, and Hearing Services in Schools*, *20* (1989): 400–406.

Hodson, B., *Computer Assessment of Phonological Processes.* Danville, Ill.: Interstate Printers and Publishers, 1985.

Hodson, B., and E. Paden, *Targeting Intelligible Speech: A Phonological Approach to Remediation* (2nd ed.). Austin, Tex.: PRO-ED, 1991.

Hoffman, P. R., J. A. Norris, and J. Monjure, "Comparison of process targeting and whole language treatments for phonologically delayed preschool treatment." *Language, Speech, and Hearing Services in Schools*, *21* (1990): 102–109.

Holm, J., *Pidgins and Creoles, Volume I: Theory and Structure.* Cambridge: Cambridge University Press, 1988.

Holm, J., *Pidgins and Creoles, Volume II: Reference Survey.* Cambridge: Cambridge University Press, 1989.

Howell, J., and E. Dean, *Treating Phonological Disorders in Children: Metaphon—Theory to Practice.* San Diego, Calif.: Singular Publishing Group, 1991.

Jimenez, B. C., "Acquisition of Spanish consonants in children aged 3–5 years, 7 months." *Language, Speech, and Hearing Services in Schools*, *18*(4) (1987): 357–363.

Krauss, M., "The world's languages in crisis." *Language*, *68*(1) (1992): 4–10.

Ladefoged, P., *A Course in Phonetics* (3rd ed.). Fort Worth, Tex.: Harcourt Brace Jovanovich Publishers, 1993.

Leap, W., "American Indian languages." In C. Ferguson and S. Heath (Eds.), *Language in the USA* (pp. 116–144). Cambridge: Cambridge University Press, 1981.

Li, C., and S. Thompson, "The acquisition of tone in Mandarin-speaking children." *Journal of Child Language, 4* (1977): 185–199.

Maez, L., "Spanish as a first language." Unpublished doctoral dissertation, University of California, Santa Barbara, 1981.

Maez, P., "Phonological analysis of Spanish utterances of highly unintelligible Mexican-American children." Unpublished master's thesis, San Diego State University, 1983.

Morgan, R., "Structural sketch of Saint Martin Creole." *Anthropological Linguistics, 1*(8) (1959): 20–24.

Muyksen, P., and N. Smith, "The study of pidgin and creole languages." In J. Arends, P. Muyksen, and N. Smith (Eds.), *Pidgins and Creoles: An Introduction* (pp. 3–14). Amsterdam: John Benjamins, 1995.

Muyksen, P., and T. Veenstra, "Haitian." In J. Arends, P. Muyksen, and N. Smith (Eds.), *Pidgins and Creoles: An Introduction* (pp. 153–164). Amsterdam: John Benjamins, 1995.

Nelson, L., "Establishing production of speech sound contrasts using minimal 'triads'." *The Clinical Connection, 8*(4) (1995): 16–19.

Nichols, P., "Creoles of the USA." In C. Ferguson and S. Heath (Eds.), *Language in the USA* (pp. 69–91). Cambridge: Cambridge University Press, 1981.

O'Grady, W., M. Dobrovolsky, and M. Aranoff, *Contemporary Linguistics: An Introduction* (2nd ed.). New York: St. Martin's Press, 1993.

Oller, D. K., and R. Eilers, "Similarity of babbling in Spanish- and English-learning babies." *Child Language, 9* (1982): 565–577.

Pandolfi, A. M., and M. O. Herrera, "Producción fonologica diastratica de niños menores de tres anos (Phonological production in children less than three-years-old)."*Revista Teorica y Aplicada, 28* (1990): 101–122.

Perez, E., "Phonological differences among speakers of Spanish-influenced English." In J. Bernthal and N. Bankson (Eds.), *Child Phonology: Characteristics, Assessment, and Intervention with Special Populations* (pp. 245–254). New York: Thieme Medical Publishers, 1994.

Pollock, K., and N. Keiser, "An examination of vowel errors in phonologically disordered children." *Clinical Linguistics and Phonetics, 4* (1990): 161–178.

Poplack, S., "Dialect acquisition among Puerto Rican bilinguals." *Language in Society, 7* (1978): 89–103.

Seymour, H., and C. Seymour, "A therapeutic model for communicative disorders among children who speak Black English Vernacular." *Journal of Speech and Hearing Disorders, 42* (1977): 247–266.

Seymour, H., and C. Seymour, "Black English and Standard American English contrasts in consonantal development of four- and five-year-old children." *Journal of Speech and Hearing Disorders, 46* (1981): 274–280.

Shuy, R., "Social dialect and employability: Some pitfalls of good intentions." In L. Davis (Ed.), *Studies in Linguistics*. Birmingham, Ala.: University of Alabama Press, 1972.

So, L., and B. Dodd, "Phonologically disordered Cantonese-speaking children. *Clinical Linguistics and Phonetics, 8*(3) (1994): 235–255.

Stepanof, E. R., "Procesos phonologicos de niños Puertorriquehos de 3 y 4- sños evidenciado an ia prueba APP-Spanish (Phonological processes evidenced on the APP-Spanish by 3- and 4-year old Puerto Rican children) *Opphia, 8*(2) (1990): 15–20.

Stewart, W., "Continuity and change in American Negro dialects." In W. Wolfram and N. Clarke (Eds.), *Black-White Speech Relationships*. Washington, D.C.: Center for Applied Linguistics, 1971.

Stoel-Gammon, C., and C. Dunn, *Normal and Disordered Phonology*. Baltimore, Md.: University Park Press, 1985.

Taylor, O., "Teaching standard English as a second dialect." In O. Taylor (Ed.), *Treatment of Communication Disorders in Culturally and Linguistically Diverse Populations* (pp. 153–178). San Diego, Calif.: College-Hill Press, 1986.

Taylor, O., K. Payne, and N. Anderson, "Distinguishing between communication disorders and differences." *Seminars in Speech and Language, 8* (1987): 415–427.

Terrell, S., and F. Terrell, "Effects of speaking Black English upon employment opportunities." *Asha, 25* (1983): 27–29.

Tipton, G., "Non-cognate consonants of Mandarin

and Cantonese." *Journal of the Chinese Language Teachers Association, 10*(1) (1975): 1–13.

Tse, J., "Tone acquisition in Cantonese: A longitudinal case study." *Journal of Child Language, 5* (1978): 191–204.

U.S. Department of Commerce, Bureau of the Census, *National Data Books and Guides to Resources: Statistical Abstract of the U.S.* (115th ed.). Washington, D.C.: U.S. Government Printing Office, 1995.

Van Riper, C., *Speech Correction: Principles and Methods* (5th ed.). Englewood Cliffs, N.J.: Prentice-Hall, 1972.

Wang, W., *Languages and Dialects of Chinese.* Palo Alto, Calif.: Stanford University Press, 1989.

Wang, W., "Theoretical issues in studying Chinese dialects." *Journal of the Chinese Language Teachers Association, 25*(1) (1990): 1–34.

Wang, W., and K. Li, "Tone 3 in Pekinese." *Journal of Speech and Hearing Research, 10*(3) (1967): 629–636.

Washington, J., and H. Craig, "Articulation test performances of low-income African-American preschoolers with communication impairments."

Language, Speech, and Hearing Services in Schools, 23 (1992): 201–207.

Welker, G., *The Native Web Project.* World Wide Web: Syracuse University, 1995.

Weston, A., and J. Irwin, "Paired stimuli treatment." In P. Newman, N. Creaghead, and W. Secord (Eds.), *Assessment and Remediation of Articulatory and Phonological Disorders* (pp. 337–368). Columbus, Ohio: Merrill, 1985.

Wolfram, W., *Sociolinguistic Aspects of Assimilation: Puerto Rican English in New York City.* Arlington, Va.: Center for Applied Linguistics, 1974.

Wolfram, W., "Language variation in the United States." In O. Taylor (Ed.), *Treatment of Communication Disorders in Culturally and Linguistically Diverse Populations* (pp. 73–116). San Diego, Calif.: College-Hill Press, 1986.

Wolfram, W., "The phonology of a sociocultural variety: The case of African American Vernacular English." In J. Bernthal and N. Bankson (Eds.), *Child Phonology: Characteristics, Assessment, and Intervention with Special Populations* (pp. 227–244). New York: Thieme Medical Publishers, 1994.

Chapter **5**

Factors Related to Phonologic Disorders

NICHOLAS W. BANKSON,
James Madison University

JOHN E. BERNTHAL,
University of Nebraska–Lincoln

Introduction

In the study of phonologic disorders, an abiding concern is the identification of variables that may relate to the presence of speech sound disorders. Various factors, such as linguistic, psychosocial, speech mechanism, and speech perception have been studied in an attempt to better understand phonologic disorders. Investigators continue to be interested in the influence that biological and environmental factors have at different periods of phonologic growth and development.

For many children with phonologic disorders it is difficult, if not impossible, to determine causal factors related to speech delay. For a small percentage of children, however, causal factors related to presence of a delay may be more readily identified. Since the medical model (i.e., determination of the cause of a disorder) is sometimes employed by speech-language pathologists during phonologic evaluation, it is important that a book on phonologic disorders include a discussion of current understandings of causality as it relates to the presence of phonologic impairment.

As discussed in sections of this chapter, certain **causal factors** may precipitate, accompany, and/or maintain the presence of phonologic/articulatory disorders. For the most part, causal factors are related to impairments and/or interference with the structure and function of the speech and hearing mechanism. Since the percentage of clients in whom causal factors can be identified is relatively small, researchers have been interested in variables, called **causal correlates**, that may coexist with phonologic impairments. From 1930 to around 1970 an extensive body of literature related to causal correlates was developed. An interest in etiological research again emerged in the late 1980s. In the 1990s, interest has focused on familial aggregation of phonologic disorders. A knowledge of these correlates is helpful in our understanding of causality as it relates to phonologic impairment.

Correlational studies have been a primary method used to explore whether phonologic proficiency and selected variables covary or coexist with each other. Stated more simply, such studies seek to determine whether one variable (such as status of articulation) is related to another variable (such as intelligence). A *high* correlation between two variables implies that such variables are related to each other. For example, a high correlation between a measure of intelligence would indicate that a high number of correct articulatory responses co-occur with a high score on a measure of intelligence, and a low number of correct articulatory responses co-occur with a low score on a measure of intelligence. A *low* correlation, on the other hand, would indicate that the score obtained on an articulatory measure and the score on an intelligence measure do not covary and are not systematically related to each other. When a correlation is high, the status of one variable can sometimes be predicted from knowledge of the status of the second variable. This does not mean, however, that a causal relationship exists between the two; it simply means that they are related to each other. The frequently cited warning, "Correlation does not imply causation," speaks to precisely this issue. Correlational studies of the relationship between a single variable and articulatory status have identified topics for further study, which may lead to identification of factors that affect phonologic performance.

In correlational studies of factors related to articulation, investigators typically have looked at only a single variable (for example, age or intelligence) as it relates to articulatory status. Several investigators have used **multivariate analysis** techniques to look at the relationship between articulation status and a number of variables simultaneously. Winitz (1969) thought it "quite possible that substantial relationships between articulation and other independent variables would be forthcoming if the independent variables were examined collectively rather than singularly" (216). Arndt, Shelton, Johnson, and Furr (1977) and Prins (1962a) used multivariate analysis to identify and describe homogeneous subgroups of misarticulating children. In both investigations, a subgroup was identified by the similarity of scores on variables potentially related to articulation.

A third type of procedure used to examine factors potentially related to phonologic impairment involves comparisons between normal children and children who are phonologically delayed. When reviewing studies of this type, several points should be kept in mind. First, a statistically significant difference between a group of normal persons and a group of phonologically impaired persons on a particular variable (for example, language comprehension) does not imply a causal relationship between that variable and articulation. Other variables may account for the differences found between the articulatory-impaired and normal-speaking groups. Second, statistical significance does not imply clinical significance for two reasons: (1) group trends frequently do not reflect individual performance, and (2) relatively small quantitative differences resulting in statistically significant differences may have limited clinical utility. In a study reported by Dubois and Bernthal (1978), a small but statistically significant difference was found between two types of articulation measures (spontaneous picture naming and a delayed imitation sentence production), and yet the numerical difference in average performance, based on a 20-item task, was less than 2 items. Because of the small numerical difference, the clinical significance of such group findings might be questioned.

A fourth procedure used to examine causal-correlates is to present descriptive profiles of children who evidence developmental phonologic disorders. A recent comprehensive investigation of speech-language, prosody, and voice characteristics of children with developmental phonologic disorders was reported by Shriberg and Kwiatkowski (1994). They presented a descriptive profile on 178 children based on an assessment battery that included six general areas (i.e., hearing, speech mechanism, speech production, language comprehension, language production, case history, and behaviors). Causal-correlate profiles, which were based on an assessment that consisted of a large number of standardized and nonstandardized tasks and measures, showed a wide range of variables under each of the six major categories.

Winitz (1969) has suggested that some variables that have been studied in relation to articulation disorders may best be viewed as **macrovariables** (variables formed from several other variables). The variable of age, for example, may be understood to comprise such components as physical maturation, motor coordination, cognitive, and linguistic maturity. As Winitz has pointed out, although a macrovariable may be found to correlate with articulation, the individual components accounting for the correlation may be difficult to identify.

In addition to examining status relationships between selected factors and phonology, investigators have explored changes that may simultaneously occur between certain variables and a phonologic measure. Improvement relations are of two types: (1) changes in articulation as a function of a change in one or more other variables; and (2) changes in one or more other variables as a function of a change in articulation. For example, Williams and McReynolds (1975) reported that improvement in articulation had resulted in improved performance in speech sound discrimination. Correlational studies demonstrating that improvement in one or more variables results in improvement in articulation may have potential for clinical application.

The primary focus of this chapter is on causal correlates rather than causal variables per se. However, some variables have been clearly identified as causal factors in phonologic disorders, and thus are discussed in this chapter (e.g., hearing loss). At the present time, most of the identified causal factors are in the area of structure and function of the speech and hearing mechanism. Some of these causal factors may require surgical management; for example, a cleft of the palate. Such treatment may be a critical part of the speech remediation plan. In this first section, defects in structure and function of the speech and hearing mechanism that might interfere with the individual's phonologic productions are reviewed; that is, hearing loss, certain structural anomalies, and certain neuromotor pathologies. The second section deals with cognitive-linguistic factors, and the final section with psychosocial factors.

Structure and Function of the Speech and Hearing Mechanisms

An obvious consideration when evaluating an individual's phonologic status relates to the potential for problems that may be manifested in the structure and function of the speech and hearing mechanisms. Management decisions related to such variables are often a critical part of helping a client achieve maximal phonologic proficiency.

Hearing Loss

Among the variables influencing articulation, perhaps none is as important as the ability to hear. Lundeen (1991) reported that the prevalence of school-age children with pure tone averages greater than 25 dB HL was 2.63 percent. Through hearing, an individual is able to monitor his or her own productions as a speaker and receive incoming messages as a listener. Speakers also listen to their own productions and compare them to an internal mental storage of the intended form. When a mismatch occurs between the production and the intended form, the production is modified to better match the intended form. A distortion in the feedback the listener receives can cause productions to become slurred and distorted.

One of the most important elements underlying the production and comprehension of speech is an intact auditory system that is sensitive to the frequency range where most speech sounds occur (500 to 4000 Hz). The listener must also be able to detect the small differences that are reflective of the phonemic and phonetic characteristics of speech. Individuals with more severe hearing loss will have difficulty decoding the incoming sound signal and will perceive words differently than individuals with normal hearing mechanisms.

The deaf child faces the challenging task of learning how to produce speech by watching how sounds look on the face, how they feel through vibrations, and what he or she can perceive from a distorted auditory signal. A certain level of hearing is required to learn and maintain normal speech production. Ling (1989) summarized this relationship by noting that the more normal a person's hearing, the more natural his or her speech is likely to be.

Several aspects of hearing loss have been shown to affect speech perception and production; these include the level of hearing sensitivity, speech recognition ability, and configuration of the hearing loss. Individual hearing losses range from mild to severe or profound (greater than 70 dB HL). Labels such as *hard of hearing* and *deaf* are frequently applied to persons with varying degrees of hearing impairment.

Hearing sensitivity typically varies somewhat from one frequency to another, with speech and language differentially influenced by the frequency configuration and severity of the hearing loss. Although information recorded on an audiogram is a useful prognostic indicator of speech reception ability, predictions based solely on pure-tone measurements are not always accurate. Thus, two children with similar audiograms may not perceive speech sounds in the same way. A pure-tone audiogram cannot measure a person's ability to distinguish one frequency from another or to track formant transitions (a skill critical to speech perception). For these and other reasons (e.g., age of fitting and full-time use of amplification, concomitant factors, quality of early intervention programs), individuals with similar pure-tone audiograms can differ greatly in their understanding of speech.

A second hearing-related factor important to phonologic acquisition and maintenance is the age of onset and the age of detection of the hearing loss. If a severe loss has been present since birth, acquisition of language including phonologic, syntactic, and semantic aspects is difficult, and specialized instruction is necessary to develop speech and language.

Such instruction may rely on visual, tactile, and kinesthetic cues as well as whatever residual auditory sensation the person possesses. For a discussion of the influence of hearing loss on infants and toddlers phonologic development, see Stoel-Gammon and Kehoe (1994). Children and adults who suffer a serious loss of hearing after language has been acquired usually retain their articulation patterns for a time, but frequently their articulatory skills deteriorate. Even those assisted with amplification may find it difficult to maintain their previous level of articulatory performance.

Influence on Speech

Investigators have explored the influence of hearing loss on speech sound productions. Levitt and Stromberg (1983) observed the following vowel characteristics in individuals with hearing loss: (1) a number of vowel substitutions (e.g., tense-lax substitutions [i for ɪ], substitution of the intended vowel by a neighboring vowel in the vowel quadrilateral, or a distant vowel in the quadrilateral); (2) substitution of diphthongs for vowels (diphthongization) and vowels for diphthongs; (3) some omissions of the intended vowel or diphthong; and (4) schwa or schwa-like vowel substitutions (neutralization). Tye-Murray (1991) reported that some deaf speakers used excessive jaw movement to establish different vowel shapes instead of appropriate tongue movement. The less flexible tongue movement reduces the formation of the acoustic vowel formants (particularly the second formant) necessary to discriminate vowels.

There seems to be general agreement that consonant errors reflect difficulties with voiced-voiceless distinction, substitutions (voice-voiceless, nasal-oral, fricative-stop) omission of initial and final consonants, distortions, inappropriate nasalization of consonants, and final consonant deletions (Paterson, 1994).

In addition to segmental difficulties, the suprasegmental patterns of hearing-impaired speakers differ from those seen in normal-hearing speakers. Hearing-impaired speakers generally speak at a slower rate than normal-hearing speakers because of longer duration of both consonants and vowels, and they also use more frequent pauses and slower articulatory transitions. Stress patterns tend to be inappropriate as many hearing-impaired speakers do not distinguish duration in stressed and unstressed syllables. Finally, hearing-impaired speakers frequently use too high or too low a pitch, use inappropriate inflectional patterns, use harsh or breathy voice quality, and are hypo- or hypernasal (Dunn and Newton, 1986).

There is a great deal of variation in speech patterns of individuals with hearing impairments. There is still no comprehensive description of the speech and language of the hearing impaired because of the complexity involved in analyzing their speech. Interestingly, less information is available for individuals with mild to moderate hearing losses than for those with more severe losses.

Calvert (1982) reported that errors of articulation common to deaf children are not confined to productions of individual phonemes; errors also occur because of the phonetic context in which the phones are embedded. Calvert delineated the following common errors of articulation in the speech of the deaf (defined as those with hearing threshold levels for speech of greater than 92 dB) for whom everyday auditory communication is impossible or nearly so.

1. Errors of Omission

   a. Omission of /s/ in all contexts
   b. Omission of final consonants
   c. Omission of initial consonants

2. Errors of Substitution

   a. Voiced for voiceless consonants
   b. Nasal for oral consonants
   c. Low feedback substitutions (substitution of sounds with easily perceived tactile and kinesthetic feedback for those with less; e.g., /w/ for /r/ substitution)
   d. Substitution of one vowel for another

3. Errors of Distortion

   a. Degree of force (stop and fricative consonants are frequently made with either too much or too little force)
   b. Hypernasality associated with vowel productions
   c. Imprecision and indefiniteness in vowel articulation
   d. Duration of vowels (deaf speakers tend to produce vowels with undifferentiated duration, usually in the direction of excess duration)
   e. Temporal values in diphthongs (deaf speakers may not produce the first or the second vowel in a diphthong for the appropriate duration of time)

4. Errors of Addition

   a. Insertion of a superfluous vowel between consonants (e.g., /sʌnoʊ/ for /snoʊ/)
   b. Unnecessary release of final stop consonants (e.g., [stopʰ])
   c. Diphthongization of vowels (e.g., *mit* → [mɪʌt])
   d. Superfluous breath before vowels

Calvert further reported that in those who become deaf after acquiring speech and language, distortions and omissions occur for speech sounds characterized by low intensity and high frequency, such as /s/, /ʃ/, /tʃ/, /f/, and /θ/. In addition, such individuals may produce consonants in the final position of words with so little force that they are not heard by the listener.

There is no one-to-one correspondence between level and type of hearing loss and patterns of misarticulations. In general, however, the less severe the loss, the less speech and language are affected. Since consonants, especially those with high-frequency energy (e.g., sibilants), have less inherent intensity in their production than vowels, consonants tend to be most frequently misarticulated.

Even relatively minor fluctuating hearing losses seen in children with recurrent middle-ear problems may affect those children's speech and language acquisition. Investigators have reported that children who are experiencing otitis media with effusion usually score more poorly on articulation tests than those free of this condition. For a complete review of the literature on the relationship of otitis media to speech perception and phonology, see

Roberts and Clarke-Klein (1994). Other researchers have reported that a delay in speech and language development at 3 years and older often follows otitis media with effusion and its accompanying fluctuating hearing loss. It has been reported that many children seen for phonologic and articulation deficiencies have a history of middle-ear involvement, and children with a history of middle-ear involvement can be differentiated from those without such a history by the phonologic patterns in their speech (Shriberg and Smith, 1983; Shriberg and Kwiatkowski, 1982). Shriberg and Kwiatkowski (1982) reported that up to one third of the children with moderate to severe phonologic delays may have histories of middle-ear involvement.

Shriberg and Smith (1983) reported that children with positive histories of middle-ear involvement made sound changes (errors) in nasals and word-initial consonants more frequently than phonologically delayed children without such histories. Initial consonants were deleted (e.g., *got* → [at]), or replaced by [h] (e.g., *tie* → [haɪ]) or glottal stop replacements (e.g., *to* → [ʔu]). The other changes noted were that nasal sounds were (1) replaced by another nasal or stop (e.g., *not* → [ma] or *my* → [baɪ]; (2) replaced by denasalization (e.g., *knee* → [ñi:]); or (3) preceded or followed by an epenthetic stop (e.g., *no* → [ᵈnoʊ]). Shriberg and Smith (1983) suggested that it may be possible to differentiate children who have a positive history of middle-ear involvement from those who do not on the basis of the phonologic patterns in their speech. Churchill, Hodson, Jones, and Novak (1985) reported that deletion of the stridency feature was the distinguishing characteristic of children with middle-ear involvement.

Paden, Novak, and Beiter (1987) attempted to identify differences between children with frequent or persistent middle-ear problems who later required phonologic intervention from those who did not. They reported no distinguishing phonological patterns in their subjects with a history of middle-ear involvement. They concluded that children with similar hearing thresholds and length of middle-ear involvement differed widely in their mastery of phonological skills. They also suggested that guidelines based on a number of variables—for example, the percentage of deviancy from age norms on velars, deletions of postvocalic obstruents, liquid durations, age of initial diagnosis of middle-ear problems, length of time the middle-ear problem persisted, and severity of the hearing impairment—could be developed to aid in the identification of 18- to 36-month-old children with a history of middle-ear involvement who are at risk phonologically. In a subsequent study, Paden, Matthies, and Novak (1989) attempted to identify which young children, 19 to 35 months, who were delayed in phonologic development and had otitis media with effusion were at risk for continued phonologic delay even when pressure equalization tubes were inserted. They reported that of the original group they studied, 24 percent, even with aggressive medical treatment, did not attain normal phonologic development by age 4. It can be inferred from this finding that with aggressive medical treatment most children who are prone to have middle-ear problems will catch up with their peers without intervention but about 25 percent will not. A statistical procedure called *discriminant analysis* indicated that the best predictors between children who would likely achieve normal phonology by age 4 and those who would not were four variables:

1. Velar deviations
2. Cluster reduction

3. Score on the retest four months following insertion of tubes
4. A time period of six months or more between initial diagnosis of otitis media and the first significant remission of this condition

Roberts, Burchinal, Koch, Footo, and Henderson (1988) studied 55 children in a longitudinal study and reported no significant relationship between otitis media during the first 3 years of life and the subsequent use of phonologic processes and/or consonant errors during the preschool years. They concluded that "the magnitude of any adverse speech outcome associated with early childhood middle-ear problems is small and more likely to be evident when children are school age" (431). Although there is disagreement in the literature about the role early middle-ear involvement has on speech development, a history of middle-ear problems may be a contributing factor to later speech difficulties. Because middle-ear involvement has the potential to adversely affect speech development, the speech of children with reoccurring otitis media should be periodically monitored.

Roberts and Clarke-Klein (1994), summarizing the literature on otitis media with effusion and later speech processing and production, concluded that these investigations were characterized by conflicting results and that further studies are needed concerning the relationship between a history of otitis media in childhood and later phonologic development. They suggested that phonologic development in these subjects needs to be followed from early infancy through the elementary school years.

Intelligibility

In evaluating the speech intelligibility of the hearing impaired, the listeners, the stimulus material, and the context for evaluation should be taken into account. As a listener becomes familiar with the speech of the hearing impaired, understanding improves and most listeners develop this familiarity in a short time.

Judgments of speech intelligibility have also been shown to vary with the samples on which they are based. For example, one-syllable words do not provide the linguistic redundancy available in sentence productions. Judgments based on utterances produced spontaneously may differ from judgments based on speech samples involving reading or elicited through questions. Judgments based on live speech may differ from those based on tape recordings.

Monson (1983) studied 10 hearing-impaired adolescents and reported that:

1. Subjects used simple sentences with few consonant clusters and few polysyllabic words and were more intelligible when using less complicated syntax than when using more complex sentences.
2. Experienced listeners understood more than inexperienced listeners.
3. Sentences presented within a verbal context were more intelligible than those presented out of context.
4. Sentences where the speaker was both seen and heard were better understood than those which were only heard.

Wolk and Schildroth (1986), in a study of intelligibility of hearing-impaired speakers, indicated that the greater the degree of hearing loss the less the intelligibility. They further indicated, however, that this relationship did not hold when the student's method of communication was considered (i.e., those who used oral communication were 73 percent intelligible, those who used sign language were 4.8 percent intelligible, and those who used both were 24.7 percent intelligible).

Speech Sound Perception

Speech-language pathologists have long been interested in a possible relationship between the perception (often referred to as discrimination) and production of speech sounds. Phonemic perception is a form of auditory perception in which the listener and/or speaker distinguishes the sound contrasts used in a language. Linguistic or phonemic perception also includes the storing and accessing of sounds for the recognition of words that are heard. From a clinical perspective, this skill includes the ability to detect differences between sounds in the language and error productions that may be substituted for those sounds. Clinicians have been interested in determining whether or not production errors are related to errors in perception of speech sounds. Numerous investigations have been conducted to ascertain the relationship between production and perception in children with normal phonologic development and children with delayed phonologic development.

As was stated in our discussion of phonologic acquisition (see Chapter 2), some scholars view phonemic perception as essentially completed by the time the normally developing child has acquired the first 50 words. If this assumption is correct, it follows that the child's speech sound production errors can be ascribed primarily to difficulties in motor (articulatory) control and/or phonologic organization, rather than perception. If, however, the acquisition and development of speech sound perception continues at least into the preschool and even the early school years, as other scholars argue, then some production errors may be the result of a mismatch between the adult form of the word and the child's perception and underlying representation (storage) of the word. In other words, some children's production errors may be related to phonemic perception. Finally, many treatment programs include auditory discrimination tasks, on the assumption that such tasks help the child to learn the adult phonologic system.

Before discussing studies concerning the relationship between production and perception, it is useful to recall some of the previously reviewed data on auditory perception in normal infants and young children. In Chapter 2, evidence was presented that infants can perceive most contrasts used in the phonology of their language at the time they begin to speak. Indeed, experiments have shown that infants under 1 year of age are able to discriminate between speech sounds (Eimas, Siqueland, Jusczyk, and Vigorito, 1971; Butterfield and Cairns, 1974). Apparently, within the first few months of life infants perceive differences in the acoustic signal as categorical differences similar to those serving as phonemic contrasts in adult languages. Speech sound perception experiments also suggest that as children begin to speak words, they do not perceive all of the relevant phonologic contrasts. This finding may perhaps be best explained by the fact that studies of infant perception require only that the subject note changes in the acoustic signal, whereas linguistic or phonemic perception involves an active attention to contrasting speech sounds and sequences in order to identify, store, and recognize distinct lexical items. The skills required for nonlinguistic discrimination (same-different distinctions) tested in investigations of infant perception are very different from those required to distinguish and store lexical items.

Perceptual discrimination experiments with preschoolers, beginning with children at approximately age 2, have shown that young children can make most of the phonologic distinctions in English. Barton (1976), who attempted to determine whether normal 2-year-olds had full or partial linguistic perception (see Chapter 2), reported that his subjects were not able to make all of the perceptions required on the experimental tasks but were able to perceive sounds they were not producing. He concluded that his subjects' perception was more advanced than their production and suggested that they may have had full or nearly full perception at this early age. He also pointed out that word familiarity influenced the children's performance on perceptual tasks: children made more errors on the perception of new or unfamiliar words than on words they knew well.

As discussed in Chapter 3, perceptual errors may result from a partially correct internal representation that becomes more accurate with increased exposure to the adult speech models. If a child fails to notice the discrepancy between his or her initial internal representation and the adult form, then a perceptually based error may exist.

The study of young children's perceptual skills has continued to be of interest to both clinicians and researchers. The extent to which the findings based on children with normal perceptual and production skills are applicable to the phonologically delayed population is unclear since it is not certain that inferences can be drawn from normal to phonologically delayed speakers. Locke (1980) suggested that a difference may exist between the role of perception in the acquisition of phonologic errors and its role in the maintenance of a phonologic disorder.

Clinical research on speech sound perception and its relationship to articulation disorders has sought to determine (1) if a relationship exists, (2) the relationship between general and phoneme-specific measures of discrimination and production as well as that between external and internal monitoring, and (3) the relationship between perceptual training and production.

Relationship between Phonologic Disorders and Speech Sound Discrimination

The possibility of a relationship between articulation disorders and speech sound (auditory) perception was first investigated in the 1930s. This early perceptual research, referred to as speech sound discrimination research, relied primarily on general measures of speech sound discrimination, which required the subject to judge whether word or nonsense pairs verbally presented by the examiner were the same or different. There was generally no attempt to compare the specific phoneme production errors with the specific perception errors the subject might have made.

Travis and Rasmus (1931) found that on a discrimination test of 366 paired nonsense-syllable items, groups of normal subjects performed significantly better than groups with mild articulation disorders. Other researchers comparing the discrimination skills of normal speakers and speakers with articulation errors (Kronvall and Diehl, 1954; Clark, 1959) reported similar findings; that is, that normal speakers had significantly better skills, and several investigators found a positive correlation between performance on an articulation test and performance on a test of speech sound discrimination (Reid, 1947b; Carrell and Pendergast, 1954).

A number of studies, however, found no relationship between discrimination and speech sound productions. In a study similar to that of Travis and Rasmus, Hall (1938) reported no significant differences in discrimination skill between normal speakers and two groups of speakers with mild and severe articulatory disorders. Hansen (1944), who studied discrimination and articulation in a college-age population, also reported little relationship between the two variables; likewise, Mase (1946), Prins (1962b), Garrett (1969), and Veatch (1970) found no significant differences in speech sound discrimination skills between children with articulation disorders and normal speakers.

Sherman and Geith (1967) suggested that one reason for the equivocal findings may have been that experimental groups were chosen on the basis of articulatory proficiency rather than speech sound discrimination performance, and consequently etiologies associated with articulatory-impaired students may not have been limited to individuals with poor speech sound discrimination skills. To control for perceptual skill, Sherman and Geith administered a 50-item speech sound discrimination test to 529 kindergarten children and then selected from this group 18 children with high discrimination scores and 18 with low scores. These two groups were given a 176-item picture-articulation test. The authors reported that children with high speech sound discrimination scores obtained significantly higher articulation scores than the group with lower discrimination scores. They concluded that poor speech sound discrimination skill may be causally related to poor articulation performance.

Schwartz and Goldman (1974) investigated the possible effects on performance by young children of the type of discrimination task required and found that their subjects consistently made more errors when stimulus words were presented in a paired-comparison context (*goat* and *coat*; *coat* and *boat*) than when target words were included in carrier phrase and sentence contexts (as in, "The man brought a *coat*"). They also found that when background noise was present during stimulus presentation performance was poorer, particularly for the paired-comparison words. The authors urged speech-language pathologists to test discrimination with tasks that are meaningful and familiar to children, and under the kind of listening conditions the child is likely to encounter in his or her environment.

After reviewing the articulation and discrimination literature, Weiner (1967) attributed the variations in findings to the fact that (1) different types of discrimination tasks were used; (2) subjects of different age levels were used; and (3) subjects reflected varying degrees of articulatory defectiveness from one study to another. He further concluded that speech sound discrimination is a developmental skill, which ceilings at about 8 years, and that a positive relationship exists between auditory discrimination problems and more severe articulation difficulties at age levels below 9 years. After reviewing the studies on the relationship between auditory discrimination and articulation performance, Winitz (1984) reported that "with few exceptions, children with functional articulation disorders show lower discrimination scores relative to children who do not have articulation disorders" (22). He also identified a number of factors that may account for the absence of more consistent reports of a positive relationship between articulatory performance and speech sound discrimination measures: (1) a lack of relevance of the discrimination test items, (2) a lack of consideration of the child's specific articulation errors, and (3) a lack of consideration of phonetic context in which the production error occurs.

Relationship between General and Phoneme-Specific Measures; External and Internal Monitoring

In most of the investigations cited above, discrimination was tested through general speech sound discrimination measures—that is, tasks comprised of items sampling a wide variety of sound contrasts (e.g., *s*un-*b*un, *k*ey-*t*ea, *s*hoe-*z*oo) and designed to examine the subject's overall capacity to distinguish among a large number of speech sounds in a variety of phonetic contexts. Investigators (Spriestersbach and Curtis, 1951; Locke, 1980) have pointed out that in testing speech sound perception of articulatory-impaired clients, the critical issue is the clients' ability to discriminate the sound or segments that they misarticulate. Although clients may not have a general problem with speech sound discrimination, they may have phoneme-specific perceptual difficulties on sounds they misarticulate. Perceptual testing should involve stimuli that focus on the children's production errors.

Locke (1980) recommended going a step further, urging that measures of sound perception should not only be phoneme specific, but also context specific. He argued that perceptual tasks should reflect the child's production errors and reflect those phonetic environments (words) in which error productions occur and include both the error productions and the target productions.

Locke studied children's ability to discriminate sounds they produced in error when those sounds were reproduced and contrasted with the correct sound by the adult examiner. Specifically, 131 children were tested on a perceptual task in which the examiner produced imitations of the subject's error productions, and the subjects were then required to judge whether the examiner's productions were correct productions of the target word. Locke reported that 70 percent of the children correctly perceived the correct and incorrect forms of the target words, thus indicating that many children could correctly discriminate sounds made by an adult, that they produced in error. About one-third of the contrasts misproduced were also misperceived, but the misperceptions were not evenly distributed across all misproductions. Although the substitution of one voiceless fricative for another accounted for 49 percent of the production errors, these contrasts accounted for 89 percent of the misperceptions.

In a study of 14 2-year-old children, Eilers and Oller (1976) found some perceptual confusions in word and nonsense pairs where production of one segment was substituted for another. Yet other common production errors were discriminated by most of their subjects. They concluded that some production errors may be related to perceptual difficulties and others to motor constraints.

Strange and Broen (1980) compared 21 children between the ages of 2 and 11 on their production and perception of word-initial /w/, /r/, and /l/. They concluded from their data that both perception and production of phonemic contrasts develop gradually and that perception of a contrast usually preceded its production.

Velleman (1983) collected data from children aged 3 to 5 on a production task that included naming of pictures and objects in a play situation and the imitation of nonsense syllables. She then tested the children's perception of /s/ and /θ/—/s/ because it is easy to perceive and /θ/ because it is not "acoustically salient" and is thus relatively difficult to perceive—and computed a correlation between the two tasks. The data confirmed her hypothesis that some frequently occurring production errors in children's speech are easier to perceive than others. Since contrasts involving /s/ were relatively easily perceived,

Velleman inferred that the late acquisition of /s/ could be ascribed to motor constraints. In contrast, the /θ/ versus /f/ contrast is a difficult distinction to make and, as she predicted, only children with high perception scores (over 80 percent) obtained high production scores on these phonemes. More errors were made on both perception and production in the case of /s/, and there was no significant correlation between the two measures.

In summary, some speech sound contrasts remain difficult to discriminate as late as 3 years or older, even in normal developing children. There does not, however, appear to be a correlation between many of the production errors seen in children and measures of speech sound perception.

An additional testing variable frequently considered in phoneme-specific discrimination testing is the source of the speech production that the subject is required to judge. When the task involves discrimination of a stimulus presented from an external source, such as speech productions from another person or recorded stimuli, it is termed **external discrimination** or **monitoring**. External discrimination can also include **external self-discrimination**, of which listening to and making judgments of tape-recorded samples of one's own speech is an example.

When the discrimination or perceptual task involves a judgment of one's own live, on-going speech sound productions, it is called **internal discrimination** or **internal monitoring**. During internal discrimination, the speaker has available both air- and bone-conducted auditory cues.

Studies of speech sound discrimination skills of young children with delayed phonologic development have indicated that subjects frequently were able to make external judgments of sound contrasts involving their error sounds (Locke and Kutz, 1975; Chaney and Menyuk, 1975). In a study employing phoneme-specific discrimination tasks, Aungst and Frick (1964) utilized the *Deep Test of Articulation* (McDonald, 1964), in which the /r/ was tested in 58 productions, to study the relationship between /r/ production and four measures of speech sound discrimination. Three of the discrimination tasks were designed by the investigators to assess subjects' discrimination of their own /r/ productions as they occurred in a set of 30 words. These discrimination tasks required each subject to (1) make an immediate right-wrong judgment of his or her /r/ production after speaking each word, (2) make right-wrong judgments of his or her /r/ productions after such productions had been audio recorded and played back, and (3) make same-different judgments of his or her /r/ productions as they followed the examiner's correct productions presented via audio tape recording.

The fourth discrimination task was the *Templin Test of Auditory Discrimination* (Templin, 1957), a general test of external discrimination. The subjects were children, 8 years or older, who made articulation errors only on /r/. The authors reported high correlations for relationships among their three discrimination tasks but low correlations between each of those tests and the Templin general discrimination measure. Moderate correlation coefficients of .69, .66, and .59 were obtained between each of the three phoneme-specific discrimination tasks and scores on the *Deep Test* for /f/. In contrast, the Templin discrimination test scores (a general discrimination measure) did not correlate well with the articulation measure. These findings indicate some relationship between performance on the *Deep Test* and the phoneme-specific discrimination measures but not between the *Deep Test* and the general test of discrimination.

Lapko and Bankson (1975) also compared external and internal monitoring with consistency of articulation, as measured by the *Deep Test of Articulation*, in a group of 25 kindergarten and first-grade children exhibiting misarticulations of /s/. All measures were phoneme-specific to /s/. They reported a significant correlation (r = .55) between the child's ability to discriminate his or her own productions of /s/ and the consistency of misarticulation of /s/. In other words, those subjects with the higher number of correct productions on the Deep Test of Articulation also had higher scores on the measure of internal discrimination. Such a correlation was not obtained between external monitoring tasks and articulation consistency as measured on the *Deep Test of Articulation.*

Wolfe and Irwin (1973) and Stelcik (1972) provided further evidence of a positive correlation between articulatory skill and self-monitoring (internal monitoring) of error sounds. But the results of other investigations (Woolf and Pilberg, 1971; Shelton, Johnson, and Arndt, 1977) have indicated that the findings in such studies may be influenced by such factors as the consistency of misarticulation, type of discrimination task used to test internal monitoring, and nature of the stimulus items.

After reviewing the findings of Aungst and Frick (1964) regarding the correlation between self-monitoring and production of /r/ and the findings of Lapko and Bankson (1975) regarding /s/, Shelton, Johnson, and Arndt (1977) concluded that "the self-discrimination testing procedures that are in use do not, by themselves, allow precise prediction of articulation behavior of individual subjects" (715). In other words, the finding that self-monitoring discrimination measures are significantly related to performance on the deep test does not necessarily imply that clinical instruction should focus on self-monitoring skills.

Some experimenters feel that more information about external monitoring is required before appropriate self-monitoring tasks can be developed. Hoffman, Stager, and Daniloff (1983) suggested that current phoneme-specific, external discrimination tasks may not be sensitive to allophonic variations that might be perceived by misarticulating children. For example, the prevocalic voicing contrast that a misarticulating child perceives and produces may not be within the perceptual boundary of an adult phoneme and, consequently, not perceived by the adult; what the child may perceive as a contrast between adult allophones of /z/ may not be perceived by the adult listener because both allophones are within the adult's perceptual boundary of /z/. Such sound variations may be used by some children to contrast forms that are not used in a contrastive manner by adults. It would follow that an adult examiner would evaluate such contrasts as a mismatch between the child's production and the adult standard. These authors have suggested that "meaningful subgroups of misarticulating children may be found to manipulate subphonemic, that is allophonic, acoustic cues in nonstandard manners and thus lead to their identification as misarticulations" (214).

Discrimination Improvement and Articulatory Productions

The influence of discrimination training on production has also been considered by investigators. Historically, clinicians routinely conducted some type of discrimination training, or "ear training," as a precursor to production training; however, that is not currently the case. Investigators have attempted to determine whether or not a functional relationship exists between articulation and discrimination and more specifically, whether or not discrimination training affects production.

Sonderman (1971) reported an investigation designed to assess (1) the effect of speech sound discrimination training on articulation skills, and (2) the effect of articulation training on speech sound discrimination skill. Holland's speech sound discrimination program (1967) and the *S-Pack* (Mowrer, Baker, and Schutz, 1968) were administered in alternate sequence to two matched groups of 10 children between 6 and 8 years old, all of whom produced frontal lisps. Four measures were administered to obtain pre-training and post-training profiles for each child: (1) the *Wepman Test of Auditory Discrimination* (a general test of external monitoring skills), (2) a /s/ specific discrimination test, (3) an examiner-designed general articulation test, and (4) the criterion test from the *S-Pack* (a deep test of the /s/). Improvement in both discrimination and articulation scores was obtained from both discrimination training and articulation training, regardless of the sequence in which the two types of training were conducted. These findings must be cautiously interpreted since articulatory improvement did not necessarily mean that speech sound errors were corrected. Rather, shifts from one type of error to another (e.g., omission to substitution; substitution to distortion) were regarded as evidence of improvement.

Williams and McReynolds (1975) explored the same question that Sonderman did. Two subjects were first given production training followed by a discrimination probe, then discrimination training followed by a production probe. Two additional subjects received the discrimination training first and the production training second. The probe measures, administered to determine if changes occurred in one modality after training in the other, indicated that production training was effective in changing both articulation and discrimination; in contrast to Sonderman (1971), however, Williams and McReynolds (1975) found that discrimination training was effective in changing only discrimination and did not generalize to production.

Shelton, Johnson, and Arndt (1977) explored the influence of articulation training on discrimination performance. One group of subjects received articulation training on the /r/ and a second group on the /s/, and pre- and post-discrimination probes, consisting of 40 items specifically related to the error sound, were administered. Results indicated that both groups of subjects improved in articulation performance, but no improvement was noted in discrimination performance. The authors suggested that the variance between their results and those of other investigators presumably could be accounted for by one or more unidentified subjects or procedural variables.

Rvachew (1994) studied the influence of various types of speech perception training that were administered concurrently with traditional speech sound training. Twenty-seven (27) preschoolers with phonologic impairment who misarticulated /s/ were randomly assigned to three groups each of which received one of the following types of discrimination training: (1) listening to a variety of correctly and incorrectly produced versions of the word *shoe*; (2) listening to the words *shoe* and *moo*; and (3) listening to the words *cat* and *Pete*. Following six weekly treatment sessions, children who received types 1 and 2 training demonstrated superior ability to articulate the target sound in comparison to those who received approach 3. Rvachew (1994) suggested that "speech perception training should probably be provided concurrently with speech production training" (355).

Another group of investigators (Koegel, Koegel, and Ingham, 1986; Koegel, Koegel, Van Voy, and Ingham, 1988) has looked at a related topic and examined the relationship between self-monitoring skills and response generalization into the natural environment. School-age children were provided specific training in self-monitoring of the speech productions. These investigators reported that generalization of correct articulatory responses of the target sounds did not occur until a self-monitoring task was initiated in the treatment program. They concluded that such self-monitoring was required for generalization of the target sounds in the natural environment to occur.

An effort was made by Gray and Shelton (1992) to replicate these findings. They employed self-monitoring procedures, which differed slightly from those employed in the studies by Koegel and colleagues (1986, 1988) with eight elementary school subjects. Results of their study did not replicate the positive treatment effects found by Koegel and colleagues (1986,1988). The authors indicated that different subject, treatment, and environmental variables may have accounted for different outcomes.

Summary

A relationship appears to exist between speech sound perception and articulation in subjects with impaired phonology although the precise nature of the relationship has not been determined. Self-monitoring of error productions would appear to be an important skill for normal articulation, but instruments to assess such a skill are lacking. Further data are needed to better understand the relationship between discrimination errors and articulation disorders. Although the efficacy of speech sound discrimination training as a predecessor to production training has yet to be established, when perceptual deficiencies are present, perceptual training would seem appropriate. There is also some indication that it may be of value for perceptual training to accompany production training.

Minor Structural Variations of the Speech Mechanism

Speech clinicians are frequently required to make judgments about the structure and/or function of the lips, teeth, tongue, and palate. These oral structures can vary significantly among individuals. Investigators have attempted to identify relationships between articulatory status and structural variations of the oral mechanism, which can range from minor deviations to gross structural anomalies. Although a cause-and-effect relationship between articulation deviations and minor variations in oral structures has not been established, individuals with significant deformities of the orofacial region (such as patients who have undergone ablative surgery) may experience articulatory effects. Articulation deviations thought to be more directly associated with structural anomalies will be discussed later in this chapter.

Lips

Approximation of the lips is required for the formation of the bilabial phonemes /b/, /p/, and /m/; lip rounding is required for various vowels and the consonants /w/ and /hw/. An impairment that would inhibit lip approximation or rounding might result in misarticulation of these sounds. Fairbanks and Green (1950) examined various dimensions of the lips in 30 adult speakers with superior consonant articulation and 30 with inferior consonant articulation and reported no differences on various lip measurements between the two groups.

Teeth

Several English consonants require intact dentition for correct production. Labiodental phonemes (/f/ and /v/) require contact between the teeth and lower lip for their production, and linguadental phonemes require interdental tongue placement for /ð/ and /θ/ productions. The tongue tip alveolars (/s/, /z/) require that the airstream pass over the cutting edge of the incisors.

Researchers investigating the relationship between deviant dentition and consonant production have examined the presence or absence of teeth, position of teeth, and dental occlusion. **Occlusion** refers to the alignment of the teeth when the jaws are closed, and **malocclusion** refers to the imperfect or irregular position of the teeth when jaws are closed. Lay terms to describe different types of occlusion include terms as open bite and overjet. Examples of different types of occlusion may be seen in Figure 5.1.

Bernstein (1954) identified malocclusions in children with normal and defective speech but did not find a higher incidence of malocclusion in children with articulation problems than in children with normal articulation skills. He found that articulation defects were generally not related to malocclusion, except in the case of the open bite (the bite is opened— that is, the teeth do not come together from the first or second molar on one side to the same tooth on the opposite side). Fairbanks and Lintner (1951) examined molar occlusion, occlusion of the anterior teeth, and anterior spaces in 60 adults, 30 of whom were judged to have superior articulation skills and 30 with inferior articulatory skills. They found that neutrocclusion (normal jaw relationship with a slight malocclusion in the anterior segments)

Normal Occlusion

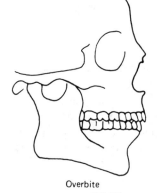

Overbite

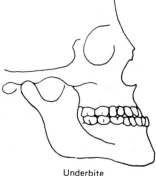

Underbite

FIGURE 5.1   Examples of types of occlusions.

tended to predominate in the group of superior speakers, and distocclusion (malocclusion with retrusion of the mandible) and mesiocclusion (malocclusion with protrusion of the mandible) tended to occur more often in the group of speakers with production errors. When data on the subjects were divided according to (1) no marked dental deviation and (2) one or more marked dental deviations, the authors found that marked dental deviations occurred significantly more frequently in the inferior speakers than in the superior ones. Open bite was present in the inferior speaking group but not in the superior speaking group.

Although speakers with normal articulatory skills tend to have a lower incidence of malocclusion than speakers with articulatory errors, malocclusion itself does not preclude normal articulation. Subtelny, Mestre, and Subtelny (1964) found malocclusion to coexist with both normal and defective speech. They also noted that during /s/ production, normal speakers with malocclusion (distocclusion) tended to position the tongue tip slightly to the rear of the lower incisors when compared to normal speakers with normal occlusion.

Starr (1972) reported several clinical observations concerning dental arch relationships and speech production skills. He stated that an articulation problem is highly probable in individuals with a short or narrow maxillary (upper) arch and a normal mandibular (lower) arch. The consonants likely to be affected by such conditions are /s, z, ʃ, tʃ, f, v, t, and d/. He further noted that rotated teeth and supernumerary (extra) teeth do not generally present significant speech problems.

Another area of interest to investigators has been the influence of *missing teeth* on articulation. Bankson and Byrne (1962) examined the influence of missing teeth in kindergarten and first-grade children on the production of /s/, /ʃ/ and /f/ in the word-initial, medial, and final positions, and /z/ in the word-medial position. Initially, subjects were identified either as children who had correct articulation with their teeth intact or as children who had incorrect articulation with their teeth intact. After four months, articulation skills were reassessed and the number of missing central or lateral incisors tabulated. A significant relationship was found between presence or absence of teeth and correct production of /s/, but not of /f/, /ʃ/, or /z/. However, some children maintained correct production of /s/ despite the loss of incisors.

Snow (1961) examined the influence of missing teeth on consonant production in first-grade children. Subjects were divided into two groups: those with normal incisors and those with missing or grossly abnormal incisor teeth. The consonants examined were /f/, /v/, /θ/, /ð/, /s/, and /z/. Although Snow found that a significantly larger proportion of children with dental deviations misarticulated consonants, she also found that three quarters of the children with defective dentition did not misarticulate these sounds. In contrast to Bankson and Byrne, who noted significant differences only for /s/, Snow found significant differences for all phonemes. Snow suggested that although dental status may be a crucial factor in sound productions for some children, it does not appear to be significant for most.

Tongue

The tongue is generally considered the most important articulator for speech production. Tongue movements during speech production include tip elevation, grooving, and protrusion. The tongue is relatively short at birth, growing longer and thinner at the tip with age.

Ankyloglossia, or "tongue-tie," are terms used to describe a restricted lingual frenum. At one time, it was commonly assumed that an infant or child with ankyloglossia should have his or her frenum clipped to allow greater freedom of tongue movement and better articulation of tongue tip sounds, and frenectomies (clipping of the frenum of the tongue) were performed relatively frequently. However, McEnery and Gaines (1941) examined 1,000 patients with speech disorders and identified only 4 individuals with abnormally short frenums. Their most extreme case of a short frenum was a 10-year-old boy, whose only articulation error was a /w/ for /r/ substitution; the error was corrected following speech instruction. The authors recommended against surgery for ankyloglossia because of the possibility of hemorrhages, infections, and scar tissue. It can be inferred from these data that a short frenum is only rarely the cause of an articulation problem.

Fletcher and Meldrum (1968) examined the relationship between length of the lingual frenum and articulation. They compared two groups of sixth-grade students, 20 with limited lingual movement and 20 with greater lingual movement, and reported that subjects with restricted lingual movement scored within normal limits on a measure of articulation but tended to have more articulation errors than the group with greater lingual movement.

Although too large a tongue (**macroglossia**) or too small a tongue (**microglossia**) might be expected to affect articulation skills, there appears to be little relationship between tongue size and articulation although these variables have not been adequately investigated. The tongue is a muscular structure capable of considerable change in length and width and thus, regardless of size, is generally capable of the mobility necessary for correct sound productions.

Hard Palate

The relationship between articulation disorders and variations in hard palate dimensions has received limited attention. Fairbanks and Lintner (1951) measured the hard palates of a group of young adults with superior consonant articulation and a group with inferior consonant articulation. They reported no significant differences in cuspid width, molar width, palatal height, and maximum mouth opening. Bloomer and Hawk (1973) pointed out that removal of any part of the maxilla, if not restored surgically or prosthetically, creates a serious problem for the speaker. Articulation problems related to structural anomalies of the palate will be discussed in the following section.

Major Structural Variations of the Speech Mechanism

Speech-language clinicians should recognize that significant anomalies of the oral structures are frequently associated with specific speech problems. Oral structural anomalies may be congenital or acquired. Cleft lip and/or palate is perhaps the most common congenital anomaly of the orofacial complex. Acquired structural deficits may result from trauma to the orofacial complex or surgical removal of oral structures secondary to oral cancers. For individuals with orofacial anomalies, the course of habilitation or rehabilitation often includes surgical and/or prosthetic management, and therefore, the speech clinician must work closely with various medical and dental specialists. See Leonard (1994) for more information concerning characteristics of speakers with glossectomy and other oral/oropharyngeal ablation.

Lips

Surgical repair of clefts of the lip can result in a relatively short immobile upper lip. Although this might be expected to adversely affect articulation skills, there is little evidence that this anomaly causes a speech problem for most speakers. Bloomer and Hawk (1973) reported the effects of ablative surgery on production of labial phonemes in a patient who underwent surgical removal of the external and internal nasal structures for treatment of cancer. Although surgery resulted in a relatively immobile and shortened upper lip, the patient maintained good overall speech intelligibility, producing labiodental approximations for all bilabial consonants. The development of compensatory articulatory gestures to achieve acoustically acceptable speech production is very common in many patients with structural anomalies.

Tongue

As we mentioned in addressing minor structural variations, the tongue is a muscular structure capable of considerable changes in length and width. Because the tongue is such an adaptable organ, speakers are frequently able to compensate for extensive amounts of the tongue missing and still maintain intelligible speech. Clinical investigators have repeatedly reported intelligible speech production following partial glossectomies (surgical removal of the tongue) (see Leonard, 1994). One such case study (Backus, 1940) recorded the speech pattern of a 10-year-old boy with an undersized tongue after excision of the tongue tip and the left half of the tongue. Initially, the child's articulation was characterized by numerous consonant substitutions, but after a period of treatment, he was able to produce all consonants with little identifiable deviation.

For many patients, however, speech production is affected in varying degrees when part of the tongue is excised. Skelly, Spector, Donaldson, Brodeur, and Paletta (1971) reported pre-treatment and post-treatment intelligibility scores for 25 glossectomy (14 total, 11 partial) patients. Intelligibility judgments were based on single-word productions audio tape-recorded and played back to listeners. Intelligibility scores for those who underwent partial glossectomy ranged from 6 to 24 percent on the pre-test and from 24 to 46 percent on the post-test. Intelligibility scores for those who underwent total glossectomy ranged from 0 to 8 percent prior to treatment and from 18 to 24 percent after treatment. The investigators noted that the compensatory articulatory patterns of the two groups differed. Partial glossectomy patients utilized the residual tongue stump to modify articulation; total glossectomy patients made mandibular, labial, buccal, and palatal adjustments.

Massengill, Maxwell, and Picknell (1970) reported that speech intelligibility in three patients decreased as the amount of tongue excised increased. The patients demonstrated minimal difficulty in verbal communication, though speech distortion was present. Skelly and colleagues (1971) reported that unilateral tongue excision required fewer speech adaptations than tongue tip excisions.

Leonard (1994) reported a study where listeners were asked to evaluate consonants produced by 50 speakers with various types of glossectomy. Results indicated that fricatives and plosives were most frequently judged to be inaccurate, while nasals and semivowels appeared more resistant to perceptual disruption.

Hard Palate

Oral cancers often require surgical removal of the diseased tissues. The removal of any part of the maxilla, if not restored surgically or prosthetically, creates a serious problem for the speaker. Majid, Weinberg, and Chalian (1974) examined speech intelligibility following prosthetic obturation of surgically acquired maxillary defects. Six adults—three women and three men—recorded speech with and without maxillary prosthetic obturators. Without the dental prosthesis, average intelligibility scores ranged from 40 to 80 percent and with it from 92 to 98 percent. The authors concluded that normal intelligibility is a realistic treatment goal for patients with acquired maxillary defects.

Clefts of the hard palate are surgically repaired, typically within the first 12 to 24 months of life. Scarring associated with the surgery has not been found to interfere with articulatory production.

Soft Palate

The relationship of the soft palate (velum) to articulation has been a topic of considerable research, much of it focusing on the sphincteral closure of the velopharyngeal port and the effect of velopharyngeal competence on articulation. **Velopharyngeal competence** refers to the valving that takes place to separate the nasal cavity from the oral cavity during non-nasal speech production. Inadequate velopharyngeal closure is frequently associated with (1) hypernasal resonance of vowels, vocalic consonants, and glides and liquids; (2) reduced or diminished intraoral breath pressure during production of pressure consonants (i.e., fricatives, stops, and affricates); and (3) nasal air emission accompanying production of pressure consonants (e.g., substitutions of glottal stops for stop consonants and pharyngeal fricatives for sibilants). Although velopharyngeal incompetence is often associated with individuals with clefts of the soft palate, some speakers without clefting also demonstrate such incompetence—for example, individuals with dysarthria related to neurogenic paresis or paralysis of the velopharyngeal muscles (Johns and Salyer, 1978).

As stated above, the pharyngeal fricative and the glottal stop are two examples of compensatory articulatory gestures associated with velopharyngeal valving problems. The glottal stop is characterized by interruption of the airstream at the glottis, resulting in a glottal click, or coughlike sound. Glottal stops are generally substituted for stops, particularly velar stops, as well as fricatives and affricates. The pharyngeal fricative is produced with the source of friction in the pharyngeal area and is frequently substituted for fricatives and affricates. The presence of hypernasality, nasal emission of air, weak consonants, glottal stops, and pharyngeal fricatives are all signs of velopharyngeal valving difficulties.

When the oral cavity communicates in some way with the nasal cavity, for example, through palatal fistulae (openings), or following ablative surgery or velopharyngeal incompetence, varying degrees of hypernasality will usually result. On the other hand, hyponasality (denasality) may result when the nasopharynx or nasal cavity is obstructed during speech production. Inflammation of the mucous membranes of the nasal cavity or a deviated septum may also cause hyponasality.

Nasopharynx

The nasopharyngeal tonsils (adenoids) are located at the upper or superior pharyngeal area. Hyperthrophied (enlarged) adenoids may compensate for a short or partially immobile velum, by assisting in velopharyngeal closure. Thus, their removal may result in hyper-nasality. But the adenoids may become sufficiently enlarged as to constitute a major obstruction of the nasopharynx, resulting in hyponasal speech. Enlarged adenoids may also interfere with Eustachian tube function in some individuals.

Summary

Although individuals with oral structural deviations frequently experience articulation problems, the relationship between structural deficits and articulation skills is not very predictable. The literature cites many instances of individuals with structural anomalies who have developed compensatory gestures to produce acoustically acceptable speech. Why some individuals are able to compensate for relatively gross abnormalities and others are unable to compensate for lesser deficits has not been resolved. A speech-language clinician who evaluates or treats individuals with oral structural anomalies must work collaboratively with various medical and dental specialists during speech habilitation or rehabilitation. For an excellent review of the speech characteristics and treatment of individuals with glossectomy and other oral/oropharyngeal ablation, see Leonard (1994).

Oral Sensory Function

Some treatment approaches include the practice of calling the client's attention to sensory cues. For example, McDonald's (1964) sensorimotor therapy includes having the client identify oral cavity contacts and movements that occur during speech. Bordon (1984) indicated the need for awareness of *kinesthesis* (sense of movement and position) during therapy. Almost any phonetic placement technique used to teach speech sounds usually includes a description of articulatory contacts and movements necessary for the production of the target speech sound. If one assumes that oral sensory and kinesthetic feedback play a role in the development and ongoing monitoring of articulatory gestures, the relationship between oral sensory function and speech sound productions may have potential clinical implications.

The investigation of *somesthesis* (sense of movement, position, touch, and awareness of muscle tension) has focused on (1) temporary sensory deprivation during oral sensory anesthetization (nerve block anesthesia) to determine the effect of sensory deprivation on speech production and (2) the assessment of oral sensory perception such as two-point discrimination or oral form discrimination to see if such sensory perception was related to articulatory skill. Considerable research into oral sensory functioning was conducted in the 1960s using a variety of methods to assess oral tactile sensitivity in order to understand if a relationship existed between these sensory tasks and articulation performance. Later research examined articulation of individuals during periods of temporary sensory deprivation, sometimes referred to as **oral blockade**.

Netsell (1986) has suggested that it is likely that adults are not consciously aware of specific speech movements during running speech. He also speculated that children may not be aware of articulatory movements during the acquisition period. If Netsell is correct, the clinician who attempts to utilize somesthetic senses in monitoring running speech may be asking the client to respond to information that is not available at a conscious level without instruction.

Oral Tactile Sensitivity

Early investigators of oral sensory function attempted to explore the sensitivity or threshold of awareness of oral structures to various stimuli. Ringel and Ewanowski (1965) studied oral tactile sensitivity utilizing an esthesiometer, a device used in the measurement of two-point discrimination. They examined discrimination sensitivity of various structures in a normal population and found that the maximal to minimal awareness hierarchy for two-point stimulation (awareness of two points rather than one) was tongue tip, finger tip, lip, soft palate, alveolar ridge, and that the midline of structures tended to be more sensitive than the lateral edges.

Fucci and associates (Arnst and Fucci, 1975; Fucci, 1972) have measured the threshold of vibrotactile stimulation of structures in the oral cavity in both normal and speech-disordered individuals. These investigators found that subjects with misarticulations tended to have poorer oral sensory abilities than normal speaking subjects.

Oral Form Recognition

Oral sensory function has also been investigated extensively through form recognition tasks. Ringel, Burk, and Scott (1970) speculated that form identification (**oral stereognosis**) may provide information on nervous system integrity since the recognition of forms placed in the mouth was assumed to require integrity of peripheral receptors for touch and kinesthesis as well as central integrating processes. Most form recognition tasks require the subject to match forms placed in the oral cavity with drawings of the forms, or to make same-different judgments. Subjects tend to improve on such tasks until adolescence when they ceiling-out on the task. Stimuli for such testing are typically small, plastic, three-dimensional forms of varying degrees of similarity, such as triangles, rectangles, ovals, and circles.

Investigators who have studied the relationship between oral form recognition and articulation performance have reported inconsistent results. Arndt, Elbert, and Shelton (1970) did not find a significant relationship between oral form recognition and articulation performance in a third-grade population. But Ringel, House, Burk, Dolinsky, and Scott (1970) reported significant differences on an oral form-matching task between normal-speaking elementary school children and children with articulation errors. They noted that children with severe misarticulations made more form-recognition errors than children with mild articulation problems.

Some researchers have investigated the relationship between production of specific phonemes and oral sensory function. McNutt (1977) found that children who misarticulated /r/ did not perform as well as the normal speakers on oral form perception tasks; there were, however, no significant differences between the normal speakers and the children who misarticulated /s/.

Bishop, Ringel, and House (1973) compared oral form-recognition skills of deaf high school students who were orally trained (taught to use speech), and those who were taught to use sign language. The authors noted skill differences that favored the orally trained students and postulated that "while a failure in oroperceptual functioning may lead to disorders of articulation, a failure to use the oral mechanism for speech activities, even in persons with normal orosensory capabilities, may result in poor performance on oroperceptual tasks" (257).

Locke (1968) examined the relationship between articulation skills and oral form-recognition scores from a different perspective. Rather than comparing the performance of normal-speaking children with those of children who demonstrated articulation errors, he compared the performance on an articulation learning task of 10 normal children with high form-recognition scores with that of 10 normal children with low form-recognition scores. Each subject was required to imitate three German sounds heard on a tape recording of a native German speaker. Locke found that the group with high form-perception scores obtained significantly better production scores on two of the three consonant sounds than the group with low form-identification scores.

McDonald and Aungst (1970) pointed out that an individual can have good articulation skills despite poor oral form-recognition scores. They cited the case of a 21-year-old neurologically impaired male who articulated normally yet demonstrated difficulty in oral form identification and in two-point discrimination on the tongue.

Oral Anesthetization

The relationship between speech sound productions and oral sensory functions has also been examined through sensory deprivation. To study the role of oral sensation during speech, researchers have induced temporary states of oral sensory deprivation through the use of oral nerve-block and topical anesthetization. Then they have compared speech under normal conditions with speech under anesthetization on a variety of dimensions, such as overall intelligibility, vowel and consonant articulation, rate, phoneme duration, and physiological and acoustic characteristics.

Gammon, Smith, Daniloff, and Kim (1971) examined the articulation skills of eight adult subjects reading 30 sentences under four conditions: (1) normal, (2) with masking noise present, (3) nerve-block anesthesia, and (4) nerve-block anesthesia with masking noise. They noted few vowel distortions under any of the conditions and a 20 percent rate of consonant misarticulation (especially fricatives and affricates) under anesthesia and under anesthesia with noise. Scott and Ringel (1971) studied the articulation of two adult males producing lists of 24 bisyllabic words under normal and anesthetized conditions. They noted that articulatory changes caused by sensory deprivation were largely nonphonemic in nature and included loss of retroflexion and lip-rounding gestures, less tight fricative constrictions, and retracted points of articulation contacts.

Prosek and House (1975) studied four adult speakers reading 20 bisyllabic words in isolation and in sentences under normal and anesthetized conditions. Although intelligibility was maintained in the anesthetized condition, speech rate was slowed and minor imprecisions of articulation were noted. The authors reported that, when anesthetized, speakers produced consonants with slightly greater intraoral air pressure and longer duration than under the normal nonanesthetized condition.

In summary, studies involving anesthetization found that speech remained intelligible although subjects did not speak as accurately under this condition as they did under normal conditions. However, the subjects in these studies were adult speakers with normal articulation skills prior to the sensory deprivation. It is unclear if reduced oral sensory feedback might interfere with the acquisition of speech or affect remediation.

Oral Sensory Function and Articulation Learning

Jordan, Hardy, and Morris (1978) studied the influence of tactile sensation as a feedback mechanism in articulation learning. Their subjects were first-grade boys, nine with good articulation skills and nine with poor articulation skills. Subjects were fitted with palatal plates equipped with touch-sensitive electrodes and taught to replicate four positions of linguapalatal contact, with and without topical anesthesia. Children with poor articulation performed less well on tasks of precise tongue placement than children with good articulation. Subjects with poor articulation were able to improve their initially poor performance when given specific training on the tongue placement tasks.

Wilhelm (1971) and Shelton, Willis, Johnson, and Arndt (1973) used oral form-recognition materials to teach form recognition to misarticulating children and reported inconsistent results. Wilhelm reported articulation improved as oral form recognition improved. Shelton and colleagues reported results that did not support that finding. Ruscello (1972) reported that form-recognition scores improved in children undergoing treatment for articulation.

Summary

The role of normal oral sensory function or somesthetic feedback in the development and maintenance of speech production is complex. Despite efforts to identify the relationship between oral sensory status and articulatory performance, conclusive findings are lacking. A review of the literature, however, has revealed the following:

1. Many methods have been used to measure oral sensory perception: that is, form recognition, touch-pressure threshold, two-point discrimination, and oral vibrotactile thresholds.
2. Oral form recognition improves with age through adolescence.
3. The role of oral sensory information in the acquisition of phonology is unclear.
4. Individuals with poor articulation tend to achieve slightly lower scores on form-perception tasks than their normal-speaking peers. However, some individuals with poor form-identification skills have good articulation.
5. Investigators who have anesthetized oral structures reported that intelligibility is generally maintained during sensory deprivation but less accuracy in articulation was noted.
6. Although research has indicated that some individuals with articulation problems may also have oral sensory deficits, the neurological mechanisms underlying the use of sensory information during experimental conditions may differ from those operating in normal running speech.
7. Information concerning oral sensory function has not been shown to have clinical applicability or a place in treatment.
8. It is important to distinguish between the effects of sensory deprivation in individuals who have already developed good speech skills and the effects in individuals with defective articulation.
9. The effects of long-term sensory deprivation have yet to be explored.

Motor Abilities

Because speech is a motor act, researchers have explored the relationship between articulation and motor skills, investigating performance on general motor tasks as well as oral and facial motor tasks.

General Motor Skills

Studies focusing on the relationship between general motor skills and articulatory abilities have yielded inconsistent and inconclusive results. However, individuals with articulation problems have not been shown to have significant retardation in general motor development.

Oral-Facial Motor Skills

Speech is a dynamic process that requires the precise coordination of the oral musculature. During ongoing speech production, fine muscle movements of the lips, tongue, palate, and jaw constantly alter the dimensions of the oral cavity. An assessment of the client's oral motor skills is typically a part of an articulatory evaluation. Tests of diadochokinetic rate or maximum repetition rate (rapid repetition of syllables) have been used most frequently to evaluate oral motor skills. Diadochokinetic rate is established either with a *count by time* procedure, in which the examiner counts the number of syllables spoken in a given interval of time, or a *time by count* measurement, in which the examiner notes the time required to produce a designated number of syllables. The advantage of the time by count measurement is that few operations are required since the examiner need only listen to the syllable count and turn off the timing device when the requisite number of syllables is produced. Performance is then compared to normative data. The syllables most frequently used to assess diadochokinetic rates are /pʌ/, tʌ/, and /kʌ/ in isolation and the sequence /pʌtʌ/, /tʌkʌ/, /pʌkʌ/, /pʌtʌkʌ/. There is some evidence that diadochokinetic rates improve with age. Fletcher (1972) examined diadochokinetic rates in children ages 6 to 13 years using a count by time procedure. He reported that children increased the number of syllables produced in a given unit of time at each successive age from 7 to 13 years. Data reported by Canning and Rose (1974) indicated that adult values for maximum repetition rates were reached by 9- to 10-year-olds, whereas Fletcher's data show a convergence after age 15. A better understanding of the relationship between oral motor skills and articulation skills in individuals without apparent neurological involvement is of interest to speech clinicians since individuals with speech problems who perform well on oral motor tasks are not uncommon.

McNutt (1977) and Dworkin (1978) examined diadochokinetic rates of children with specific misarticulations and of their normal-speaking peers. McNutt examined the rate of alternating syllable productions (e.g., /dʌgə/) in children with normal articulation, children with /s/ misarticulation, and children with /r/ misarticulation. Both groups of children with misarticulations were noted to be slower than normal speakers in syllable production rates. Dworkin examined lingual diadochokinetic rates for the syllables /tʌ/, /dʌ/, /kʌ/, and /gʌ/, in normal speakers and frontal lisping speakers aged 7 to 12 years. The mean rate of utterances of the syllables tested was significantly lower in the disordered group.

Some researchers have questioned the usefulness of rapid syllable repetition tasks and their relationship to articulation skills because the movements of articulation are produced by the simultaneous contraction of different groups of muscles rather than the alternating contraction of opposed muscles (McDonald, 1964). Wintz (1969) also pointed out that because normal speakers have a history of success with speech sounds, they may have an advantage over subjects with misarticulations on diadochokinetic tasks. Tiffany (1980) pointed out that little is known about the significance of scores obtained on diadochokinetic tasks and thus "such measures appear to lack a substantial theoretical base" (895). The one exception to this generality relates to those children that might be considered to evidence developmental verbal dyspraxia (discussed elsewhere in this chapter). Poor performance in diadochokinetic tasks is often reflective of syllable sequencing problems evident in other speech tasks.

Summary

Individuals with articulation problems have not been shown to exhibit significantly depressed motor coordination on tasks of general motor performance. The relationship between oral motor skills and articulation skills in functional articulation disorders remains uncertain. Although individuals with defective articulation have been found to perform more poorly on diadochokinetic tasks than their normal-speaking peers, these results cannot be accurately interpreted until the relationship between diadochokinetic tasks and the ability to articulate sounds in context is clarified. Children with developmental verbal dyspraxia are one subgroup of the "functional" disorders population for whom poor diadochokinetic performance is of diagnostic significance in terms of identifying the problem.

Tongue Thrust

The term **tongue thrust** refers to habitual or frequent resting or pushing of the tongue against the lingual surface area of the incisors or cuspids, or protrusion between the upper and lower anterior teeth (Hanson, 1994). Proffit (1986) points out that tongue thrust is something of a misnomer since it implies that the tongue is thrust forward forcefully, when in reality such individuals do not seem to use more tongue force against the teeth than non-thrusters. Rather, *tongue thrust swallow* implies a directionality of tongue activity in swallowing. Other terms sometimes used to describe these behaviors include *reverse swallow*, *deviant swallow*, and *infantile swallow*. These terms should be avoided because of their inherent faulty implications (Mason, 1988). The most salient features of a tongue thrust swallow pattern, according to Mason and Proffit (1974), include one or more of these conditions:

1. ... during the initiation of a swallow, a forward gesture of the tongue between the anterior teeth so that the tongue tip contacts the lower lip;
2. During speech activities, fronting of the tongue between or against the anterior teeth with the mandible hinged open (in phonetic contexts not intended for such placements); and
3. At rest, the tongue carried forward in the oral cavity with the mandible hinged slightly open and the tongue tip against or between the anterior teeth (116).

Everyone starts out life as a tongue thruster because at birth the tongue fills the oral cavity, making tongue fronting obligatory. Sometime later, prior to about 5 years, most children replace an anterior tongue-gums/teeth seal during swallowing with a superior tongue-palate seal (Hanson, 1988b).

Tongue thrust during swallow and/or tongue fronting at rest can usually be identified by visual inspection. Mason (1988) has pointed out that two types of tongue fronting should be differentiated. The first is described as a **habit** and is seen in the absence of any morphological structural delimiting factors. The second is **obligatory** and may involve factors such as airway obstruction or enlarged tonsils with tongue thrusting being a necessary adaptation to maintain the size of the airway to pass food during swallow. Oral myofunction therapy for obligatory tongue fronting has been questioned by Shelton (1989) because of the poor prognosis for change.

Hanson (1988a) suggested that a better description for these tongue position and movement behaviors would be "oral muscle pattern disorders." Orthodontists and speech-language pathologists have been interested in tongue thrusting and a forward tongue resting posture because of the perception that tongue function can cause certain types of (1) malocclusion problems, (2) altered patterns of facial development, and (3) articulation problems. The type of articulation disorder associated with tongue thrust and malocclusion is a frontal lisp characterized by anterior tongue placement for /s/ and /z/. Some children who evidence tongue thrusting also manifest articulatory errors. The number of lisps is higher in children who evidence tongue thrusting than for children who do not evidence such behavior. Sometimes tongue thrust is also associated with anterior placement for /ʃ/, /tʃ/, /dʒ/, /ʒ/, /t/, /d/, /l/, and /n/.

Impact of Tongue Thrust on Dentition

The current view is that the resting posture of the tongue affects the position of the teeth and jaws more than does the tongue function during swallowing (tongue thrust) or speaking (Proffit, 1986). Tongue thrusting may play a role in maintaining or influencing an abnormal dental pattern when an anterior resting tongue position is present. If the position of the tongue is forward (forward resting position) and between the anterior teeth at rest, this condition can impede normal teeth eruption and can result in an anterior open bite. However, tongue thrusting patients, in the absence of an anterior tongue resting position, are not thought to develop malocclusions. The pressure or force on dentition associated with tongue thrust during speaking and swallowing are of short duration and do not exert enough force on the dentition to cause problems of dental occlusion. Mason (1988) pointed out that individuals who exhibit a tongue thrust pattern and forward tongue posture create morphological conditions that can potentially lead to dental occlusion problems and would be much more likely to develop a malocclusion than when only a tongue thrust is present.

Tongue Thrust and Presence of Articulation Errors

Investigators have reported that articulation errors, primarily sibilant distortions, occur more frequently in children who evidence tongue thrust than in those who do not. Fletcher, Casteel, and Bradley (1961) studied 1,615 school children aged 6 to 18 and found that children who demonstrated a tongue thrust swallow pattern were more likely to have associated sibilant distortions than children who did not. They also reported that subjects with normal swallow patterns demonstrated a significant decrease in sibilant distortion with age, whereas tongue thrusters did not.

Palmer (1962) found that clients referred for marked tongue thrusting nearly always demonstrated a sibilant "difference" but that the difference was perceived as only a slight lisp. He reported that such differences also occurred on /t/, /d/, and /n/.

Jann, Ward, and Jann (1964) examined the relationship among speech defects, tongue thrusting, and malocclusion in children in the early primary grades and reported a high incidence of /s/, /z/, and /l/ variations in children with tongue thrust swallow patterns.

Subtelny, Mestre, and Subtelny (1964) used radiographic techniques to examine the relationship between normal and abnormal oral morphology and /s/ production. Their subjects, 81 adolescents and adults, were divided into three groups: (1) normal speakers with normal occlusion, (2) normal speakers with severe malocclusion, and (3) abnormal speakers with severe malocclusion. In contrast to earlier investigators, these authors found that the incidence of tongue thrusting and malocclusion in normal speakers was comparable to that in abnormal speakers. This finding is consistent with the reported developmental decrease in the reverse swallow pattern.

Dworkin and Culatta (1980) studied the relationships among protrusive tongue strength, open bite, and articulation in 141 children. They reported no significant difference among their group in tongue strength.

Treatment Issues

Hanson (1994), in a review of the 15 studies that examined the effectiveness of tongue thrust therapy, reported that 14 of the investigators indicated that swallowing and resting patterns were altered successfully. Most studies reviewed patients at least one year following the completion of treatment. Only one study of five subjects (Subtelny, 1970) found therapy to be ineffective in correcting the disorders.

Other support for tongue thrust intervention has often come from clinical reports by clinicians who conduct oral myofunctional therapy. For example, Hilton (1984) stated: "In my experience, many tongue-fronting children who begin speech articulation therapy without having had the early sensorimotor and stretching activities of myotherapy . . . begin with an unnecessary handicap . . . I provide every tongue-fronting speech articulation case these initial oral awareness, control, and flexibility exercises prior to initiation of the place-feature oriented therapy . . ." (51).

The official statement adopted by the ASHA Legislative Council (ASHA, 1991) on the role of the speech-language pathologist in assessment and management of oral myofunctional disorders includes the statement: "Investigation, assessment, and treatment of oral myofunctional disorders are within the purview of speech-language pathology" (7). This statement, as well as others quoted below, shows that ASHA's view of tongue thrust and oral myofunctional therapy changed considerably from the skepticism about this group of disorders reflected in the 1974 joint statement and endorsement by the American Speech-Language-Hearing Association, the American Dental Association, and the American Association of Orthodontists.

1991 Position Statement

It is the position of the American Speech-Language-Hearing Association (ASHA) that:

1. Oral myofunctional phenomena, including abnormal fronting (tongue thrust) of the tongue at rest and during swallowing, lip incompetency, and sucking habits, can be identified reliably. These conditions co-occur with speech misarticulations in some patients.
2. Tongue fronting may reflect learned behaviors, physical variables, or both.

3. Published research indicates that oral myofunctional therapy is effective in modifying disorders of tongue and lip posture and movement.

4. Investigation, assessment, and treatment of oral myofunctional disorders are within the purview of speech-language pathology.

5. The speech-language pathologist who desires to perform oral myofunctional services must have the required knowledge and skills to provide a high quality of treatment. The provision of oral myofunctional therapy remains an option of individual speech-language pathologists whose interests and training qualify them.

6. Evaluation and treatment should be interdisciplinary and tailored to the individual. The speech-language pathologist performing oral myofunctional therapy should collaborate with an orthodontist, pediatric dentist, or other dentists, and with medical specialists such as an otolaryngologist, pediatrician, or allergist, as needed.

7. Appropriate goals of oral myofunctional therapy should include the retraining of labial and lingual resting and functional patterns (including speech). The speech-language pathologist's statements of treatment goals should avoid predictions of treatment outcome based on tooth position or dental occlusal changes.

8. Basic and applied research is needed on the nature and evaluation of oral myofunctions and the treatment of oral myofunctional disorders (7).

The ad hoc committee report (ASHA, 1989) on the labial-lingual posturing function developed the above statement based on the following concepts relative to oral myofunctional phenomena as they relate to communication disorders:

1. All infants exhibit a tongue thrust swallow as a normal performance.

2. This pattern changes with growth and maturation to the extent that many different swallow patterns can be identified from infancy to adulthood.

3. At some time in development, a tongue protrusion swallow is no longer the norm and can be considered undesirable or as a contributing and maintaining factor in malocclusion, lisping, or both.

4. A related condition that has a stronger link to malocclusion is a forward resting posture of the tongue. . . . This is consistent with orthodontic theory and research that long-acting forces against the teeth result in tooth movement whereas short-acting (intermittent) forces are not as likely to cause tooth movement.

5. There is descriptive evidence that during the course of oral myofunctional therapy some individuals have corrected or controlled a tongue thrust swallow and an anterior resting posture.

6. Diagnostic attention should be directed toward determining whether a tongue thrust swallow and a forward tongue resting posture coexist in a given patient. When these conditions coexist, a greater link to malocclusion would be expected than from a tongue thrust swallow alone. However, there is insufficient evidence to show that a forward tongue posture and tongue thrust swallow are more detrimental than a tongue forward resting posture alone. There is also some evidence that a tongue forward resting posture or tongue thrust swallow and lisping coexist in some persons. Correction of tongue function or posture may facilitate correction of the lisp or the interdentalization of the /t/, /d/, /n/, and /l/ phonemes.

7. In normal development, slight separation of the lips at rest ("lip incompetence") is normal in children. With growth, the lips typically achieve contact at rest in the teenage years. Some individuals, however, persist in a lips-apart posture after development has advanced sufficiently to permit lip closure. Such individuals may be candidates for treatment.

8. There is some evidence that lip exercises can be successful in facilitating a closed-lip posture.

9. Sucking habits (e.g., finger, thumb, tongue, lips) can influence dental development. When tongue thrusting and thumb sucking coexist with dental problems, developmental correction of the tongue thrust would not be expected until the thumb, finger, or sucking habit ceases.

10. Other variables besides learning influence tongue posture. They include posterior airway obstruction, which may involve tonsils, adenoids, nasal blockage, high posterior tongue position with a short mandibular ramus, or a long soft palate. Many morphologic features or combinations of features can reduce oral isthmus size and obligate the tongue to rest forward. Diagnostic procedures should distinguish such patients from those with other forward tongue postures or functions. The obligatory tongue forward posture group would seem unlikely candidates for myofunctional therapy in the absence of medical treatment. Any indicated remedial medical procedures are usually carried out prior to consideration of myofunctional therapy.

Summary

1. The current position of the American Speech-Language-Hearing Association as stated in the 1991 position statement on the clinical entity of tongue thrust as well as the management of oral myofunctional disorders was modified significantly from the 1974 statement.

2. Existing data support the idea that abnormal labial-lingual posturing function can be identified, including abnormal fronting (tongue thrust) of the tongue at rest and during swallowing, lip incompetency, and sucking habits.

3. A forward tongue resting posture has the potential, with or without a tongue thrust swallow, to be associated with malocclusions.

4. There is some evidence that an anterior tongue resting posture or a tongue thrust swallow and lisping coexist in some persons.

5. Oral myofunctional therapy can be effective in modifying disorders of tongue and lip posture and movement.

6. Assessment and treatment of oral myofunctional disorders that may include some nonspeech remediation are within the purview of speech-language pathology but should involve interdisciplinary collaboration.

7. Research is needed on the nature and evaluation of oral myofunctions and the treatment of such disorders.

Neuromotor Disorders

Speech production at a motor level requires muscle strength, speed of movement, appropriate range of excursion, accuracy of movement, coordination of multiple movements, motor steadiness, and muscle tone (Darley, Aronson, and Brown, 1975). Damage that impairs one or more of these neuromuscular functions may affect motor speech production. Motor speech disorders are not only disorders of articulation but also frequently involve other components of speech production, including phonation, respiration, or velopharyngeal function. Neuromotor speech disorders more typically occur in adults than children, since they are often associated with strokes or other forms of brain injury. Cerebral palsy is one example of a condition that results in neuromotor-based speech disorders in children.

Neurologists and speech-language pathologists have sought to understand the possible relationship between the clinical (behavioral) responses associated with neurologically impaired individuals and the site and extent of the neurological lesions (brain damage). The reason for such inquiry is to identify some potential commonality across patients in the specific brain damage and the concomitant cognitive language impairment.

Although entire books are devoted to motor speech disorders, the following offers a brief introduction to this topic:

Dysarthria

Dysarthria is a speech problem caused by neuromuscular impairment. It may result from a lesion of the central or peripheral nervous system that involves the pathways subserving the speech mechanism (Darley, Aronson, and Brown, 1969). Because this disorder has varying characteristics that can be caused by different types of lesions at different locations in the brain, the term *dysarthrias* is, perhaps, more accurate than *dysarthria*.

Dysarthrias are caused by a paralysis, weakness, or incoordination of the speech musculature, which may result from localized injuries to the nervous system, various inflammatory processes, toxic metabolic disorders, vascular lesions of the brain, degenerative disorders of the nervous system, or be associated with a brain tumor. The most significant characteristic of dysarthric speech is reduced intelligibility. Dysarthric speech can involve disturbances in respiration, phonation, articulation, resonance, and prosody. Phonemes misarticulated in spontaneous speech are also likely to be misarticulated in other situations, such as reading and imitation tasks.

Table 5.1 lists the six types of dysarthrias and the most prominent deviant speech characteristics associated with each. The most common of these characteristics is the production of imprecise consonants.

Apraxia

Apraxia is a motor speech disorder also caused by brain damage, but it is differentiated from the dysarthrias and described as a separate clinical entity. Apraxia of speech is characterized by an impairment of motor speech programming with no weakness, paralysis, or incoordination of the speech musculature. Whereas dysarthrias frequently affect all motor speech processes—respiration, phonation, articulation, resonance, and prosody—apraxia primarily affects articulatory abilities with secondary prosodic alterations.

A description of some of the clinical characteristics of this disorder has been provided by Darley, Aronson, and Brown (1975):

> Apraxia of speech is characterized by highly variable articulation errors embedded in
> a pattern of speech made slow and effortful by trial-and-error gropings for the desired

articulatory postures. The off-target productions are usually complications of articulatory performance, that is, substitutions (many of them unrelated to the target phoneme), additions, repetitions, and prolongations. Less frequently, the errors are simplifications, that is, distortions and omissions. Errors are most often on consonants occurring initially in words, predominately on those phonemes and clusters of phonemes requiring more complex muscular adjustment. Errors are exacerbated by increase in length of word and the linguistic and psychologic "weight" of a word in the sentence. They are not significantly influenced by auditory, visual, or instructional set variables. Islands of fluent, error-free speech highlight the marked discrepancy between efficient automatic-reactive productions and inefficient volitional-purposive productions (267).

Some clients who demonstrate apraxia of speech (**verbal apraxia**) also demonstrate similar difficulty in volitional oral nonspeech tasks, a behavior described as **oral apraxia**

TABLE 5.1 Dysarthrias and Associated Speech Deviations

Type	Discrete Neurological Group	Relative Prominence of Speech Deviations
Flaccid dysarthria— (disorders of the lower motor neuron)	bulbar palsy	1. hypernasality 2. imprecise consonants 3. breathiness (continuous)
Spastic dysarthria— (disorders of the upper motor neuron)	pseudobulbar palsy	1. imprecise consonants 2. monopitch 3. reduced stress
Ataxic dysarthria— (disorders of the cerebellar system)	cerebellar lesions	1. imprecise consonants 2. excess and equal stress 3. irregular articulatory breakdown
Hypokinetic dysarthria— (disorders of the extra-pyramidal system)	Parkinsonism	1. monopitch 2. reduced stress 3. monoloudness
Hyperkinetic dysarthria— (disorders of the extra-pyramidal system)	chorea	1. imprecise consonants 2. prolonged intervals 3. variable rate
	dystonia	1. imprecise consonants 2. distorted vowels 3. harsh voice quality
Unilateral upper motor neuron— (disorders on right or left side)	pseudobulbar palsy	1. imprecise articulation 2. hypernasality 3. slow-labored rate
Mixed dysarthrias—	amyotrophic lateral sclerosis with relative prominence in pseudobulbar palsy and bulbar palsy	1. imprecise consonants 2. hypernasality 3. harsh voice quality

Source: Adapted from F. Darley, A. Aronson, and J. Brown, *Motor Speech Disorders* (Philadelphia: W.B. Saunders, 1975).

(Darley, 1970; De Renzi, Pieczuro, and Vignolo, 1966). For example, an individual may protrude his or her tongue during eating but may be unable to perform this act voluntarily. Although oral apraxia often coexists with verbal apraxia, this is not always the case.

Johns and Darley (1970) compared apraxic and dysarthric speakers on tasks involving spontaneous speaking and reading at a "self-chosen rate" and at a rapid rate. They reported that (1) apraxic speakers were less consistent than dysarthric speakers in their articulatory errors; (2) apraxics made fewer articulation errors and were more intelligible when reading at rapid rates rather than slow rates; (3) apraxics performed better on the spontaneous speaking tasks than on the reading tasks; (4) dysarthrics made fewer errors and were more intelligible when speaking at slow rates rather than fast rates; and (5) distortions accounted for 65 percent of the errors made by dysarthrics but only 10 percent of the errors made by apraxic speakers; substitutions accounted for 50 percent of the errors made by apraxic speakers but only 10 percent of the errors made by dysarthric speakers. Speech sound errors seen in apraxia have usually been identified as sound substitution errors and thereby differentiated from the speech sound distortions seen in dysarthrics. Itoh and Sasanuma (1984) have argued, however, that some of the substitutions seen in apraxia can better be described as distortions, and thus apraxia may be characterized by both substitution and distortion errors. Lapointe and Wertz (1974) described patients who demonstrated a "mixed" articulation disorder consisting of a combination of apraxic and dysarthric speech characteristics.

Developmental Verbal Dyspraxia

A speech sound production disorder, often considered to be neurologically based, is developmental verbal dyspraxia. This disorder is seen in a small percentage of those children who are often labeled as having a "developmental phonological disorder." Such disorders have often been associated with some type of congenital neuromotor impairment in the absence of dysarthria. The labels **developmental verbal dyspraxia** (DVD) and **developmental apraxia of speech** (DAS) are sometimes used to identify this subcategory of children. While the literature in this area is almost exclusively focused on children, Haynes, Johns, and May (1978) have suggested that the syndrome of conditions commonly associated with this disorder may persist to adulthood.

Descriptions of this unique subgroup of phonologically impaired children have existed for some time. Morley (1957), along with other Europeans, was among the first to call attention to this type of developmental speech disorder and to describe this subgroup of articulatory impaired youngsters. During the 1970s, the diagnostic label **developmental apraxia/dyspraxia** came into prominence in the United States to identify a particular subcategory of children who traditionally were identified as having "functional" articulation disorders (disorders of unknown etiology), but whom clinicians suspected as having a subtle motor or neurological basis to their phonological errors.

As stated earlier, apraxia in the adult population is viewed as a motor speech disorder associated with lesions of the nervous system and characterized by an impairment of motor speech programming (i.e., select, plan, organize, and initiate a motor pattern) with no weakness, paralysis, or incoordination of the speech musculature (Darley, 1970; Darley, Aronson, and Brown, 1975). The term *apraxia* has been borrowed from the adult literature to identify a somewhat behaviorally similar, but etiologically dissimilar phenomenon in children. Thus, the term *developmental verbal dyspraxia* or *developmental apraxia* has come to refer to children with articulation errors who also have difficulty with volitional or imitative production of speech sounds and sequences. These symptoms may or may not be accompanied by symptoms of oral apraxia.

Although DVD is widely discussed and a body of literature has developed that addresses the description, assessment, and treatment of the disorder, some controversy has historically persisted over the existence of such a disorder. Some have suggested that it is inappropriate to consider DVD as a "diagnostic entity" of phonologically impaired children since the symptoms attributed to the syndrome are not consistent enough in occurrence or unique enough to support such a designation. In spite of this concern, however, most clinical phonologists acknowledge the existence of such a diagnostic category.

Characteristics of DVD

Rosenbek and Wertz (1972) and Yoss and Darley (1974) conducted early studies that sought to document the characteristics of DVD. More recently, Velleman and Strand (1994) summarized the literature and presented the following features, the presence of which are often felt to be diagnostic:

1. Persistent speech difficulty and/or unintelligibility, including vowel misarticulations, poor or reduced production of consonants, increase in errors as length or complexity of utterance increases, and two and three phoneme features in error
2. Inconsistent errors with some awareness of errors as they occur
3. Difficulty sequencing phonemes, especially in diadochokinesis tasks
4. Groping/silent posturing and difficulties in performing volitional oral movements and sequences of movements
5. Inconsistent timing and control of nasality and prosody
6. Slow progress in therapy

In addition, the following exclusionary features are often used to describe this population:

1. No apparent organic conditions
2. No muscle weakness
3. IQ within normal limits
4. Receptive language within normal limits
5. Normal hearing

Guyette and Diedrich (1981), presenting an earlier extensive review of the literature related to DVD, concluded that (1) there is little agreement on which symptoms or behaviors are important in diagnosis of the disorder; (2) there is a paucity of data to support agreed-upon symptoms; and (3) even when data are available, there is no clear specification of how these data can be used in identifying children.

In spite of the arguments against the validity of the DVD syndrome, however, the diagnosis is supported by clinicians and researchers, including those with a primary concern for neurologically based communication impairments. For those clinicians working with children who are perceived to evidence dyspraxic characteristics, several concepts may be useful in guiding professional actions.

1. Jaffe (1986) has pointed out that DVD appears to be a syndrome in which all symptoms and signs need not be present to diagnose the disorder, nor must one typical sign or symptom be present to establish the diagnosis.
2. Velleman and Strand (1994) point out that the controversy about this disorder centers around the characterization of DVD as a purely motoric disorder with some linguistic symptoms versus a linguistic disorder affecting motor speech. They have further stated that "the existence of a subgroup of children with phonological disorders who demonstrate multiple articulation errors, effortful speech and slow progress in remediation is rarely questioned, but the nature, etiology prognosis and remediation of this disorder have been the subject of debate for a century" (110).
3. It has been suggested (Crary and Towne, 1984) that clinicians should work to better describe the basic motor properties of the deficits seen in dyspraxic children—in other words, keep better records of children's performances on both speech and nonspeech tasks (for both those who are and are not perceived as evidencing motor articulation problems). In this way, we can refine our descriptions and make comparisons among clients.
4. One way to support the presence of a diagnostic category is to demonstrate that particular remediation procedures are effective in ameliorating symptoms. Documenting progress (single subject research designs can be useful in this regard) in response to particular intervention procedures can be helpful in testing the viability of the DAS diagnosis.
5. Love (1992) suggested that "despite the serious questions raised about the etiology, pathology, and validity of the reported signs and symptoms of the DVD syndrome, it remains an appropriate and useful diagnostic category of childhood motor speech disability" (95). He further suggested that DVD "provides substantial assistance in the differential diagnosis of the most prevalent speech disorder encountered by the speech-language pathologist—a developmental phonologic disorder, or so called 'functional articulation disorder.' The appropriate identification of children with phonologic disorders whose etiology is likely neurogenic rather than learned or idiopathic provides added explanatory power to the understanding, assessing, and managing of a select group of children with severe and often unyielding articulation defects that make them special problem cases for the speech-language pathologist" (98).

Chapter 8 presents suggestions for assessment and treatment of developmental verbal dyspraxia.

Cognitive-Linguistic Factors

A second category of variables that have been studied relative to a possible relationship to phonologic productions is that of cognitive-linguistic factors. Historically, the field of communication sciences and disorders has been interested in the relationship between intelligence and the presence of speech sound productions. In more recent years investigators have sought to describe the relationship between disordered phonology and performance on other types of language tasks. Knowledge of the relationship between phonology and these variables is not only useful in determining the type of intervention program that may be most efficacious, but also helps to provide us with a better understanding of overall language behavior.

Intelligence

When identifying factors related to the presence of phonological disorders, one might assume intelligence to be a relevant variable. The relationship between intelligence (as measured by IQ tests) and articulation disorders has been a subject of interest for many years, and of several investigations. Reid (1947a, 1947b) studied the intelligence level of 38 elementary and junior high school students identified as having disordered articulation. Mental ages were obtained from school records and the *California Test of Mental Maturity*. The authors reported that articulation proficiency could not be predicted from intelligence scores when the IQ was 70 or above. Winitz (1959a, 1959b), in his investigation of 150 children, reported similarly low positive correlations between scores obtained on the *Wechsler Intelligence Scale for Children* and the *Templin-Darley Articulation Screening Test*. Thus, in terms of the relationship between intelligence and articulation in children of normal intelligence, data indicated that one is not a good predictor of the other.

A second perspective on the relationship between intelligence and phonology may be gleaned from studies of the phonological status of developmentally delayed individuals. Prior to 1970, a number of studies were conducted to explore the prevalence of articulation disorders in developmentally delayed individuals. Typical of these studies are those of Wilson (1966), Schlanger (1953), and Schlanger and Gottsleben (1957). Wilson used the *Hejina Articulation Test* in his study of 777 mentally retarded children whose chronological ages ranged from 6 to 16 years. He reported that 53.4 percent of the children evidenced articulation disorders. Errors of substitution, omission, and distortion tended to decrease as the mental ages of the children increase. Wilson (1966) concluded that "there is a high incidence of articulatory deviation in an educable mentally retarded population, and the incidence and degree of severity is closely related to mental-age levels" (432). Wilson's findings also indicated that articulatory skills which continue to improve until approximately age 8 in the normal population continue to show improvement well beyond that age in the retarded population.

Schlanger (1953) and Schlanger and Gottsleben (1957) reported similar findings to Wilson in their studies of articulation in the mentally retarded. Schlanger investigated 74 children in a residential school; the children's mean chronological age (C.A.) was 12;1, and their mean mental age (M.A.), 6;8. Of the 74 children, 56.7 percent were found to have articulation disorders. In their study of 400 randomly selected residents at a training school with a chronological age mean of 28;9 and a mean mental age of 7;8, Schlanger and Gottsleben reported that 78 percent presented articulation delays ranging from slight to severe. Individuals with Down's syndrome or whose etiologies were based upon central nervous system impairment demonstrated the most pronounced speech delay.

A review of specific phonologic errors (Bleile, 1982, Smith and Stoel-Gammon, 1983; Sommers, Reinhart, and Sistrunk, 1988) suggests that speech development and error patterns of persons with mental retardation are not qualitatively different from those of young normally developing children. Kumin, Council, and Goodman (1994) reported a great deal of variability in the age at which sounds emerge in the speech of children with Down's syndrome. They also stated that these children do "not appear to follow the same order as the norms for acquisition for typically developing children" (300), and also that emergence of some sounds were as much as five years later than the age in which normally developing children acquire a sound.

Shriberg and Widder (1990) indicated that findings from nearly four decades of speech research in mental retardation can be summarized as follows:

1. Persons with mental retardation are likely to have articulation errors.
2. The most frequent type of articulation error is likely to be deletions of consonants.
3. Articulation errors are likely to be inconsistent.
4. The pattern of articulation errors is likely to be similar to that of very young children or children with "functional" articulation delays.

Several investigators have explored the phonological characteristics of Down's syndrome (DS) individuals, a genetically controlled subset of the mentally retarded population. Sommers, Reinhart, and Sistrunk (1988) reported that among the phonological errors evidenced by DS children ages 13 to 22 years, some were phonemes frequently seen in error in 5- and 6-year-olds of normal intelligence (i.e., /r/, /r/ clusters, /s/, /s/ clusters, /z/, /θ/, and /v/). The authors indicated that these errors would appear to support the assertion that the phonological development of children with DS follows the same general pattern as that of normal children. However, they also reported that DS children evidenced errors not typically seen in normal 5- and 6-year-olds (i.e., deletion of alveolar stops and nasals). They also reported that imitative and spontaneous single-word picture-naming responses of their subjects failed to identify many of the omission errors found in connected speech samples of their subjects.

Rosin, Swift, Bless, and Vetter (1988) studied the articulation of DS children as part of a study of overall communication profiles in this population. They compared a group of 10 DS male subjects (x C.A. = 14;7 years) with a control group of mentally retarded subjects, and two control groups of normals representing two age levels (x C.A. 6;1, 15;5). They reported that as M.A. increased across subjects, intelligibility on a language sample increased. The DS group was also significantly different from the mentally retarded and the younger age normal group (the older group was not compared) in terms of the percent of consonants correctly articulated on the *Goldman-Fristoe Test of Articulation.*

In addition to the speech measures mentioned above, Rosin and colleagues (1988) also included other language measures, an oral motor evaluation, and aerodynamic measures in their assessment. They reported that the DS group had more difficulty with production measures as demands for sequencing increased (e.g., consonant-vowel repetitions, length of words). The DS group needed a significant amount of cueing in order to articulate the target /pataka/, and had more variable intraoral pressure when producing /papapaps/. The mean length of utterance of the DS group was also significantly shorter. The authors indicated that these findings are in accord with observations of others and suggested that sequencing underlies both oral motor control and language problems evidenced in DS subjects.

Summary

Investigators concur that there is a low positive correlation between intelligence and articulatory function within the range of normal intelligence, and thus it can be inferred that intellectual functioning is of limited importance as a contributing factor to articulatory skill, and can be viewed as a poor predictor of articulation. On the other hand, a much higher correlation has been found between intelligence and articulation in the mentally retarded population. The articulatory skills in individuals with Down's syndrome reflect error patterns similar to those seen in young normally developing children; however, they also evidence errors that are considered deviant or unusual.

Language Development

Because phonology is one component of a child's developing linguistic system, there has been a natural interest in the relationship between phonologic development and development of other aspects of language (i.e., morphology/syntax, semantics, pragmatics). Of particular interest to clinical phonologists has been the extent to which delay or disorders in phonology may co-occur with delay or disorder in other aspects of language.

Whitaker, Luper, and Pollio (1970) reported that children with articulation disorders were also impaired in language skills involving knowledge of phonological rules, form classes, and sentence structure. Subjects ranged in age from 6;1, to 7;7 and included both an articulation disorders group and a normal control group. All subjects in the disorders group failed to meet the cutoff score for 7-year-old children on the *Templin-Darley Articulation Screening Test*. The authors reported that the disordered group appeared to be developing language in the normal sequence but at a retarded rate.

Shriner, Holloway, and Daniloff (1969) compared the language skills of a normal control group with those of a group of 30 children between the ages of 5 and 8 who were considered to have severe articulation disorders (had at least seven articulatory errors and scored one standard deviation below the mean on the *Templin-Darley Tests of Articulation*). Subjects in the articulatory-defective group used significantly shorter and less complex utterances in their spontaneous conversation than members of the control group.

The relationship between articulation disorders and language comprehension was explored by Marquardt and Saxman (1972) using two groups of kindergarten children; one group performed one standard deviation or more below the norm for that age on the *Templin-Darley Tests of Articulation*, and the other (the control group) produced no more than one defective sound. The investigators administered the *Test of Auditory Comprehension of Language* and found that the impaired group made significantly more language comprehension errors than the control group. A correlation of scores obtained on both measures revealed that children who made the greatest number of articulation errors also made the greatest number of errors in language comprehension.

Gross, St. Louis, Ruscello, and Hull (1985) studied the language skills of three groups of school-age subjects: (1) a group with multiple articulation errors; defined as those with at least two errors in the final position; with /l/, /r/, and /s/ not included in this consideration; (2) a group with residual articulation errors; defined as two or more positional errors for at least one of the following phonemes: /l/, /r/, and /s/. Consonant cluster errors on these phonemes were allowed, but subjects could have no other phonemic errors; and (3) a normal control group. A total of 144 subjects from grades 1, 3, 5, and 7 were included in this retrospective study. The investigators reported that mean language structural scores for completeness and complexity were significantly lower for the multiple error group than the residual error and control groups. Scores for length of utterances were not significantly different among groups. The total number of language errors reduced progressively from multiple error to residual error to control groups.

Research investigations such as those cited above, which have attempted to explore the correlation between certain aspects of language and phonology, have generally reported a moderate correlation between phonologic and language disorders. After reviewing literature related to the language-phonology relationship, Tyler and Watterson (1991) indicated that one might expect to find disorders of language and phonology co-occurring in 60 to 80 percent of the young children who have been identified as having a disorder of one type or the other. Shriberg and Kwiatkowski (1994) reported that based on 178 children with developmental phonological disorders that between 50 and 70 percent of the children will have productive language involvement and 10–40 percent will also have a delay in language comprehension.

Some investigators have attempted to further study and explain the interaction between phonology and other aspects of language, especially syntax. A common perception is that language is organized "from the top down"—in other words, a speaker goes from pragmatic intent, to semantic coding, to syntactic structure, to phonologic productions. Thus, higher-level linguistic formulations may ultimately be reflected in a child's phonologic productions. If this theory is accurate, it might be expected that the more complex the syntax, the more likely a child is to evidence linguistic breakdown, which may then be evidenced in phonologic productions. Schmauch, Panagos, and Klich (1978) conducted a study in which 5-year-old children with phonologic and language problems were required to produce certain nouns (drawn from phonologic inventories) in three syntactic contexts; that is, an isolated noun phrase, a declarative sentence, and a passive sentence. These investigators reported a 17 percent increase in articulatory errors between the noun phrase and each of the sentence contexts. They also reported that later developing consonants were those most influenced by syntactical complexity and that error productions reflected quantitative rather than qualitative changes.

A follow-up study of the top-down notion was conducted by Panagos, Quine, and Klich (1979). In this study, 5-year-old children were required to produce 15 target consonants in noun phrases, declarative sentences, and passive sentences; consonants appeared in the initial and final word-positions of one- and two-syllable words. Syntax was again found to significantly influence articulatory accuracy, as did number of syllables in target words. Word position did not influence phonologic accuracy. The authors further reported that two sources of complexity—phonologic (including difficulty with later developing consonants as well as specific contexts) and syntactic—combined additively to increase the number of phonologic errors. From the easiest context (final word position, one-syllable word, noun phrase) to the hardest (final word position, two-syllable word, passive sentence), there was a 36 percent increase in articulatory errors. The effects of grammatical complexity on articulatory accuracy were cumulative.

A second perspective on the language-phonology relationship suggests that linguistic influences operate "from the bottom up." In this view, language expression is regulated by feedback (internal and external) from phonologic performance. Feedback from phonologic performance is needed to maintain syntactic processing and accuracy, especially when errors occur and must be corrected.

Panagos and Prelock (1982) conducted a study to test the hypothesis that phonologic structure influences children's syntactic processing. Ten children with language disorders were required to produce sentences containing words with varying syllable complexity; that is, **simple**: "The (CV) kid (CVC) pushed (CVCC) the (CV) car (CVC) in (VC) the (CV) room (CVC)," and **complex**: "The (CV) chocolate (CVCVCVC) is (VC) in (VC) the (CV) napkin (CVCCVC)." In addition, sentence complexity was varied from unembedded ("The girl washed the doll in the tub") to right embedded ("The cook washed the pot the boy dropped") to center embedded ("The lady the uncle liked sewed the coat"). The results of the study supported the hypothesis. When subjects repeated sentences containing words of greater syllable complexity, they made 27 percent more syntactic errors. In addition to this bottom-up influence, Panagos and Prelock (1982) also reported that syntactic complexity further compounded production difficulties. From the unembedded to the center embedded, there was a 57 percent increase in phonologic errors.

These findings support the view that a simultaneous top-down–bottom-up relationship exists between language and phonology. Another way of expressing this concept is to consider that children with disordered language-phonology have a limited encoding capacity; and the more this capacity is strained at one level or another, the greater the probability of delay in one component or more of language. It should be pointed out that the study by Panagos and Prelock (1982), as well as others in a series of experimental studies, employed elicited imitation tasks, and thus complexity of utterances was controlled by the investigators. It can be argued that with this type of performance task, structural simplifications are expected outcomes. Elicited imitation tasks do not reflect the conditions present when a child is engaged in conversation, and thus we cannot assume that constraints of the nature demonstrated by Panagos and Prelock can predict behavior in a conversational context (Paul and Shriberg, 1984).

In an investigation by Paul and Shriberg (1982) designed to study phonologic productions as they relate to particular morphophonemic structures, continuous speech samples were obtained in 30 speech-delayed children. They found that in over half their subjects general syntactic delays accompanied delayed phonologic development. They also reported that certain of their subjects were able to produce complex morphosyntactic contexts spontaneously, which did not result in phonologic simplifications. In other words, some of their subjects were able to maintain a similar level of phonologic production in spite of producing more complex syntactic targets. They suggested (Paul and Shriberg, 1984) that children may "do things other than phonologic simplification in an attempt to control complexity in spontaneous speech" (319). They summarized by indicating that some speech-delayed children are sometimes able to allocate their limited linguistic resources to realize phonologic targets consistent with their linguistic knowledge in the context of free speech, even though at other times they may use avoidance strategies or other means of reducing the encoding load.

A *synergistic view* of language (Schwartz, Leonard, Folger, and Wilcox, 1980; Shriner et al., 1969) assumes a complex interaction and interdependency of various aspects of linguistic behaviors including language and phonology. Experimental evidence for this view was provided by Matheny and Panagos (1978), who looked at the effects of syntactic programming on phonologic improvement and the effects of phonologic programming on syntactic improvement in school-age children. Syntactic training resulted in both phonologic and syntactic improvement, and phonologic intervention resulted in significant gains in syntactic development as well as phonologic performance. Similar findings were reported by Hoffman, Norris, and Monjure (1990). Based on a study of two siblings from a set of triplets, they reported that language-based therapy not only resulted in improvement in syntax-morphology but also in phonology. Phonologic instruction, however, resulted only in improvement in phonology but not syntax morphology. These findings have not been supported in the research of Tyler and Watterson (1991) or Fey, Cleave, Ravida, Long, Dejmal, and Easton (1994) who reported that language-focused intervention did not impact phonologic errors.

Results of the experimental treatment studies identified above reinforce the complexity of the language-phonology interaction. Tyler and Watterson (1991) reported that subjects with a severe overall language and phonological disorder made improvements in language when presented with language therapy; however, gains were not made in phonology (they actually reported a tendency for performance to become worse). On the other hand, subjects with mild-moderate but unequal impairments in phonology and language, improved in both areas when presented with phonologic therapy. The authors suggested that a language-based intervention program may not result in improvement in phonologic as well as other language skills for children whose disorders are severe and comparable in each domain. However, children with less severe problems in one or both domains may benefit from therapy with either a language or phonology focus.

Fey and colleagues (1994) conducted an experimental treatment program with 26 subjects, ages 44–70 months, with impairments in both grammar and phonology. Eighteen children received language intervention (grammar facilitation) in accord with one or another of two designated teaching approaches and eight children served as controls. Results indicated that despite a strong effect for intervention on the children's grammatical output, there were no direct effects on the subjects' phonologic productions. The authors indicated that trying to improve intelligibility by focusing on grammar is not defensible for children in the age and severity range of their subjects. They further indicated that for most children who have impairments in both speech and language, intervention will need to be focused on both areas. While this study only examined one form of language intervention that anticipated phonologic effects, these data provide strong evidence that in children aged 4–6 treatment approaches should address phonologic problems directly if changes in phonologic performance are to be expected. Clearly, further developmental and clinical studies are needed to clarify the interactions between phonology and other aspects of language. The influences of age, severity, and specific treatment approaches need further study. Perhaps studies where these variables are manipulated will lend a better understanding of the relationship between phonology and language.

Summary

Research has shown that younger children with severe phonologic disorders are more likely to evidence language problems than those with mild-moderate delay and that up to 80 percent of moderate to severely involved phonologically delayed children are likely to also have language delay. Language and phonology may be related in what has been termed a synergistic relationship. Investigators face the challenge of further defining the intricacies of the relationship between phonology and other linguistic behaviors in terms of both development and clinical management of disorders. It also appears that for children with moderate to severe phonologic delay, direct phonologic intervention is the treatment strategy of choice for the phonologic component.

Academic Performance

The relationship between phonologic disorders and educational problems is of interest to clinicians working with school-age children since oral language skills are fundamental to the development of many academic skills such as reading and spelling. Because the use of sounds in symbolic lexical units is a task common to learning to speak, read, and write, researchers for many years have studied the co-occurrence of reading and articulation disorders, and have discussed possible common factors underlying the acquisition of literacy and other language-related skills.

Hall (1938) compared 21 children with functional articulation disorders with a normal control group on the *Gates Silent Reading Test* and the *Iowa Silent Reading Test* and reported no significant differences in silent reading achievement between the two groups. Everhart (1953) also used the *Gates Reading Test* and reported no significant relationship between articulatory disorders and reading ability, although boys with normal articulation tended to obtain higher reading scores than the overall group of children with articulation disorders.

The relationship between reading readiness and articulation development in children with and without defective articulation was studied by Fitzsimons (1958) and Weaver, Furbee, and Everhart (1960). Fitzsimons used the *Metropolitan Reading Readiness Test* to determine the status of reading readiness and reported that below grade-level scores were more frequent among children with articulation disorders than among those with normally developing articulation. Weaver and colleagues (1960) reported a significant relationship between articulatory performance and reading readiness as well as between articulatory performance and reading scores.

Flynn and Byrne (1970) took a different approach to exploring the relationship between articulation disorders and reading. They compared articulatory performance of 52 advanced and 42 delayed third-grade readers on the *Templin-Darley Tests of Articulation*. Those who scored 4.2 or higher on the *Iowa Test of Basic Skills* were classified as advanced readers; those who scored 2.2 or lower as delayed readers. The authors reported no significant difference between the two groups in articulation test scores.

Lewis and Freebairn-Farr (1991) conducted a cross-sectional study designed to examine the performance of individuals with a history of a preschool phonologic disorder on measures of phonology, reading, and spelling. Groups of subjects included at least 17 individuals from each of the following categories: preschool, school age, adolescence, and adulthood. Normal comparison groups at each age level were also tested. Significant differences between the disordered and normal groups were reported on the reading and spelling measures for the school-age group, and on the reading measure for the adult group. Although the reading and spelling measures for the adolescent group and the spelling measure for the adult group did not reach significance, the trend was for the individuals with histories of disorders to perform more poorly than normals. Data also indicated that subjects who evidenced a phonologic disorder accompanied by additional language problems performed more poorly on measures of reading and spelling than subjects with phonologic disorders only. The authors indicated that children evidencing phonologic impairment are at risk for reading and spelling problems in school and may have special educational needs.

Felsenfeld, McGue, and Broen (1995) conducted a comparison study of the children of 24 adults with a documented history of a phonologic-language disorder that persisted from childhood until at least grade 11 (proband group), and 28 adults who were known to have had normal articulation abilities as children (control group). Included among the comparison variables were several categorized under "educational performance." Results revealed that 28 percent of the children of the proband group repeated at least one grade, compared to 0 percent from the control group. Likewise, 22 percent of the proband children compared to 4 percent of the controls had received academic tutoring. Speech treatment had been received by 33 percent of the proband group and 0 percent of the controls. They also reported that half of the school-age children who were receiving speech treatment were also either participating in remedial academic services and/or had repeated a grade.

While interest has traditionally focused on the co-occurrence of reading-spelling and phonologic disorders in children, more recently there has also been interest in children's ability to process phonology as part of various reading tasks. More specifically, some reading-disabled students may lack awareness of individual sounds, have difficulty dividing words into sounds, and recalling sound-symbol relationships (phonologic awareness). Catts (1986) found that reading-disabled children may have problems with these linguistically oriented tasks and yet not reflect phonologic impairments.

Researchers have attempted to apply phonologic concepts to aid in the understanding of reading and spelling disorders. This activity is based on the assumption that acquisition of speaking, reading, and writing skills involves the analysis of sounds in lexical units, which may be related to underlying cognitive-linguistic processes. In particular, the concepts of phonologic processes and underlying internal knowledge of the sound system have been employed to aid in understanding the development of spelling and reading skills (Hoffman and Norris, 1989).

Liberman and Shankweiler (1985), in a discussion of the phonologic basis of literacy, indicated that reading success was related to the degree to which children were aware of "underlying phonologic structure" and that poor readers often were unable to segment words into their phonologic constituents. They suggested that a relationship exists between children's readiness for reading and spelling and their metalinguistic awareness of the internal structure of words.

Catts (1991) suggested that speech-language pathologists working in school systems should seek to develop programs designed to facilitate "phonologic awareness" in children, particularly those at risk for reading disabilities. Catts suggested that "phonologic awareness" activities might include activities designed to increase awareness of syllables, phonemes, manner of phoneme production, and sound positions in words. Activities to accomplish these goals could include sound play, rhyming, alliteration, and segmentation tasks. This topic is discussed in greater detail in Chapter 8.

Hoffman and Norris (1989) analyzed spelling errors of 45 elementary school children for evidence of phonologic process patterns. They reported that many of the spelling errors involved both syllable reduction and feature changes similar to the sound simplifications seen in the speech of young children with normal speech development. They further indicated that even though children had acquired normal speech, they exhibited spelling errors similar to those seen in the speech simplifications of younger children. Hoffman (1990) related specific types of developmental spelling patterns to stages of normal phonologic acquisition. For example, "precommunicative spellings" (seemingly random selection of letters of the alphabet to represent words), were described as parallel to the random sound productions of babbling. "Semiphonetic spellings" (letters used to represent sounds, but only some of the sounds are represented, e.g., *E* for *eagle*), were described as parallel to the stage where children delete syllables or segments and substitute sound classes for one another. He also indicated that because the speech-language pathologist is the school-based professional who has the most detailed knowledge of sound perception and production, phonologic organization, stages of acquisition, and methods of phonologic description, he or she is in a good position to serve as a resource to teachers regarding the application of phonologic concepts to the understanding of spelling errors.

Summary
Research investigations that have focused on the co-occurrence of phonologic and reading disorders indicate a possible relationship between these in some children. Data indicate that young children with severe phonologic and/or other language disorders are at risk for academic problems, and there may be a familial propensity for such difficulties. More recently interest has focused on the role of "phonologic awareness" in the development of reading and spelling skills. Parallels have been made between the use of phonologic processes and stages in the acquisition of oral language and acquisition of reading and spelling skills. It has been suggested that speech-language pathologists are in a unique position to offer assistance to the classroom teacher in their efforts to assist children at risk for reading and/or spelling problems.

Psychosocial Factors

Psychosocial factors represent a third cluster of variables that have long fascinated clinicians in terms of their potential relationship to phonology. Age, gender, family history, and socioeconomic status have been studied in an effort to better understand factors that may precipitate or otherwise be associated with phonologic impairment.

Age

Chapters 2 and 3 reviewed the literature on phonologic acquisition. Investigations of phonologic development have revealed that children's articulatory and phonologic skills continue to improve until approximately 8 years of age, by which time the normal child has acquired most aspects of the adult sound system. In fact, it appears that by age 4 normally developing children have articulation that closely resembles that of adults (Hodson and Paden, 1981).

Speech-language pathologists use normative information concerning phonologic development as a guide in case selection and for determining treatment goals. Clinicians should keep in mind that the order in which sounds are incorporated into speech varies from child to child and does not necessarily follow a specific sequence. There is no indication that one sound is dependent on any other for its development.

Speech-language pathologists have shown a particular interest in the effect of maturation on children identified as having phonologic disorders. Roe and Milisen (1942) sampled 1,989 children in grades 1 through 6 and found that the children's mean number of articulation errors decreased between grades 1 and 2, grades 2 and 3, and grades 3 and 4. In contrast, the difference in the mean number of errors between grades 4 and 5 and grades 5 and 6 was not significant. The authors concluded that maturation was responsible for improvement in articulation performance between grades 1 and 4 but was not an appreciable factor in articulation improvement in grades 5 and 6.

Sayler (1949) assessed articulation in 1,998 students in grades 7 through 12 as they read sentences orally. His findings indicated a slight decrease in the mean number of articulation errors at each subsequent grade level, but because the improvement in speech sound productions was so small, he concluded that maturation does not appear to be an appreciable factor in improvement in the secondary grades. Children in upper elementary and secondary grades appear to be more consistent in their phonologic patterns than children in the lower elementary grades.

Factors that relate to phonologic variations during the school years include refinement of the timing of sequential articulatory gestures, the influence of reading and spelling, and peer influence (Vihman, Chapter 3 of this book). These factors would only result in, at most, minor phonologic variations within this age group.

Summary

Acquisition by a child of the adult speech sound system has been shown to be related to maturation. There is a direct correlation between improvement in articulation skills and age through approximately age 8. In other words, the probability of a child outgrowing a phonologic delay is much higher prior to than after age 9 in normally developing children.

Gender

Child development specialists have long been interested in contrasts between males and females in phonologic acquisition, and, likewise, speech-language pathologists have investigated the relationship between gender and articulation status. Research in this area has focused on (1) a comparison of phoneme acquisition in males and females, and (2) a comparison of the incidence of phonologic disorders in males and females.

Dawson (1929) examined the articulatory skills of 200 children from grades 1 through 12 on six measures of articulation. He reported that until approximately age 12, girls were slightly superior to boys in their articulatory skills. Templin (1963) reported similar findings: "In articulation development, girls consistently are found to be slightly accelerated . . . in all instances the differences are relatively small and often are not statistically significant" (13).

Smit, Hand, Freilinger, Bernthal, and Bird (1990) conducted a large-scale normative study of phonologic development in children ages 3 through 9 from Iowa and Nebraska. They reported that the Iowa-Nebraska girls appeared to acquire sounds at somewhat earlier ages than boys through age 6. The differences reached statistical significance only at age 6 and younger, and not in every preschool age group.

Speech surveys conducted by Hall (1938), Mills and Streit (1942), Morley (1952), Everhart (1960), and Hull, Mielke, Timmons, and Willeford (1971) indicated that the incidence of articulation disorder was higher in males than females, regardless of the age group studied. Smit and colleagues (1990) stated that "it is a well-known fact that boys are at much greater risk than girls for delayed speech, and this propensity continues to be reported" (790). Kenney and Prather (1986), who elicited multiple productions of frequent error sounds, reported significant differences favoring girls in the age range 3 through 5. Contrary to the above findings, Winitz (1959a) reported no significant differences between the articulatory skills of 75 males and 75 females entering kindergarten.

After a review of the literature on articulatory differences between the sexes, Perkins (1977) and Winitz (1969) both concluded that gender is a minor variable in the development of articulatory skill.

Summary

The sex of a child does not appear to be a significant factor in phonologic acquisition. It should be recognized, however, that at certain ages females tend to be slightly ahead of males in phonologic acquisition, and significantly more male than female children are identified as being phonologically delayed.

Family Background

Researchers have been interested in the influence of family background, both environmental and biological, and how it may affect a child's speech and language development. In the paragraphs below we will review literature related to family background and phonology organized around three topics: (1) socioeconomic status, (2) family transmission, and (3) sibling influences.

Socioeconomic Status

The socioeconomic status of a child's family, as measured by parents' educational background, parental occupation, income, and location of family residence, is a significant part of the child's environment. Since some behavioral deficiencies occur more frequently in lower socioeconomic environments, socioeconomic status has been of interest to speech-language clinicians as a possible factor in language development.

Everhart (1953, 1956) explored the variable of parental occupational status in an investigation of the relationship between articulation and other developmental factors in children. In speech surveys of children in grades 1 through 6, those classified as having articulation disorders were compared to children with normal articulation development with respect to parental occupation. No significant differences were found, and Everhart concluded that the occurrence of articulation disorders in children was not related to parental occupation. Winitz (1959a, 1959b) also reported no significant relationships between ratings of socioeconomic status and scores obtained from an articulation screening test on 150 kindergarten children.

Templin (1957) analyzed developmental language data from children aged 3 to 8 years in terms of parental occupation and reached a somewhat different conclusion. She used the *Minnesota Scale for Parental Occupations* to categorize parental occupation. At each age level, children whose parents were in the upper occupational group had fewer misarticulations than the children in the lower occupational group. In particular, 4-, $4\frac{1}{2}$-, and 7-year-old children whose parents were in the lower occupational group had significantly more articulation errors than those whose parents were in the upper group. Templin concluded that parental occupation seemed to be a factor in children's articulation skill until about age 4 but that parental occupation no longer seemed to influence articulation development by the time children were 8 years old.

Weaver, Furbee, and Everhart (1960) also investigated the relationship between parental occupation and articulation proficiency in 592 first-grade children and found that a greater number of children with normal articulation skills came from homes in the upper occupational group, whereas more children with articulation errors came from homes in the lower occupational group. The poorest articulation proficiency, as judged by number of articulation errors, was found among children from the two lowest occupational classes.

Prins (1962a) found no significant correlation between articulation and socioeconomic level for 92 articulatory defective children between the ages of 2 and 6 years. Likewise, Smit and colleagues (1990) in the Iowa-Nebraska normative study reported that socioeconomic level did not have a significant relationship to articulatory performance. After an extensive review of the literature on the relationship between articulation and socioeconomic status, Winitz (1969) concluded that "more misarticulating children and more articulatory errors are found in the lower socioeconomic groups than in the upper socioeconomic groups. However, when a correlational index is used, the relationship is low or nonsignificant" (147).

Familial Tendencies
It is not uncommon for speech-language pathologists to observe a family history for developmental speech and language disorders. While information of this nature is often noted in diagnostic reports, until the 1980s few systematic attempts were made to study phonologic disorders as they related to family history. Neils and Aram (1986) obtained reports from the parents of 74 preschool language-disordered children and indicated that 46 percent reported that other family members had histories of speech and language disorders. Of this group, 55 percent were reported to have articulation disorders, the most prevalent type of familial disorder reported. Shriberg and Kwiatkowski (1994) reported data from sixty-two 3- to 6-year-old children with developmental phonologic disorders. They found that 39 percent of the children had one member of the family with the same speech problem, while an additional 17 percent (total = 56 percent) had more than one family member with the same speech problem.

Two twin studies have been reported that contribute to our understanding of familial influences, including genetic factors that may relate to phonologic disorders. Matheny and Bruggeman (1973) studied 101 same-sex twin sets, 22 opposite-sex twin sets, and 94 siblings between the ages of 3 and 8 years. An articulation screening test was administered to each child. Monozygotic twins' articulation screening correlated more closely with each other than did dizygotic twins' scores. The authors concluded that there is a strong hereditary influence on articulation status. In addition, sex differences were found to favor females. Locke and Mather (1987) examined speech sound productions in 13 monozygotic and 13 dizygotic twin sets. They reported more phonetic concordance in the monozygotic than the dizygotic twins.

Lewis, Ekelman, and Aram (1989) examined the familial basis of phonologic disorders by comparing sibling articulation status for a group of children identified as evidencing a severe phonologic disorder, and a group whose siblings reflected abnormal phonologic development. Phonologic measures included the *Natural Process Analysis*, repetition of 50 multisyllabic words, and the *Screening Test for Developmental Verbal Apraxia*. In addition, language, gross and fine motor skills, and reading were assessed. Family histories of communication disorders and/or learning disabilities were noted. Results revealed that the siblings of the disordered children performed more poorly than control siblings on phonology and reading measures. Disordered subjects' phonologic skills correlated positively with those of their siblings, whereas controls' scores did not. Families of disordered children reported significantly more members with speech and language disorders and dyslexia than did families of controls. Sex differences were reflected in the incidence but not in the severity or type of disorder present. The authors concluded that their findings suggested a familial basis for at least some forms of severe phonologic disorders.

One of the most comprehensive studies of the familial basis of phonologic impairments was conducted by Felsenfeld and colleagues (1995). These investigators utilized speech and academic development data involving 400 normally developing children that was gathered between 1960 and 1972 by Templin and Glaman (1976). From this large sample, two follow-up groups were identified consisting of 24 adults with a history of a moderate phonologic-language disorder as children, and a control group of 28 adults with a documented history of normal articulation development. Results demonstrated that in comparison to the children of controls, the children of the "disordered" subjects performed significantly more poorly on all tests of articulation and expressive language functioning and were significantly more likely to have received articulation treatment. There was, however, no evidence that specific misarticulations or phonologic processes could be identified with the "disorders" families.

It may be inferred from the studies reviewed above that genetic or biological inheritance factors may precipitate phonologic impairment, yet it is often difficult to separate environmental from genetic/biological influences. A study that examined environmental influences was reported by Parlour and Broen (1991). Their research was predicated on the possibility that individuals who themselves experienced significant speech and language disorders as children are likely to become adults who will provide a less than optimal cultural or linguistic milieu for their own families.

Parlour and Broen collected follow-up family data of adults with and without a childhood history of delayed phonologic development. Both groups of subjects were originally part of the large normative study that was conducted by Mildred Templin (1968), 28 years earlier. The group who had displayed a moderate to moderately severe phonologic disorder in early elementary school was comprised of 24 individuals. The control group was comprised of 28 adults who had evidenced average or better articulation during the same time period. Two environmental measures, the *Preschool HOME Scale* and the *Modified Templin Child-Rearing Questionnaire*, were employed to ascertain qualitative aspects of a child's environment including physical, emotional, and cognitive support available to preschool children, and child-rearing practices. These two measures included direct observation of the examiner, parental reports, and parental responses to a written questionnaire.

The two groups performed in a generally comparable manner for all of the environmental domains sampled, with one exception, **acceptance**, which assessed disciplinary practices. Parlour and Broen (1991) reported that families with a history of phonologic disorders were more reliant on physical punishment than were control families. In terms of future research efforts, the authors suggested that although differences were generally not significant between the groups, the disordered group received lower mean scores than controls on each of the Home subscales, suggesting that some subtle differences may have been present, particularly for domains involving the use of punishment, learning, and language stimulation.

Sibling Influence

Another factor of interest to investigators of phonologic acquisition has been sibling number and birth order. Since the amount of time that parents can spend with each child decreases with each child added to a family, some clinicians have questioned whether sibling status is related to articulatory development. Koch (1956) studied the relationships between certain speech and voice characteristics in young children and siblings in two-child families. In this study, 384 children between 5 and 6 years old were divided into 24 matched subgroups matched individual by individual on the basis of age, socioeconomic class, and residence. Data on speech and voice characteristics consisted of teachers' ratings. Koch reported that firstborn children had better articulation than secondborn, and the wider the age difference between a child and his or her sibling, the better the child's articulation. Likewise, Davis (1937) reported that children without siblings demonstrated superior articulatory performance to children with siblings and to twins. On the other hand, Wellman, Case, Mengert, and Bradbury (1931) did not find a significant relationship between the number of siblings and level of articulation skill for 3-year-olds.

Twins have been reported to present unique patterns of speech sound acquisition (Perkins, 1977; Powers, 1971; Winitz, 1969). From birth, twins receive speech stimulation not only from others within their environment but also from each other. Powers (1971) indicated that the "emotional ties of twins, too, are likely to be closer than those of singled siblings, which further augments their interdependence in speech" (868). It is not uncommon for twins to reflect common phonologic patterns and use similar phonologic processes. Schwartz, Leonard, Folger, and Wilcox (1980) reported, however, that in the very early stages of phonologic acquisition (the first 50 words), similarities in phonemes used, including phonologic patterns and lexical items, were not present. Unique patterns of speech occasionally found in twins 2 years and older that have little resemblance to adult models and are meaningful only to the twins are termed *idioglossia*.

Summary

Little relationship exists between socioeconomic and articulation status based on available reports. Although greater numbers of misarticulating children tend to be found in lower socioeconomic groups (especially children under 4 years), socioeconomic status does not appear to contribute to the presence of a phonologic disorder.

Studies of phonologic development in twins, as well as in families with a history of phonologic impairment, suggest some sort of familial propensity toward the presence of such a disorder.

Investigations examining phonologic status and sibling relationships are limited, but findings have been fairly consistent. Firstborn and only children exhibit significantly better articulation performance than children with older siblings or twins. The age span between siblings also appears to affect phonologic proficiency, with better articulation associated with wider age differences. One can speculate that the firstborn or only child receives better speech models and greater stimulation than the child who has older siblings. The possibility also exists that older siblings produce "normal" developmental phonologic errors and, thus at points in time present imperfect speech models to younger siblings. Unique patterns of sound productions have been found in twins; reasons for these patterns are speculative and tend to focus on the stimulation each twin receives from the other. Differences in phonology have, however, been reported, even in very young twins.

Personality

The relationship between personality characteristics and phonologic behavior has been investigated to determine if particular personality patterns are likely to be associated with phonologic disorders. Researchers have examined not only the child's personality traits but also those of the child's parents, using various assessment tools.

In a review of research in phonologic disorders and personality, Spriestersbach (1956) criticized the term *personality* as vague and argued that numerous obstacles are confronted when trying to test a construct that has such divergent definitions. He concluded that "the contribution of research to an understanding of the relationship between articulatory defects and personality is largely negative" (334).

Bloch and Goodstein (1971) concluded, in a later review of similar literature spanning a 10-year period, that evidence of personality differences exists between parents of children who present articulatory deficits and parents of children with normal articulation. They noted that studies of the personality traits and emotional adjustment of individuals with articulatory disorders have shown contradictory findings and attributed this to two major problems with the investigations: (1) the criteria for defining articulatory impaired has varied from one study to the next, and (2) the tools or instruments used to assess personality and adjustment have varied in their validity and reliability.

In a causal-correlates profile based on 178 children with developmental phonologic disorders, Shriberg and Kwiatkowski (1994) presented data on psychosocial inputs (parental behaviors) and psychosocial behaviors (child characteristics) that were descriptive of this population. Twenty-seven (27) percent of the parents were judged to be either somewhat or considerably ineffective in terms of behavioral management, and 17 percent were either somewhat or considerably overconcerned about their child's problem. An even smaller percentage of parents indicated that it was their perception that their child had difficulty with initial acceptance by peers. Over half the children (51 percent) were described as somewhat too sensitive (easily hurt feelings), and an additional 14 percent were described as overly sensitive (very easily hurt feelings). They reported that their descriptive data indicated that "a significant number of children with developmental phonologic disorders experience psychosocial difficulties" (1115). They indicated, however, that one cannot be completely certain that sampling biases did not inflate the magnitudes of the findings, or whether the subjects would differ significantly from data in a nonspeech-delayed group.

Parlour and Broen (1991) studied environmental factors in the homes of 24 adults who as children evidenced moderate to moderately severe phonologic disorders, and a control group of adults who as children evidenced average or better articulation. Two environmental measures, the *Preschool HOME Scale* and the *Modified Templin Child-Rearing Questionnaire*, were used to study and rate aspects of the home presumed to reflect the quality of physical, emotional, and cognitive support available to a preschool child. While the findings for the two groups were generally similar, mean scores for the group with a history of phonologic disorders were lower than for the normal group. A significant difference between the two groups was found in disciplinary practices, suggesting that "disorders" families were more reliant on physical punishment than were control families.

Summary

While certain personality characteristics have been linked to some children with developmental phonologic impairments, no clear picture of personality variance from normals has emerged in this population. Likewise, certain parental/home variables have been associated with this population, but the strength of that association is unclear. Further studies involving normal–disordered child comparisons are necessary before a definitive statement regarding this causal-correlate can be made.

Conclusion

The speech-language pathologist must have a basic knowledge of factors related to phonologic disorders in order to assess phonologic status, plan remediation programs, and counsel clients and their parents. Despite the large body of literature reflecting investigations of variables potentially related to articulation impairments, many questions remain unanswered. One truth that emerges from the literature, however, is the absence of any one-to-one correspondence between the presence of a particular etiological factor and the nature of most individuals' phonologic status. Prediction of cause-effect relationships represents a scientific ideal, but determination of such relationships in the realm of human behavior, including communication disorders, is extremely difficult.

References

American Speech-Language-Hearing Association, "Report of ad hoc committee on labial-lingual posturing function." *Asha, 31* (1989): 92–94.

American Speech-Language-Hearing Association, "The role of the speech-language pathologist in management of oral myofunctional disorders." *Asha, 33* (suppl. 5) (1991): 7.

Arndt, W., M. Elbert, and R. Shelton, "Standardization of a test of oral stereognosis." In J. Bosman (Ed.), *Second Symposium on Oral Sensation and Perception*. Springfield, Ill.: Charles C Thomas, 1970.

Arndt, W., R. Shelton, A. Johnson, and M. Furr, "Identification and description of homogeneous subgroups within a sample of misarticulating children." *Journal of Speech and Hearing Research, 20* (1977): 263–292.

Arnst, D., and D. Fucci, "Vibrotactile sensitivity of the tongue in hearing impaired subjects." *Journal of Auditory Research, 15* (1975): 115–118.

Aungst, L., and J. Frick, "Auditory discrimination ability and consistency of articulation of /r/." *Journal of Speech and Hearing Disorders, 29* (1964): 76–85.

Backus, O., "Speech rehabilitation following excision of tip of the tongue." *American Journal of the Disabled Child, 60* (1940): 368–370.

Bankson, N., and M. Byrne, "The relationship between missing teeth and selected consonant sounds." *Journal of Speech and Hearing Disorders, 24* (1962): 341–348.

Barton, D., "The role of perception in the acquisition of phonology." Ph.D. Dissertation, University of London, 1976.

Bernstein, M., "The relation of speech defects and malocclusion." *American Journal of Orthodontia, 40* (1954): 149–150.

Bishop, M., R. Ringel, and H. House, "Orosensory perception, speech production and deafness." *Journal of Speech and Hearing Research, 16* (1973): 257–266.

Bleile, K., "Consonant ordering in Down's Syndrome," *Journal of Communicative Disorders, 15* (1982): 275–285.

Bloch, R., and L. Goodstein, "Functional speech disorders and personality: A decade of research," *Journal of Speech and Hearing Disorders, 36* (1971): 295–314.

Bloomer, H., and A. Hawk, "Speech considerations: Speech disorders associated with ablative surgery of the face, mouth and pharynx—ablative approaches to learning." In *Asha Report #8: Orofacial Anomalies*. Washington, D.C.: Asha, 1973.

Bordon, G., "Consideration of motor-sensory targets and a problem of perception." In H. Winitz (Ed.), *Treating Articulation Disorders: For Clinicians by Clinicians*. Austin, Tex.: Pro-Ed, 1984.

Butterfield, E., and G. Cairns, "Discussion-summary of infant reception research." In R. Schiefulbusch

and L. Lloyd (Eds.), *Language Perspectives: Acquisition, Retardation and Intervention*. Baltimore, Md.: University Park Press, 1974.

Calvert, D., "Articulation and hearing impairments." In L. Lass, J. Northern, D. Yoder, and L. McReynolds (Eds.), *Speech, Language and Hearing*. Vol. 2. Philadelphia: Saunders, 1982.

Canning, B., and M. Rose, "Clinical measurements of the speech, tongue and lip movements in British children with normal speech." *British Journal of Disorders of Communication, 9* (1974): 45–50.

Carrell, J., and K. Pendergast, "An experimental study of the possible relation between errors of speech and spelling." *Journal of Speech and Hearing Disorders, 19* (1954): 327–334.

Catts, H. W., "Speech, production/phonological deficits in reading-disordered children." *Learning Disabilities, 19* (1986): 504–508.

Catts, H. W., "Facilitating phonological awareness: role of speech-language pathologists." *Language, Speech, and Hearing Services in Schools, 22* (1991): 196–203.

Chaney, C., and P. Menyuk, "Production and identification of /w, l, r/ in normal and articulation-impaired children." Paper presented at the convention of the American Speech and Hearing Association, Washington, D.C., 1975.

Churchill, J., B. Hodson, B. Jones, and R. Novak, "A preliminary investigation comparing phonological systems of speech disordered clients with and without histories of recurrent otitis media." Paper presented at the convention of the American Speech-Language-Hearing Association, Washington, D.C., 1985.

Clark, R., "Maturation and speech development." *Logos, 2* (1959): 49–54.

Crary, M., and R. Towne, "The asynergistic nature of developmental verbal dyspraxia." *Australian Journal of Human Communication Disorders, 12* (1984): 27–28.

Darley, F., "Apraxia of speech: Description, diagnosis and treatment." Paper presented at the convention of the American Speech and Hearing Association, New York, 1970.

Darley, F., A. Aronson, and J. Brown, "Differential diagnostic patterns of dysarthria." *Journal of Speech and Hearing Research, 12* (1969): 246–269.

Darley, F., A. Aronson, and J. Brown, *Motor Speech Disorders.* Philadelphia: Saunders, 1975.

Davis, E., "The development of linguistic skills in twins, singletons with siblings, and only children from age five to ten years." *Institute of Child Welfare Monograph Series, 14,* Minneapolis: University of Minnesota Press, 1937.

Dawson, L., "A study of the development of the rate of articulation." *Elementary School Journal, 29* (1929): 610–615.

De Renzi, E., A. Pieczuro, and L. Vignolo, "Oral apraxia and aphasia." *Cortex, 2* (1966): 50–73.

Dubois, E., and J. Bernthal, "A comparison of three methods for obtaining articulatory responses." *Journal of Speech and Hearing Disorders, 43* (1978): 295–305.

Dunn, C., and L. Newton, "A comprehensive model for speech development in hearing-impaired children." *Topics in Language Disorders: Hearing Impairment: Implications from Normal Child Language, 6* (1986): 25–46.

Dworkin, J., "Protrusive lingual force and lingual diadochokinetic rates: A comparative analysis between normal and lisping speakers." *Language, Speech, and Hearing Services in Schools, 9* (1978): 8–16.

Dworkin, J., and R. Culatta, "Tongue strength: Its relationship to tongue thrusting, open-bite, and articulatory proficiency." *Journal of Speech and Hearing Disorders, 45* (1980): 227–282.

Eilers, R. E., and D. K. Oller, "The role of speech discrimination in developmental sound substitutions." *Journal of Child Language, 3* (1976): 319–329.

Eimas, P., E. Siqueland, P. Jusczyk, and J. Vigorito, "Speech perception in infants." *Science, 171* (1971): 303–306.

Everhart, R., "The relationship between articulation and other developmental factors in children." *Journal of Speech and Hearing Disorders, 18* (1953): 332–338.

Everhart, R., "Paternal occupational classification and the maturation of articulation." *Speech Monographs, 23* (1956): 75–77.

Everhart, R., "Literature survey of growth and developmental factors in articulation maturation." *Journal of Speech and Hearing Disorders, 25* (1960): 59–69.

Fairbanks, G., and E. Green, "A study of minor organic deviations in 'functional' disorders of articulation; 2. Dimension and relationships of the lips." *Journal of Speech and Hearing Disorders, 15* (1950): 165–168.

Fairbanks, G., and M. Lintner, "A study of minor organic deviations in functional disorders of articulation." *Journal of Speech and Hearing Disorders, 16* (1951): 273–279.

Felsenfeld, S., M. McGue, and P.A. Broen, "Familial aggregation of phonological disorders: Results from a 28-year follow-up." *Journal of Speech and Hearing Research, 38* (1995): 1091–1107.

Fey, M. E., P. L. Cleave, A. I. Ravida, S. H. Long, A. E. Dejmal, and D. L. Easton, "Effects of grammar facilitation on the phonological performance of children with speech and language impairments." *Journal of Speech and Hearing Research, 37* (1994): 594–607.

Fitzsimons, R., "Developmental, psychosocial and educational factors in children with nonorganic articulation problems." *Child Development, 29* (1958): 481–489.

Fletcher, S., "Time-by-count measurement of diadochokinetic syllable rate." *Journal of Speech and Hearing Research, 15* (1972): 763–780.

Fletcher, S., R. Casteel, and D. Bradley, "Tongue thrust swallow, speech articulation and age." *Journal of Speech and Hearing Disorders, 26* (1961): 201–208.

Fletcher, S., and J. Meldrum, "Lingual function and relative length of the lingual frenulum." *Journal of Speech and Hearing Research, 11* (1968): 382–399.

Flynn, P., and M. Byrne, "Relationship between reading and selected auditory abilities of third-grade children." *Journal of Speech and Hearing Research, 13* (1970): 731–740.

Fucci, D., "Oral vibrotactile sensation: An evaluation of normal and defective speakers." *Journal of Speech and Hearing Research, 15* (1972): 179–184.

Gammon, S., P. Smith, R. Daniloff, and C. Kim, "Articulation and stress juncture production under oral anesthetization and masking." *Journal of Speech and Hearing Research, 14* (1971): 271–282.

Garrett, R., "A study of children's discrimination of phonetic variations of the /s/ phoneme." Ph.D. Dissertation, Ohio University, 1969.

Gray, S. I., and R. L. Shelton, "Self-monitoring effects on articulation carryover in school-age children." *Language, Speech, and Hearing Services in Schools, 23* (1992): 334–342.

Gross, G., K. St. Louis, D. Ruscello, and F. Hull, "Language abilities of articulatory-disordered school children with multiple or residual errors." *Language, Speech, and Hearing Services in Schools, 16* (1985): 174–186.

Guyette, R., and W. Diedrich, "A critical review of developmental apraxia of speech." In N. Lass (Ed.), *Speech and Language: Advances in Basic Research and Practice*, Vol. 5 (pp. 1–48). New York: Academic Press, 1981.

Hall, M., "Auditory factors in functional articulatory speech defects." *Journal of Experimental Education, 7* (1938): 110–132.

Hansen, B., "The application of sound discrimination tests to functional articulatory defectives with normal hearing." *Journal of Speech Disorders, 9* (1944): 347–355.

Hanson, M. L., "Orofacial myofunctional disorders: Guidelines for assessment and treatment." *International Journal of Orofacial Myology, 14* (1988a): 27–32.

Hanson, M. L., "Orofacial myofunctional therapy: Historical and philosophical considerations." *International Journal of Orofacial Myology, 14* (1988b): 3–10.

Hanson, M. L., "Oral myofunctional disorders and articulatory patterns." In J. Bernthal and N. Bankson (Eds.), *Child Phonology: Characteristics, Assessment, and Intervention with Special Populations* (pp. 29–53). New York: Thieme Medical Publishers, 1994.

Haynes, S., D. Johns, and E. May, "Assessment and

therapeutic management of an adult patient with developmental apraxia of speech and orosensory perceptual deficits." *Tejas, 3* (1978): 6–9.

Hilton, L., "Treatment of deviant phonologic systems: Tongue thrust." In W. Perkins (Ed.), *Phonological-articulatory Disorders*. New York: Thieme- Stratton, 1984.

Hodson, B., and E. Paden, "Phonological processes which characterize unintelligible and intelligible speech in early childhood." *Journal of Speech and Hearing Disorders, 46* (1981): 369–373.

Hoffman, P., "Spelling, phonology, and the speech pathologist: A whole language perspective." *Language, Speech, and Hearing Services in Schools, 21* (1990): 238–243.

Hoffman, P., and J. Norris, "On the nature of phonological development: Evidence from normal children's spelling errors." *Journal of Speech and Hearing Research, 32* (1989): 787–794.

Hoffman, P., J. Norris, and J. Monjure, "Comparison of process targeting and whole language treatments of phonologically delayed children. *Language, Speech, and Hearing Services in Schools, 21* (1990): 102–109.

Hoffman, P., S. Stager, and R. Daniloff, "Perception and production of misarticulated /r/." *Journal of Speech and Hearing Disorders, 48* (1983): 210–214.

Holland, A., "Training speech sound discrimination in children who misarticulate. A demonstration of teaching machine technique in speech correction." Project No. 5007. Washington, D.C.: U.S. Department of Health, Education and Welfare, 1967.

Hull, F., P. Mielke, R. Timmons, and J. Willeford, "The national speech and hearing survey: Preliminary results." *Asha, 13* (1971): 501–509.

Itoh, M., and S. Sasanuma, "Articulatory movements in apraxia of speech." In J. Rosenbek, M. McNeil, and A. Aronson (Eds.), *Apraxia of Speech: Physiology, Acoustics, Linguistics, Management*. San Diego: College-Hill Press, 1984.

Jaffe, M., "Neurological impairment of speech production: Assessment and treatment." In J. Costello and A. Holland (Eds.) *Handbook of Speech and Language Disorders* (pp. 157–186). San Diego: College Hill Press, 1986.

Jann, G., M. Ward, and H. Jann, "A longitudinal study of articulation, deglutition and malocclusion." *Journal of Speech and Hearing Disorders, 29* (1964): 424–435.

Johns, D., and F. Darley, "Phonemic variability in apraxia of speech." *Journal of Speech and Hearing Research, 13* (1970): 556–583.

Johns, D., and K. Salyer, "Surgical and prosthetic management of neurogenic speech disorders." In D. Johns (Ed.), *Clinical Management of Neurogenic Communicative Disorders*. Boston: Little, Brown, 1978.

Jordan, L., J. Hardy, and H. Morris, "Performance of children with good and poor articulation on tasks of tongue placement." *Journal of Speech and Hearing Research, 21* (1978): 429–439.

Kenny, K., and E. Prather, "Articulation in preschool children: Consistency of productions." *Journal of Speech and Hearing Research, 29* (1986): 29–36.

Koch, H., "Sibling influence on children's speech." *Journal of Speech and Hearing Disorders, 21* (1956): 322–329.

Koegel, L. K., R. L. Koegel, and J. C. Ingham, "Programming rapid generalization of correct articulation through self-monitoring procedures." *Journal of Speech and Hearing Disorders, 51* (1986): 24–32.

Koegel, R., L. Koegel, K. Van Voy, and J. Ingham, "Within-clinic versus outside-of-clinic self-monitoring of articulation to promote generalization." *Journal of Speech and Hearing Disorders, 53* (1988): 392–399.

Kronvall, E., and C. Diehl, "The relationship of auditory discrimination to articulatory defects of children with no known organic impairment." *Journal of Speech and Hearing Disorders, 19* (1954): 335–338.

Kumin, L., C. Council, and M. Goodman, "A longitudinal study of emergence of phonemes in children with Down syndrome." *Journal of Communication Disorders, 27* (1994): 293–303.

Lapko, L., and N. Bankson, "Relationship between auditory discrimination, articulation stimulability and consistency of misarticulation." *Perceptual and Motor Skills, 40* (1975): 171–177.

Lapointe, L., and R. Wertz, "Oral-movement abilities and articulatory characteristics of brain-injured adults." *Perceptual Motor Skills, 39* (1974): 39–46.

Leonard, R. J., "Characteristics of speech in speakers with oral/oralpharyngeal ablation." In J. Bernthal and N. Bankson (Eds.), *Child Phonology: Characteristics, Assessment, and Intervention with Special Populations* (pp. 54–78). New York: Thieme Medical Publishers, 1994.

Levitt, H., and H. Stromberg, "Segmental characteristics of speech of hearing-impaired children: Factors affecting intelligibility." In I. Hochberg, H. Levitt, and M. Osberger (Eds.), *Speech of the Hearing Impaired*. (pp. 53–73) Baltimore, Md.: University Park Press, 1983.

Lewis, B., B. Ekelman, and D. Aram, "A familial study of severe phonological disorders." *Journal of Speech and Hearing Research, 32* (1989): 713–724.

Lewis, B., and L. Freebairn-Farr, "Preschool phonology disorders at school age, adolescence, and adulthood." Paper presented at the convention of the American Speech-Language-Hearing Association, Atlanta, 1991.

Liberman, I., and D. Shankweiler, "Phonology and problems of learning to read and write." *Remedial and Special Education, 6* (1985): 8–17.

Ling, D., *Foundations of Spoken Language for Hearing-Impaired Children*. Washington, D.C.: Alexander Graham Bell Association for the Deaf, 1989.

Locke, J. L., "Oral perception and articulation learning." *Perceptual and Motor Skills, 26* (1968): 1259–1264.

Locke, J. L., "The inference of speech perception in the phonologically disordered child, part I: A rationale, some criteria, the conventional tests." *Journal of Speech and Hearing Disorders, 4* (1980): 431–444.

Locke, J. L., and K. Kutz, "Memory for speech and speech for memory." *Journal of Speech and Hearing Research, 18* (1975): 179–191.

Locke, J., and P. Mather, "Genetic factors in phonology. Evidence from monozygotic and dizygotic twins." Paper presented at the convention of the American Speech-Language-Hearing Association, New Orleans, 1987.

Love, R., *Childhood Motor Speech Disability*. New York: Macmillan, 1992.

Lundeen, C., "Prevalence of hearing impairment among school children." *Language, Speech, and Hearing Services in Schools*, 22 (1991): 269–271.

Majid, A., B. Weinberg, and B. Chalian, "Speech intelligibility following prosthetic obturation of surgically-acquired maxillary defects." *Journal of Prosthetic Dentition*, 32 (1974): 87–96.

Marquardt, T., and J. Saxman, "Language comprehension and auditory discrimination in articulation deficient kindergarten children." *Journal of Speech and Hearing Research*, 15 (1972): 382–389.

Mase, D., "Etiology of articulatory speech defects." *Teacher's College Contribution to Education*, no. 921. New York: Columbia University, 1946.

Mason, R. M., "Orthodontic perspectives on orofacial myofunctional therapy." *International Journal of Orofacial Myology*, 14 (1988): 49–55.

Mason, R., and W. Proffit, "The tongue-thrust controversy: Background and recommendations." *Journal of Speech and Hearing Disorders*, 39 (1974): 115–132.

Massengill, R., S. Maxwell, and K. Picknell, "An analysis of articulation following partial and total glossectomy." *Journal of Speech and Hearing Disorders*, 35 (1970): 170–173.

Matheny, A., and C. Bruggeman, "Children's speech: Heredity components and sex differences." *Folia Phoniatrica*, 25 (1973): 442–449.

Matheny, N., and J. Panagos, "Comparing the effects of articulation and syntax programs on syntax and articulation improvement." *Language, Speech, and Hearing Services in Schools*, 9 (1978): 57–61.

McDonald, E. T., *Articulation Testing and Treatment: A Sensory Motor Approach*. Pittsburgh, Penn.: Stanwix House, 1964.

McDonald, E. T., and L. Aungst, "Apparent impedence of oral sensory functions and articulatory proficiency." In J. Bosma (Ed.), *Second Symposium on Oral Sensation and Perception*. Springfield, Ill.: Charles C Thomas, 1970.

McEnery, E., and F. Gaines, "Tongue-tie in infants and children." *Journal of Pediatrics*, 18 (1941): 252–255.

McNutt, J., "Oral sensory and motor behaviors of children with /s/ or /r/ misarticulations." *Journal of Speech and Hearing Research*, 20 (1977): 694–703.

Mills, A., and H. Streit, "Report of a speech survey, Holyoke, Massachusetts." *Journal of Speech Disorders*, 7 (1942): 161–167.

Monson, R., "The oral speech intelligibility of hearing-impaired talkers." *Journal of Speech and Hearing Disorders*, 48 (1983): 286–296.

Morley, D., "A ten-year survey of speech disorders among university students." *Journal of Speech and Hearing Disorders*, 17 (1952): 25–31.

Morley, M. E., *The Development and Disorders of Speech in Childhood*, (1st ed.). London: Livingston, 1957.

Mowrer, D., R. Baker, and R. Schutz, "Operant procedures in the control of speech articulation." In H. Sloane and B. MacAulay (Eds.), *Operant Procedures in Remedial Speech and Language Training*. Boston: Houghton Mifflin, 1968.

Neils, J., and D. Aram, "Family history of children with developmental language disorders." *Perceptual and Motor Skills*, 63 (1986): 655–658.

Netsell, R. A., *A Neurobiologic View of Speech Production and the Dysarthrias*. Boston, Mass.: College-Hill Press, 1986.

Paden, E. P., M. L. Matthies, and M. A. Novak, "Recovery from OME-related phonologic delay following tube placement." *Journal of Speech and Hearing Disorders*, 54 (1989): 94–100.

Paden, E. P., M. A. Novak, and A. L. Beiter, "Predictors of phonological inadequacy in young children prone to otitis media." *Journal of Speech and Hearing Disorders*, 52 (1987): 232–242.

Palmer, J., "Tongue-thrusting: A clinical hypothesis." *Journal of Speech and Hearing Disorders*, 27 (1962): 323–333.

Panagos, J., M. Quine, and R. Klich, "Syntactic and phonological influences on children's articulation." *Journal of Speech and Hearing Research*, 22 (1979): 841–848.

Panagos, J., and P. Prelock, "Phonological constraints on the sentence productions of language disordered children." *Journal of Speech and Hearing Research*, 25 (1982): 171–176.

Parlour, S., and P. Broen, "Environmental factors in familial phonological disorders: Preliminary home scale results." Paper presented at the annual convention of the American Speech-Language-Hearing Association, Atlanta, 1991.

Paterson, M., "Articulation and phonological disorders in hearing-impaired school-aged children with severe and profound sensorineural losses." In J. Bernthal and N. Bankson (Eds.), *Child Phonology: Characteristics, Assessment, and Intervention with Special Populations* (pp. 199–224). New York: Thieme Medical Publishers, 1994.

Paul, R., and L. D. Shriberg, "Associations between phonology and syntax in speech delayed children." *Journal of Speech and Hearing Research, 25* (1982): 536–546.

Paul, R., and L. D. Shriberg, "Reply to Panagos and Prelock [Letter]." *Journal of Speech and Hearing Research, 27* (1984): 319–320.

Perkins, W., *Speech Pathology: An Applied Behavioral Science*. St. Louis: Mosby, 1977.

Powers, M., "Functional disorders of articulation-symptomatology and etiology." In L. Travis (Ed.), *Handbook of Speech Pathology and Audiology*. Engelwood Cliffs, N.J.: Prentice-Hall, 1957, 1971.

Prins, D., "Analysis of correlations among various articulatory deviations." *Journal of Speech and Hearing Research, 5* (1962a): 151–160.

Prins, D., "Motor and auditory abilities in different groups of children with articulatory deviations." *Journal of Speech and Hearing Research, 5* (1962b): 161–168.

Proffit, W. R., *Contemporary Orthodontics*. St. Louis, Mo.: C.V. Mosby, 1986.

Prosek, R., and A. House, "Intraoral air pressure as a feedback cue in consonant production." *Journal of Speech and Hearing Research, 18* (1975): 133–147.

Reid, G., "The etiology and nature of functional articulatory defects in elementary school children." *Journal of Speech and Hearing Disorders, 12* (1947a): 143–150.

Reid, G., "The efficiency of speech re-education of functional articulatory defectives in elementary school." *Journal of Speech and Hearing Disorders, 12* (1947b): 301–313.

Ringel, R., K. Burk, and C. Scott, "Tactile perception: Form discrimination in the mouth." In J. Bosma (Ed.), *Second Symposium on Oral Sensation and Perception*. Springfield, Ill.: Charles C Thomas, 1970.

Ringel, R., and S. Ewanowski, "Oral perception: I. Two-point discrimination." *Journal of Speech and Hearing Research, 8* (1965): 389–400.

Ringel, R., A. House, K. Burk, J. Dolinsky, and C. Scott, "Some relations between orosensory discrimination and articulatory aspects of speech production." *Journal of Speech and Hearing Disorders, 35* (1970): 3–11.

Roberts, J. E., M. R. Burchinal, M. A. Koch, M. M. Footo, and F. W. Henderson, "Otitis media in early childhood and its relationship to later phonological development." *Journal of Speech and Hearing Disorders, 53* (1988): 424–432.

Roberts, J. E., and S. Clarke-Klein, "Otitis media." In J. Bernthal and N. Bankson (Eds.), *Child Phonology: Characteristics, Assessment, and Intervention with Special Populations* (pp. 182–198). New York: Thieme Medical Publishers, 1994.

Roe, V., and R. Milisen, "The effect of maturation upon defective articulation in elementary grades." *Journal of Speech Disorders, 7* (1942): 37–50.

Rosenbek, J., and R. Wertz, "A review of fifty cases of developmental apraxia of speech." *Language, Speech and Hearing Services in Schools, 1* (1972): 23–33.

Rosin, M., E. Swift, D. Bless, and D. K. Vetter, "Communication profiles of adolescents with Down's Syndrome." *Journal of Childhood Communication Disorders, 12* (1988): 49–62.

Ruscello, D. M., "Articulation improvement and oral tactile changes in children." Thesis, University of West Virginia, 1972.

Rvachew, S., "Speech perception training can facilitate sound production learning." *Journal of Speech and Hearing Research, 37* (1994): 347–357.

Sayler, H., "The effect of maturation upon defective articulation in grades seven through twelve." *Journal of Speech and Hearing Disorders, 14* (1949): 202–207.

Schlanger, B., "Speech examination of a group of institutionalized mentally handicapped children." *Journal of Speech and Hearing Disorders, 18* (1953): 339–349.

Schlanger, B., and R. Gottsleben, "Analysis of speech defects among the institutionalized mentally retarded." *Journal of Speech and Hearing Disorders, 22* (1957): 98–103.

Schmauch, V., J. Panagos, and R. Klich, "Syntax influences the accuracy of consonant production in language-disordered children." *Journal of Communication Disorders, 11* (1978): 315–323.

Schwartz, A., and R. Goldman, "Variables influencing performance on speech sound discrimination tests." *Journal of Speech and Hearing Research, 17* (1974): 25–32.

Schwartz, R., L. Leonard, M. K. Folger, and M. J. Wilcox, "Evidence for a synergistic view of linguistic disorders: Early phonological behavior in normal and language disordered children." *Journal of Speech and Hearing Disorders, 45* (1980): 357–377.

Scott, C., and R. Ringel, "Articulation without oral sensory control." *Journal of Speech and Hearing Research, 14* (1971): 804–818.

Shelton, R., "Science, clinical art, and speech pathology." Paper presented at Kansas University, Spring 1989.

Shelton, R., A. Johnson, and W. Arndt, "Delayed judgment speech sound discrimination and /r/ or /s/ articulation status and improvement." *Journal of Speech and Hearing Research, 20* (1977): 704–717.

Shelton, R. L., V. Willis, A. F. Johnson., and W. B. Arndt, "Oral form recognition training and articulation change." *Perceptual Motor Skills, 36* (1973): 523–531.

Sherman, D., and A. Geith, "Speech sound discrimination and articulation skill." *Journal of Speech and Hearing Disorders, 10* (1967): 277–280.

Shriberg, L., and J. Kwiatkowski, "Developmental phonological disorders I: A clinical profile." *Journal of Speech and Hearing Research, 37* (1994): 1100–1126.

Shriberg, L. D., and J. Kwiatkowski, "Phonological disorders I: A diagnostic classification system." *Journal of Speech and Hearing Disorders, 47* (1982): 226–241.

Shriberg, L. D., and A. J. Smith, "Phonological correlates of middle-ear involvement in speech-delayed children: A methodological note." *Journal of Speech and Hearing Research, 26* (1983): 293–297.

Shriberg, L., and C. Widder, "Speech and prosody characteristics of adults with mental retardation." *Journal of Speech and Hearing Research, 33* (1990): 627–653.

Shriner, T., M. Holloway, and R. Daniloff, "The relationship between articulatory deficits and syntax in speech defective children." *Journal of Speech and Hearing Research, 12* (1969): 319–325.

Skelly, M., D. Spector, R. Donaldson, A. Brodeur, and F. Paletta, "Compensatory physiologic phonetics for the glossectomee." *Journal of Speech and Hearing Disorders, 36* (1971): 101–114.

Smit, A., L. Hand, J. Freilinger, J. Bernthal, and A. Bird, "The Iowa articulation norms project and its Nebraska replication." *Journal of Speech and Hearing Disorders, 55* (1990): 779–798.

Smith, B., and C. Stoel-Gammon, "A longitudinal study of the development of stop consonant production in normal and Down's Syndrome children." *Journal of Speech and Hearing Disorders, 48* (1983): 114–118.

Snow, K., "Articulation proficiency in relation to certain dental abnormalities." *Journal of Speech and Hearing Disorders, 26* (1961): 209–212.

Sommers, R., R. Reinhart, and D. Sistrunk, "Traditional articulation measures of Down's Syndrome speakers, ages 13–22." *Journal of Childhood Communication Disorders, 12* (1988): 93–108.

Sonderman, J., "An experimental study of clinical relationships between auditory discrimination and articulation skills." Paper presented at the convention of the American Speech and Hearing Association, San Francisco, 1971.

Spriestersbach, D., "Research in articulation disorders and personality." *Journal of Speech and Hearing Disorders, 21* (1956): 329–335.

Spriestersbach, D., and J. Curtis, "Misarticulation and

discrimination of speech sounds." *Quarterly Journal of Speech*, *37* (1951): 483–491.

Starr, C., "Dental and occlusal hazards to normal speech production." In K. Bzoch (Ed.), *Communicative Disorders Related to Cleft Lip and Palate*. Boston: Little, Brown, 1972.

Stelcik, J., "An investigation of internal versus external discrimination and general versus phoneme-specific discrimination." Unpublished Thesis, University of Maryland, 1972.

Stoel-Gammon, C., and M. Kehoe, "Hearing impairment in infants and toddlers: Identification, vocal development, and intervention in child phonology." In J. Bernthal and N. Bankson (Eds.), *Child Phonology: Characteristics, Assessment, and Intervention with Special Populations* (pp. 163–181). New York: Thieme Medical Publishers, 1994.

Strange, W., and P. Broen, "Perception and production of approximant consonants by 3 year olds: A first study." In G. Yeni-Komshian, J. Kavanaugh, and C. A. Ferguson (Eds.), *Child Phonology*, Vol. 2. *Perception*. New York: Academic Press, 1980.

Subtelny, J. D., "Malocclusions, orthodontic corrections and orofacial muscle adaptation." *Angle Orthod*, *40* (1970): 170.

Subtelny, J., J. Mestre, and J. Subtelny, "Comparative study of normal and defective articulation of /s/ as related to malocclusion and deglutition." *Journal of Speech and Hearing Disorders*, *29* (1964): 269–285.

Templin, M., *Certain Language Skills in Children*. Institute of Child Welfare Monograph Series 26. Minneapolis: University of Minnesota, 1957.

Templin, M., "Development of speech." *Journal of Pediatrics*, *62* (1963): 11–14.

Templin, M., *Longitudinal Study Through the 4th Grade of Language Skills of Children with Varying Speech Sound Articulation in Kindergarten*. (Final Report, Project 2220). Washington, D.C.: U.S. Department of Health, Education, and Welfare, Office of Education, 1968.

Templin, M., and G. Glaman, "A longitudinal study of correlations of predictive measures obtained in prekindergarten and first grade with achievement measures through eleventh grade" (Unpublished report no. 101). Washington, D.C.: U.S. Department of Health, Education, and Welfare, Office of Education, 1976.

Tiffany, W., "Effects of syllable structure on diadochokinetic and reading rates." *Journal of Speech and Hearing Research*, *23* (1980): 894–908.

Travis, L., and B. Rasmus, "The speech sound discrimination ability of cases with functional disorders of articulation." *Quarterly Journal of Speech*, *17* (1931): 217–226.

Tye-Murray, N., "The establishment of open articulatory postures by deaf and hearing talkers." *Journal of Speech and Hearing Research*, *34* (1991): 453–458.

Tyler, A., and K. Watterson, "Effects of phonological versus language intervention in preschoolers with both phonological and language impairment." *Child Language Teaching and Therapy*, *7* (1991): 141–160.

Veatch, J., "An experimental investigation of a motor theory of auditory discrimination." Ph.D. Dissertation, University of Idaho, 1970.

Velleman, S. L., "Children's production and perception of English voiceless fricatives." Unpublished Ph.D. Dissertation, University of Texas at Austin, 1983.

Velleman, S., and K. Strand, "Developmental verbal dyspraxia." In J. Bernthal and N. Bankson (Eds.), *Child Phonology: Characteristics, Assessment, and Intervention with Special Populations* (pp. 110–139). New York: Thieme Medical Publishers, 1994.

Weaver, C., C. Furbee, and R. Everhart, "Paternal occupational class and articulatory defects in children." *Journal of Speech and Hearing Disorders*, *25* (1960) 171–175.

Weiner, P., "Auditory discrimination and articulation." *Journal of Speech and Hearing Disorders*, *32* (1967): 19–28.

Wellman, B., I. Case, I. Mengert, and D. Bradbury, "Speech sounds of young children." *University of Iowa Studies in Child Welfare*, *5* (1931).

Whitaker, J., H. Luper, and H. Pollio, "General language deficits in children with articulation problems." *Language and Speech*, *3* (1970): 231–239.

Wilhelm, C. L., "The effects of oral form recognition training on articulation in children." Dissertation, University of Kansas, 1971.

Williams, G., and L. McReynolds, "The relationship between discrimination and articulation training in children with misarticulations." *Journal of Speech and Hearing Research*, 18 (1975): 401–412.

Wilson, F., "Efficacy of speech therapy with educable mentally retarded children." *Journal of Speech and Hearing Research*, 9 (1966): 423–433.

Winitz, H., "Language skills of male and female kindergarten children." *Journal of Speech and Hearing Research*, 2 (1959a): 377–386.

Winitz, H., "Relationship between language and non-language measures of kindergarten children." *Journal of Speech and Hearing Research*, 2 (1959b): 387–391.

Winitz, H., *Articulatory Acquisition and Behavior.* Englewood Cliffs, N.J.: Prentice-Hall, 1969.

Winitz, H., "Auditory considerations in articulation training." In H. Winitz (Ed.), *Treating Articulation Disorders: For Clinicians By Clinicians*. Baltimore: University Park Press, 1984.

Wolfe, V., and R. Irwin, "Sound discrimination ability of children with misarticulation of the /r/ sound." *Perceptual and Motor Skills*, 37 (1973): 415–420.

Wolk, S., and A. N. Schildroth, "Deaf children and speech intelligibility: A national study." In A. N. Schildroth and M. A. Karchmer (Eds.), *Deaf Children in America* (pp. 139–159). San Diego: College-Hill, 1986.

Woolf, G., and M. Pilberg, "A comparison of three tests of auditory discrimination and their relationship to performance on a deep test of articulation." *Journal of Communication Disorders*, 3 (1971): 239–249.

Yoss, K., and F. Darley, "Developmental apraxia of speech in children with defective articulation." *Journal of Speech and Hearing Research*, 17 (1974): 399–416.

Chapter 6

Phonological Assessment Procedures

NICHOLAS W. BANKSON,
James Madison University

JOHN E. BERNTHAL,
University of Nebraska–Lincoln

Phonological Sampling

Introduction

One of the unique contributions of the field of speech-language pathology to the assessment of verbal behavior is the development of **phonological assessment** instruments. For several decades, phonological/articulation assessment procedures have remained almost the exclusive domain of speech-language clinicians, although linguists, child development specialists, psychologists, pediatricians, and special educators also use such tools.

Evaluation of an individual's phonological status typically involves description of his or her speech sound production system and relating this system to the adult standard of the speaker's linguistic community. Phonological assessment is often done in the context of a communication evaluation that also includes assessment of voice quality, fluency of speech, and aspects of language including syntax, semantics, pragmatics, and discourse. In addition, such related measures as hearing testing and oral cavity examination are usually included in a comprehensive communication evaluation/assessment. As part of the evaluation, the clinician seeks to identify etiological factors that may be related to the presence and maintenance of the phonological delay/disorder. Although some authors have differentiated between phonological delay (children whose speech sound errors are similar to those found in younger normally developing children) and phonological disorders (children whose speech sound errors differ from normal developing children), in this text we will not differentiate between the two. In reality, most children with multiple misarticulations will have errors that fall into both categories.

Phonological assessment is used to:

1. Describe the phonological status of an individual and determine if his or her speech sound system is sufficiently different from normal development to warrant intervention.
2. Determine treatment direction, including target behaviors and strategies to be used in the management of the client.
3. Make predictive and prognostic statements relative to phonological change with or without intervention.
4. Monitor change in phonological performance across time.
5. Identify factors that may be related to the presence or maintenance of a phonologic disability.

The primary purposes of a phonological assessment are to determine whether an individual needs remedial instruction, and if so, the direction of treatment. To make these determinations, the clinician engages in a multistep process that involves sampling the client's speech through a variety of procedures, analyzing the data gathered, interpreting the data that have been analyzed, and then making clinical recommendations and decisions. No hard-and-fast rules dictate when intervention is warranted or the type of treatment to be recommended. State or local guidelines often dictate when a child qualifies for services in the public schools. In this chapter, we will discuss various sampling and testing procedures and discuss factors and issues that should be taken into consideration when analyzing and interpreting phonological samples.

Screening for Phonological Disorders

Phonological assessment, including analysis and interpretation of results, often requires a considerable expenditure of time. Frequently, a clinician will do a *screening* to determine if a more comprehensive phonological assessment is warranted. Screening procedures are not designed to determine the need or direction of therapy, but rather to identify individuals who merit further evaluation from those for whom further evaluation is not indicated. Typical screening situations might include (1) screening children at a preschool or "kindergarten roundup" to determine whether they have age-appropriate phonological skills, (2) screening children in grade 3 (by which time maturation should have resolved most developmental errors), (3) screening college students preparing for occupations, such as teaching or broadcast journalism, which require specific speech performance standards, and (4) screening the phonological status of clients referred for a suspected communication impairment.

In screening, individuals are not identified as candidates for therapy, but rather are simply identified as needing further assessment. Additional testing is often required before statements about the presence or absence of a phonological disorder can be made, and it is certainly required for determining the direction for treatment. Instruments used for screening consist of a limited sampling of speech sound productions, which can usually be administered in five minutes or less. Screening measures can be categorized as informal or formal. *Informal measures* are often used when people wish to develop their own screening tools in order to meet their particular needs. *Formal measures* are often employed when users desire established norms or testing methodologies that are more uniform from one location to another.

Informal Screening Measures

Informal screening measures are usually devised by the examiner and are tailored to the population being screened. While informal procedures can be easily and economically devised, they do not include standardized administration procedures or normative data, which are characteristics of formal screening measures. For example, with a group of kindergarten children, the examiner might ask each child to

1. state his or her name and address.
2. count to ten; name the days of the week.
3. tell about a television show.

If the subjects are adults, the examiner might ask them to do one or both of the following:

1. Read sentences designed to elicit several productions of frequently misarticulated sounds, such as /s/, /r/, /l/, and /θ/. For example, "I saw Sally at her seaside house; Rob ran around the orange car."
2. Read a passage with a representative sample of English speech sounds, such as the "Grandfather Passage" or the "Rainbow Passage."

Grandfather Passage.   You wish to know all about my grandfather. Well, he is nearly 93 years old, yet he still thinks as swiftly as ever. He dresses himself in an old black frock coat, usually several buttons missing. A long beard clings to his chin, giving those who observe him a pronounced feeling of the utmost respect. When he speaks, his voice is just a bit cracked and quivers a bit. Twice each day he plays skillfully and with zest upon a small organ. Except in winter when the snow or ice prevents, he slowly takes a short walk in the open air each day. We have often urged him to walk more and smoke less, but he always answers, "Banana oil." Grandfather likes to be modern in his language.

Rainbow Passage.   When the sunlight strikes raindrops in the air, they act like a prism and form a rainbow. The rainbow is a division of white light into many beautiful colors. These take the shape of a long round arch, with its path high above, and its two ends apparently beyond the horizon. There is, according to legend, a boiling pot of gold at one end. People look, but no one ever finds it. When a man looks for something beyond his reach, his friends say he is looking for the pot of gold at the end of the rainbow.

Criterion for failure of informal screening is usually determined by the examiner. An often-used rule of thumb is, "If in doubt, refer." In other words, an examiner who suspects that the client's speech sound system is not appropriate for his or her age and/or language community should refer for a more complete assessment. The examiner may also choose to determine or establish performance standards on the screening instrument that will help to indicate those referred on for further testing. Those individuals with the greatest need for additional testing and probable intervention will usually be obvious to the examiner from even a small sample of their speech and language.

Formal Screening Measures

Formal screening measures include published elicitation procedures for which normative data and/or cut-off scores are often available. These formal measures are of three types: (1) tests that are part of a single-word articulation test, (2) tests designed solely for screening phonology, and (3) tests that screen phonology as well as other aspects of language. Tests designed explicitly for screening phonology are most frequently used when screening phonology is the primary goal. Those instruments that combine phonological screening with other aspects of language screening are most commonly used for more general communication screening often conducted by child development specialists, pediatricians, and special educators.

The following are formal phonology screening tests:

Quick Screen of Phonology (QSP) (Bankson and Bernthal, 1990a). This test consists of 28 picture-naming items, with each word assessing sounds in more than one context (usually initial and final). Twenty-three phonemes plus three consonant clusters are screened. These items were selected because of their correlation with the overall performance on the *Bankson-Bernthal Test of Phonology*. Percentile ranks and standard scores are provided for children ages 3;0 through 7;11 years on the QSP.

Denver Articulation Screening Test (Drumwright, 1971). This instrument was designed specifically for screening phonological status in Anglo, African-American, and Mexican-American children. Responses are elicited imitatively. The examiner is asked to judge intelligibility on a 4-point scale, with 1 being "easy to understand" and 4 being "can't evaluate." Children are ranked "normal" to "abnormal," depending on composite articulation and intelligibility scores.

Predictive Screening Test of Articulation (Van Riper and Erickson, 1969). This test, as its title implies, was designed not only for screening but also for predicting whether or not first-grade children are likely to correct their speech sound errors without intervention. In other words, it was designed both to indicate the need for additional testing for those who fail to obtain a cut-off score and to allow the examiner to make prognostic statements about the likelihood of self-correction of speech sound errors. Stockman and McDonald (1980) reported that this test may have greater predictive value for those first graders who misarticulate specific consonant sounds (e.g., those with defective sibilant sounds or defective liquids) since those sounds occur frequently in the test.

The following tests include screening of phonology as part of a speech and language screening:

***Fluharty Speech and Language Screening Test for Preschool Children* (Fluharty, 1978).** This test was designed for children ages 2 through 6 years. The phonology portion of the test uses 15 objects to elicit 19 target sounds. Some stimulus items are designed to assess a single segment; other items assess two sounds. Cut-off scores to indicate the need for further testing are included.

***Preschool Language Scale–3* (Zimmerman, Steiner, and Pond, 1992).**   This test was designed for children ages 1 through 7. The "articulation screener" portion of the test consists of 37 items that test 18 speech sounds plus one consonant cluster. Performance levels expected for children are provided.

Summary.   Screening procedures are not designed to determine the need or direction of treatment. Rather, their purpose is to identify individuals for further testing. The criteria for failure on screening tests are often left up to the examiner. When available, standard scores and percentile ranks aid the examiner in establishing such criteria. It is not uncommon for a score one standard deviation below the mean to be used as a cut-off score. For some instruments, cut-off scores or age expectation scores are provided.

The Assessment Battery

As indicated earlier, the two major purposes of a phonological assessment are to determine the need for and direction of treatment. It is to these purposes that most of the writings, research, and testing materials on phonological disorders have been addressed. In the following pages, components of a phonological evaluation battery, with an emphasis on procedures for obtaining phonological samples, are presented. In Chapter 7 analysis and interpretation of data collected through sampling procedures are discussed. Throughout these chapters an attempt is made to synthesize the available literature and make suggestions based upon the authors' clinical experience.

Sampling procedures involved in phonological assessment are more detailed and time consuming than those described for screening. When doing testing of this nature, the clinician usually employs not just one, but rather a battery of assessment instruments and sampling procedures. A phonological evaluation typically involves phonological productions in samples of varying lengths, phonetic contexts, and in response to various elicitation procedures. This collection of samples is often referred to as an **assessment battery**, a framework for assessment based on the recognition that no one procedure provides all a clinician needs to know when making case selection decisions and determining the direction that an intervention program should take.

It is important to recognize that a variety of assessment, analysis, and interpretation procedures are used and have been found helpful. Unfortunately, not all procedures are as efficient or as scientific (data based) as we might like them to be. In the interest of professional advancement, the efficacy of our assessment practices must continue to be carefully examined.

In the pages that follow, criteria for selecting testing instruments and various types of samples that comprise a phonological assessment battery are described. Characteristics and elicitation procedures for each sample type will be presented.

Criteria for Selecting Phonological Assessment Instruments

Speech-language pathologists have traditionally used a variety of formal and informal tests to assess phonology. Although clinicians often tend to use particular assessment tools, most recognize that no one test or procedure is appropriate for all purposes. The test instruments selected should be appropriate to the individual tested and provide the information desired by the clinician. When selecting commercially available test instruments for phonological assessment, the clinician will want to consider the sample the instrument is designed to obtain, the nature of the stimulus materials, the scoring system, and the type of analysis facilitated by the instrument. A practical consideration in test selection is the amount of time required to administer the instrument and analyze the sample obtained.

Sample Obtained.   A factor to consider in selecting a test instrument is the adequacy or representativeness of the speech sample obtained: the specific consonants, consonant clusters, vowels, and diphthongs tested as well as the units in which they are produced (i.e., syllables, words, sentences). The model of stimulus presentation and sample elicitation (e.g., picture naming, imitation, delayed imitation, conversation) should also be considered in selecting instruments.

Material Presentation.   Another practical factor in selecting commercially available tests is the attractiveness, compactness, and manipulability of materials. Size, familiarity, and color of stimulus pictures and appropriateness for the client may influence the ease with which the clinician obtains responses to test stimuli. In addition, the organization and format of the scoring sheet are important for information retrieval. Tests with familiar and attractive stimulus items and score sheets that facilitate error analysis are desirable.

Scoring and Analysis.   Because the scoring and analysis procedures that accompany a test instrument determine the type of information obtained from the instrument, they are important considerations in test selection. Different assessment instruments currently available are designed to facilitate the following types of analysis: (1) phonetic and/or phoneme repertoire of English consonant and vowel sounds; (2) sound productions in a variety of contexts; (3) place, manner, voicing, and feature analysis; (4) phonological pattern/process analysis; and (5) age appropriateness of phonological productions.

Transcription and Scoring Procedures

Methods for Recording Responses.   The recording systems used by clinicians vary according to the purposes of testing, the transcription skills of the examiner, and personal preferences. The type of response recording the examiner employs will, however, determine the type of analysis the clinician is able to do with the sample obtained. In turn, the treatment approach may be significantly influenced by the type of analysis conducted.

In the least sophisticated scoring level, phonological productions are simply scored as correct or incorrect, based on the examiner's perception of whether the sound produced is within the acceptable adult phoneme boundary. This type of judgment is often the first assessment skill that clinicians learn and may be adequate for screening purposes. This type of scoring, however, is not recommended for the clinician doing a phonological assessment to determine the direction of treatment where more detail is necessary.

A second scoring level is to identify error productions as **substitutions**, **distortions**, or **omissions** (deletions). Sound substitutions are the replacement (substitution) of incorrect sounds for target segments (correct sounds), as when a child substitutes *w*abbit for *r*abbit. Sound distortions are similar to substitutions, but the replacement phone is an unacceptable allophonic variation within the perceptual boundary of a target phoneme.

The most common and useful transcription system is the *International Phonetic Alphabet* (IPA), which includes a different symbol for each phoneme. As indicated in Chapter 1, over 40 such symbols are utilized to identify the phonemes of the English language. This broad transcription system supplemented with a set of **diacritics** (narrow markers) usually provides sufficient detail for speech-language clinicians to adequately describe speech sound productions. For example, in a broad transcription of the word *key*, one would transcribe the initial segment with the symbol /k/. A more precise transcription of the initial /k/ would include the diacritic for aspiration [ʰ] following word-initial [kʰ] since aspiration occurs in production of /k/ in word-initial contexts. The aspiration modifier [ʰ] in this transcription represents one example of a diacritic. Use of diacritics, sometimes called a *close transcription system*, allows for recording specific topographical dimensions of individual segments. Such a transcription system is recommended when broad transcription does not adequately describe the errors. An example of a diacritic that reflects an error seen in disordered phonology is the following: If /t/ in the word /tɪp/ is dentalized, the diacritic for dentalization [̪] is placed under the /t/, thus [t̪ɪp]. Edwards (1986) recommended the symbols and diacritics presented in Table 6.1 for clinical use. Shriberg, Kwiatkowski, and Hoffman (1984) categorized some diacritic symbols as typically either "non-error" symbols or "error" symbols. In other words, as reflected in the preceding examples, some diacritics are most commonly used to transcribe variations in correct or standard productions, while others are more frequently used when transcribing speech sound errors.

Close transcription is particularly useful for describing the speech of individuals whose speech sound productions cannot be adequately described by broad phonetic symbols. For example, in assessing the phonological status of an individual with a cleft condition who is unable to achieve velopharyngeal closure for certain speech sounds, diacritics indicating nasal emission (s̈nail), or nasalization (bãet), may be useful in the description of the client's production of certain segments. Similarly, when assessing the articulation of an individual with impaired hearing, symbols to indicate excessive breathiness on vowels (e.g., [ɪ̤]), inappropriate vowel duration (e.g., [si:] for lengthened, [we'] for shortened), devoicing (e.g., [b̥]), and denasalization (e.g., ræet) are recommended if these characteristics are present in productions. Likewise, with developmental articulation errors characterized by lateralization (e.g., [s̪]), dentalization (e.g., [s̪], and devoicing (e.g., [n̥]), diacritics should be utilized.

Accuracy of Transcriptions.   One of the major concerns regarding transcription of responses relates to the accuracy of transcriptions. Clinicians must be concerned with whether or not their transcriptions are a valid representation of a client's productions. In making transcriptions, clinicians rely primarily upon auditory perceptual judgments. These

TABLE 6.1 Symbols and Diacritics

[x]	voiceless velar fricative, as in *Bach*
[Φ]	voiceless bilabial fricative
[ß]	voiced bilabial fricative
[¢]	voiceless lateral fricative
[pf]	voiceless labial affricative
[ts]	voiceless alveolar affricative
[dz]	voiced alveolar affricative
[ʔ]	glottal stop, as in [mʌʔi]

Stop Release Diacritics

[ʰ]	aspirated, as in [tʰap]
[⁼]	unaspirated, as in [p⁼un]
[¬]	unreleased, as in [kʰæt¬]
[ʻ]	slightly aspirated

Diacritics for Lip Shape

[w]	labialized, as in [s̫wit]
[↩ʷ]	protruded labialized
[ʌ] or [o]	unrounded
[x]	produced with lip inversion
[ɔ]	a vowel produced with lip rounding
[c]	a vowel produced with less lip rounding than usual

Diacritics for Nasality

[~]	nasalized, as in [fæ̃n]
[⸴]	denasalized
[⸕]	produced with nasal emission

Diacritics for Length

[:]	lengthened
[ʼ] or [˘]	shortened
[^] or [‿]	synchronous

Diacritics for Voicing

[ˬ]	partially voiced, as in [k̬æt]
[˳]	partially devoiced, as in [spuṇ]
[..]	produced with breathy voice (murmured)

Diacritics for Syllabicity

[ˌ]	a syllabic consonant, as in [bʌtn̩]
[‿]	a nonsyllabic vowel, as in [ðeə̯]

Diacritics for Stress

[ʼ], [ˈ], or [¹]	primary stress
[ˋ], [ˌ] or [²]	secondary stress
[ˌ] or [³]	tertiary (weak) stress

Diacritics for Tongue Position or Shape

[ᶾ] or [ʲ]	palatalized, as in [sʲu]
[ˌ]	dentalized, as in [tɛ̪n̪θ]
[~]	velarized, as in [tʰebɫ] (or pharyngealized)
[ᶜ] or [ʳ]	/r/-colored, rhotacized, or retroflexed, as in [kʰa̙]
[c] or [‿]	lateralized, as in [s̯op]
[ʊ]	markedly grooved
[⊷]	produced with a flattened tongue
[ˌ] or [¨]	centralized

TABLE 6.1 *Continued*

[ɻ] or [→]	retracted tongue, as in [s→op] or [s̠op]
[˕] or [←]	advanced tongue, as in [ʃ←u] or [ʃ̟u]
[˔] or [^]	raised tongue
[ᴛ] or [ˇ]	lowered tongue
[<]	a fronted sound
[>]	a backed sound
[˳]	derhotacized or deretroflexed
Other Diacritics	
['], [ʔ], or [.]	glottalized
[ₓ]	produced with frication
[ₗₗ]	whistled
[√]	trilled
Juncture Markers	
+	open juncture
		internal open juncture
↓	falling terminal juncture
↑	rising terminal juncture
→	checked or held juncture

Source: From M. L. Edwards. *Introduction to Applied Phonetics: Laboratory Workbook.* San Diego, Calif.: College-Hill Press, 1986, 185–187 © 1986. Used with permission.

The additional symbols listed here are part of the International Phonetic Alphabet (1978). Some diacritics are also from the IPA. Others are adapted from Bush and colleagues (1973) and Shriberg and Kent (1982). This is not an exhaustive list of additional symbols and diacritics.

judgments are sometimes supplemented with physiological measures (such as air pressure and flow information) and acoustical measures (such as that obtained from spectrographic analysis). These three types of data may not always be consistent with each other. For example, a glottal substitution for a stop in word-final position may be identified via a spectrographic analysis; and yet the glottal production may not be heard by a listener and thus will be transcribed as a deletion (omission). It must be recognized, however, that even the more objective measures of speech segments (i.e., acoustical and physiological recordings) are not devoid of human interpretation since no one-to-one correspondence exists between a phoneme production, perception, and/or acoustical and physiological measurements. For most aspects of clinical phonology, auditory perceptual judgments by the examiner form the basis for intervention decisions. Because of this, it is important for clinicians to establish the reliability of their perceptual judgments.

Interjudge Reliability.   Traditionally, clinicians have used agreement between two independent transcribers as a means of establishing reliability of judgments. *Interjudge agreement* or *reliability* is determined by the comparison of one examiner's transcriptions with those of another and is essential for reporting the results of phonologic research. In addition, for students beginning to make judgments about accuracy of phonological productions, establishing interjudge reliability with a more experienced person establishes the accuracy of judgments. A commonly used method to determine interjudge reliability, called *point-to-point agreement*, compares the clinicians' judgments on each test item. The number of items judged the same is divided by the total number of items to determine a percentage of agreement between judges. As an example, if two judges agreed on 17 of the 20 items and disagreed on 3; then, 17 divided by 20 is 0.85, which is then multiplied by 100 to obtain an interjudge reliability index of 85 percent agreement. (See Table 6.2.) Such point-to-point, or item-by-item, reliability is a stringent method for establishing agreement between judges.

Sometimes transcriptions are made by two or more examiners independently but simultaneously, with the final transcript arrived at by consensus (Shriberg, Kwiatkowski, and Hoffman, 1984). Discussion between examiners regarding what is heard takes place before a "final" judgment. This procedure, which typically involves a panel of examiners listening to tape-recorded responses, is used in difficult to judge situations. Obviously, some independence of judgment is lost in such a procedure.

In Table 6.2 the reliability index was based on correct-incorrect judgments of sound productions. It is easier to reach agreement on binary right-wrong judgments than on judgments recorded phonetically. It is even more difficult to obtain high reliability when sounds are transcribed with close phonetic transcription. An interjudge reliability figure of at least 90 percent or above on an item-by-item right-wrong comparison is usually considered suf-

TABLE 6.2   Independent Judgments by Judges A and B

Item	Judge A	Judge B
1	correct	correct
2	correct	correct
3	correct	incorrect
4	correct	incorrect
5	incorrect	incorrect
6	incorrect	incorrect
7	correct	correct
8	correct	correct
9	correct	correct
10	incorrect	correct
11	correct	correct
12	correct	correct
13	correct	correct
14	incorrect	incorrect
15	incorrect	incorrect
16	correct	correct
17	correct	correct
18	correct	correct
19	correct	correct
20	incorrect	incorrect

ficient to ensure that one person's judgments of articulatory productions are similar to another's. For more difficult transcription tasks, such as those where diacritics are used, interjudge agreement percentages will likely be considerably lower than this figure. Shriberg and Lof (1991), in a study of reliability of judgments of broad and narrow phonetic transcription, reported that for interjudge and intrajudge reliability, average agreement for broad transcriptions exceeded 90 percent, and for narrow transcriptions, between 65 and 75 percent agreement.

As inexpensive instrumentation is developed to record and analyze productions, acoustic data may serve to clarify some perceptual ambiguities.

Intrajudge Reliability.   Along with knowing that his or her judgments are in agreement with those of another examiner, the clinician will also want to know that his or her standards for judgments are consistent over time. Comparison of judgments made when scoring the same data on two separate occasions is referred to as *intrajudge reliability*. High reliability on such a measure is an indication that the examiner is consistent in his or her judgments. Tape recordings of responses are used to determine this type of reliability, since judgments are made twice of the same responses.

Connected Speech Sampling

Rationale.   All phonological evaluations should include a sample of connected speech. The ultimate objective of phonological treatment is correct production of sounds in spontaneous conversation; therefore, it is important that the examiner observe sound productions in as "natural" a speaking context as possible. Such samples allow one to transcribe phoneme productions in a variety of phonetic contexts, to observe error patterns, and, very importantly, to judge the intelligibility of the speaker in continuous discourse. Sounds produced in connected speech may also be studied in relation to other factors such as speech rate, intonation, stress, and syllable structure. This is not the case when sounds are sampled in isolated syllables or word productions. In addition, connected speech samples allow for multiple productions of sounds across lexical items.

Because spontaneous connected speech samples are the most valid or representative sample of phonological performance, some clinicians suggest that phonological analyses should almost exclusively be based on this type of sample (Shriberg and Kwiatkowski, 1980; Stoel-Gammon and Dunn, 1985; Morrison and Shriberg, 1992). Connected speech samples have the advantage of allowing the examiner to transcribe sound productions within the context of the child's vocabulary and with natural prosodic patterns. In addition, these samples can be used for other types of language analysis. Sometimes, however, there are practical problems associated with totally relying on such samples. Many individuals with severe phonological problems may be almost unintelligible, and it may be impossible or very difficult to reliably determine and/or transcribe what they are attempting to say in a conversational speech sample. Some children may be reluctant to engage in conversational dialogue with an adult they do not know. Simply eliciting single-word responses from some children may represent a challenge, even for a skilled clinician. It may also be an almost impossible task to obtain a spontaneous speech corpus that contains a truly representative sample of English phonemes.

Ingram (1989) has suggested that difficulty in obtaining a "cross-section of the sounds in English" (representative sample) may not be a critical issue. He argued that if a spontaneous sample is of "sufficient size," the child's preference for sounds is revealed. Sounds missing from the sample may reflect a "selective avoidance" by the child; that is, the child chooses not to produce them. He speculated that the "important sounds" will be produced a number of times in a spontaneous conversational speech sample and will provide a general picture of the child's phonological system. Words of caution on Ingram's speculations would suggest first, that the absence of specific sounds in a child's spontaneous speech may reflect an infrequent occurrence of those sounds in English rather than selective avoidance; and second, that even if the assumption of selective avoidance is valid, clinicians may want the benefit of information about other productions.

Elicitation Procedures.   The customary and preferred method for obtaining a sample of connected speech is to engage a client in spontaneous conversation. The clinician may talk with the client about such things as hobbies, television shows, or places the client has visited. The samples should be tape-recorded so that the clinician can play them back as often as required to accurately transcribe the client's utterances. Clinicians should make notes about topics covered and errors noted to facilitate later transcription.

Allen (1984) presented the following suggestions for recording speech-language samples:

1. *Avoid noise sources as much as possible.* By using soft toys, soft books, and cloth-covered table tops, noises can be muted considerably. By not talking while the client is talking, the voice of interest will not be obscured, and, by recording in a closed room, other environmental noises can be kept off the tape.
2. *Record in stereo.* This procedure records a wider dynamic range of voice signals and permits the use of binaural auditory acuity in later analyses.
3. *Moderately priced equipment may be entirely satisfactory for the job.* A stereo cassette recorder, two lavaliere microphones, low-priced tape, and light open-back headsets will deliver fully adequate recording and playback performance. In addition, look for output level controls; a "review" button; and direct, sturdy, and convenient connectors. Take spares of anything you can afford to buy and manage to carry.

Some clinicians have the client read a passage orally as an alternative method for obtaining a connected sample of speech. Although this procedure provides a sample of connected speech, it has been demonstrated that usually fewer errors occur in a sample obtained in this manner than in a corpus of conversational speech (Wright, Shelton, and Arndt, 1969). Moreover, clinicians frequently test children who have not yet learned to read, in which case this procedure is obviously not a viable option.

Some speech sound tests specify procedures for obtaining a sample of connected speech. For example, in the "Sounds-in-Sentences" subtest of the *Goldman-Fristoe Test of Articulation* (1969, 1986), the client listens to a story while viewing the accompanying pictures and is then asked to repeat the story. Such a *delayed imitation task* is designed to elicit particular sounds in certain phonetic contexts. A variation of the delayed imitation method is the *sentence repetition technique*, in which the clinician verbalizes a sentence containing a target sound and instructs the client to repeat it.

A more spontaneous method than either the immediate or delayed imitation technique is for the client to tell a story about a series of pictures selected to elicit target words and sounds. Dubois and Bernthal (1978) compared productions in the same word stimuli elicited through a picture-naming task, a delayed imitation task, and a storytelling task. They reported that the greatest number of errors were found on the storytelling task and the smallest number on the picture-naming task. These findings were not surprising since the task of naming single words requires different skills than the sequencing of words in phrases and sentences. Although the differences between the methods were statistically significant, the authors interpreted the differences as clinically nonsignificant. They did, however, report that some individuals varied from group trends in their production of certain sounds, depending on the task; for example, some children made significantly more errors on the delayed imitation task than on the picture-naming task.

Summary.   A connected speech sample is a crucial part of any phonological assessment battery because it allows (1) assessment of overall intelligibility, (2) determination of speech sound usage in its natural form, and (3) a database from which to judge the accuracy of individual sounds, patterns of errors, and consistency of misarticulations. The preferred method for obtaining connected speech samples is to engage the client in spontaneous conversation. If, for some reason, this cannot be accomplished, alternate procedures that can be used include: (1) conversational responses elicited via picture stimuli or objects, (2) utilization of a reading passage, and (3) telling a story following the clinician's model (delayed imitation).

Single-Word Testing

Rationale.   From the standpoint of widespread usage, analyzing phoneme productions in a corpus of single-word productions (usually elicited by having an examinee name pictures) has been a common method for assessing speech sounds. Single words provide a discrete, identifiable unit of production that examiners can usually readily transcribe. Since transcribers often are interested in observing the production of only one or perhaps two segments per word production, they are thus able to transcribe and analyze single-word samples more quickly than multiple or connected word samples. The efficiency of analyzing sound productions from single-word samples has resulted in widespread usage of such samples.

Examiners, in some instances, may be interested in transcribing all the phonemes in a single word, including vowels. It is more often the case that for a given word, only one or two consonants in particular word-positions are transcribed or scored. The most widely used descriptors of sound-positions in a word are *initial* (sound at the beginning of a word, e.g., /b/ in /bot/), *final* (sound at the end of a word, e.g., /t/ in /ræbɪt/), and *medial* (all sounds between the initial and final sounds, e.g., /ɔ/, /k/, and /ɪ/ in /wɔkɪŋ/).

In some instances, the prefixes *pre-*, *inter-*, and *post-* are each combined with the term *vocalic* to describe the location of a consonant sound within syllables. Prevocalic position refers to consonants that precede a vowel (CV) and, therefore, initiate the syllable (e.g., *s*oap, *c*at). Postvocalic position refers to consonants that follow the vowel (VC) and, therefore, terminate the syllable (e.g., soa*p*, ca*t*). Intervocalic position involves a consonant that is embedded (VCV) between two vowels (e.g., ca*m*el, ea*g*er). A singleton consonant in the initial position of a word is prevocalic. Likewise a singleton sound in word-final position is postvocalic. Fisher and Logemann (1971) indicated that a consonant in the intervocalic position serves the dual function of ending the preceding syllable and initiating the following syllable. Ingram (1981) suggested that when one consonant occurs between two vowel nuclei, such "ambisyllabic" consonants may be viewed as being shared by both syllables. The intervocalic consonant would be in the word-medial position since medial refers to somewhere between the first and the last sounds of the word. A medial consonant may stand next to another consonant and serve to initiate or terminate a syllable and, therefore, is not necessarily intervocalic. Thus, references to initial, medial, and final positions refer to location of consonants in a word, whereas the terms *prevocalic, intervocalic, postvocalic, releasor,* and *arrestor* refer to consonant position relative to syllables.

It has been suggested that speech sound productions may be influenced by the complexity of the syllables and words in which they are produced. We know that the number and juxtaposition of segments make some syllables more difficult to produce than others. The first syllable shapes to develop are generally CV, VC, and CVCV, which constitute the simplest syllable shapes.

One of the key issues in assessment concerns the correlation between phonological productions that occur in citation form (single words) and those that occur in connected speech. Most investigators have reported a positive correlation between the information obtained from naming pictures and speech sound productions in spontaneous speaking situations, although differences are frequently obtained in the two types of measures. Clinicians need to be aware that there may be relatively large differences between the two sampling procedures. Sound productions in single words may not accurately reflect the same sounds produced in a spontaneous speech context, especially in clients who have had experience with testing or been enrolled in therapy, since clients often have learned to produce certain sounds correctly in single-word responses to picture stimuli.

Jordan (1960) reported a relatively high correlation between the listener's perception of articulation adequacy in a spontaneous sample and the number of speech sound errors identified by a single-word articulation test. Although the Jordan study is frequently cited as justification for the use of a single-word test to predict performance in spontaneous speech, it should be remembered that these correlations (1) did not compare the number of errors in single-word productions with the number in spontaneous speech, and (2) were based on group trends, which may not reflect the performance of a given individual.

A second issue concerning the use of single-word test stimuli arises from the fact that speech does not occur in single words but in syllable strings. Therefore, using single words to make inferences about performance during connected speech may be questionable. Faircloth and Faircloth (1970) and Dubois and Bernthal (1978) reported differences in specific speech sound errors identified with single-word tests and those identified with conversational speech samples. In a study of natural processes, Shriberg and Kwiatkowski (1980) reported a nonsignificant correlation between responses obtained through single-word and connected speech samples. More recently, Morrison and Shriberg (1992) reported that children produced sounds more accurately in connected speech than they did in citation form testing.

Single-word testing does not provide the tester an opportunity to thoroughly evaluate the effect of context on speech sound productions (coarticulation). As discussed in Chapter 1, coarticulatory effects transcend phonetic, syllabic, and lexical (word) boundaries. Gallagher and Shriner (1975) reported that children's /s/ productions were affected by position in CCV consonant clusters. Curtis and Hardy (1959) reported that /r/ was more likely to be produced correctly in consonant clusters than in single phoneme productions. Hoffman, Schuckers, and Ratusnik (1977) reported that /r/ was influenced by factors such as lexical constraints (within vs. across word boundaries) and phonetic contexts. For example, when *r* was embedded in nonlexically constrained contexts (e.g., "the sick *r*at dies"), production was facilitated in the environment of /s/ as compared to /m/, /p/, and /t/. Variations in consonant production when sounds are elicited in consonant plus vowel contexts rather than in consonant clusters are widely recognized.

Despite reservations concerning some of the inferences that can be made about conversational speech on the basis of single word samples, most clinicians value and include single-word productions in the assessment battery. Single-word tests can provide the clinician with information concerning phonetic skills, may include all phonemes in a language, and can provide phonological data in a relatively short time. In addition, for unintelligible clients, the tester has the advantage of knowing the productions the client has attempted to say.

Elicitation Procedures. The customary way to elicit single-word productions is through the administration of a single-word articulation test (sometimes called a speech sound inventory), where a client names single words in response to picture stimuli. Single words may also be obtained by having a child name toys or objects. For young children, the clinician may simply wish to transcribe single-word productions the child produced spontaneously. Since picture-naming tests are the typical method for sampling single words, the following discussion will focus on this type of sampling procedure.

Speech sound inventories typically sample consonants, consonant clusters, and occasionally vowels and diphthongs. Consonants are usually assessed in the initial, medial, and final positions of words, for example, /s/ in *s*aw, pen*c*il, hou*s*e; /ʃ/ in *sh*oe, sta*t*ion, fi*sh* (see Figure 6.1). Some instruments elicit sounds only in the initial and final positions. The specific sounds included vary from test to test but almost always include those sounds that have a high frequency of error in children's speech. Winitz (1969) summarized data on frequently defective sounds from Roe and Milisen (1942) and Templin (1957) and indicated the following are the most frequently misarticulated sounds: /s, z, θ, ð, ʃ, ʒ, tʃ, dʒ, v, r, hw/. With the exception of the /hw/ (a phoneme that is occurring less frequently in English), these sounds are among those items usually included in single-word tests.

As stated previously, in comparison to consonants, speech sound inventories have traditionally placed little emphasis on the assessment of vowels. Undoubtedly this is a reflection of the fact that most children with phonological disorders have problems primarily with consonants. In addition, vowels are typically mastered at a relatively early age and are seldom misarticulated by children. Some speech sound tests do sample vowels (e.g., *Fisher-*

| | | | Consonants | | | | | Vowels/Dipthongs | | | | |
| | | | Sound Production | | | Errors | | | | Sound Production | Errors | |
Age	Sound	Words	I	M	F	Tongue	Lips					Comments
3.5	p	pie[1], apples[2], cup[3]						aɪ	pie[1]			
	m	monkey[4], hammer[5], comb[6]						o	comb[6]			
	w	witch[7], flowers[8]						ɪ	witch[7]			
	h	hanger[9]										
	b	book[10], baby[11], bathtub[12]						ʊ	book[10]			
	d	dog[13], ladder[14], bed[15]						ɔ	dog[13]			
	n	nails[16], bananas[17], can[18]						ə	bananas[17]			
	j	yes, thank you										
4	k	cat[19], crackers[20], cake[21]						ɚ-ə	crackers[20]			
	g	gum[22], wagon[23], egg[24]						ʌ	gum[22]			
	t	table[25], potatoes[26], hat[27]						æ	hat[27]			
	f	fork[28], elephant[29], knife[30]										
5	ŋ	hanger[31], swing[32]										
	dʒ	jars[33], angels[34], orange[35]										
6	ʃ	shoe[36], station[37], fish[38]						u	shoe[36]			
	l	lamp[39], balloons[40], bell[41]						ɛ	bell[41]			
	ʒ	measure, beige										
	v	vacuum[42], TV[43], glove[44]						ju	vacuum[42]			
	tʃ	chair[45], matches[46], sandwich[47]										
7	s	saw[48], pencil[49], house[50]						aʊ	house[50]			
	s bl	spoon[51], skates[52], stars[53]										
	z	zipper[54], scissors[55], keys[56]										
	l bl	blocks[57], clock[58], flag[59]						ɑ	blocks[57]			
	ð	(this/that)[60], feathers[60], bathe										
	r bl	brush[61], crayons[62], train[63]						e	train[63]			
8	θ	thumb[64], toothbrush[65], teeth[66]						i	teeth[66]			
	r	radio[67], carrots[68], car[69]										
	[Story][70–72] ___ voice quality ___ fluency ___ language use ___ intelligibility of connected speech								ɔɪ	boy[70]			
								ɝ-ɜ	bird[70]			
		Totals										Raw Score Total

Key: (+) *no error;* (–) *omission, sound substitution, distortion;* (i) *imitated sounds*
*Used with permission of PRO-ED.

FIGURE 6.1 Three position Speech Sound Test.

Logemann Test of Articulation Competence, Fisher and Logemann, 1971; *Templin-Darley Tests of Articulation*, Templin and Darley, 1969; *Photo Articulation Test*, Pendergast, Dickey, Selmar, and Soder, 1984).

Pollack (1991) delineated the following suggestions regarding vowel sampling:

1. Clients should be provided with multiple opportunities to produce each vowel.
2. Vowels should be assessed in a variety of different contexts, including (a) monosyllabic and multisyllabic words, (b) stressed and unstressed syllables, and (c) a variety of adjacent preceding and especially following consonants.
3. Limits for the range of responses considered correct or acceptable should be established since cultural influences may affect what is considered "correct."
4. Recommended vowels and diphthongs to be assessed include the following:

Nonrhotic

/i/	/ou/
/ɪ/	/ɔ/
/ei/	/ɑ/
/ɛ/	/ʌ/ə/
/ae/	/aɪ/
/u/	/au/
/ʊ/	/ɔi/

Rhotic

/ɝ, ɚ/	/ɔɚ/
/ɪɚ/	/ɑɚ/
/ɛɚ/	

To compensate for the lack of formal vowel assessment procedures, Pollack (1991) suggested that clinicians transcribe whole-word responses to the stimuli from commonly used articulation or phonological process tests. In order to get a comprehensive review of vowels and diphthongs, it may be necessary, however, to supplement existing stimuli with additional vowels, diphthongs, and contexts not included in standard tests.

Speech sound tests have enjoyed widespread popularity because they constitute an efficient way to sample sound productions. By focusing on particular word productions, the examiner knows what the child is attempting to say and that the client will produce (or attempt to produce) a particular set of sound productions. In contrast, with spontaneous speech samples, the examiner may not obtain a representative sample of sounds the child may be able to produce and, if intelligibility is a problem, will not know what the client has attempted to say.

A number of tests are commercially available. Despite the similarities among such tests, certain stimulus and response features differentiate one test from another. For example, one test may present items in a developmental sequence, another may organize the analysis according to place and manner of articulation. Still a third test may emphasize colored line drawings that are especially attractive to young children or include actual photographs.

Although phonological tests usually use pictures to elicit spontaneous responses, in some instances, imitation tasks are used. Studies comparing responses elicited via imitation with those elicited through spontaneous picture naming have produced inconsistent results. Investigators studying children between the ages of 5 and 8 years have reported that responses elicited via imitation tasks yield a greater number of correct responses than those elicited via spontaneous picture-naming (Siegel, Winitz, and Conkey, 1963; Smith and Ainsworth, 1967; Carter and Buck, 1958; Snow and Milisen, 1954). Other investigators who studied children ranging in age from 2 to 6 years reported no significant differences in results from elicitation via picture naming and imitation (Templin, 1947; Paynter and Bumpas, 1977).

Harrington, Lux, and Higgins (1984) studied responses to different types of picture-naming tasks and reported that children produced fewer errors when items were elicited via photographs as compared to line drawings. These data again suggest that different response elicitation procedures frequently produce different findings.

In spite of their widespread use, single-word tests have a number of limitations. Some experimenters have questioned the use of these tests because such measures do not allow children to use their "own" words but rather a set of predetermined and sometimes complex syllable and word shapes. Speech sound tests typically include both monosyllabic and multisyllabic words. The use of multisyllabic words may make more demands on a child's productions and elicit more errors than would monosyllabic words or the words used in a child's own spontaneous speech. Ingram (1976) compared young children's productions of initial fricatives and affricates in word-pairs in which the two words differed in syllable structure and/or stress. He reported that when stimulus pairs were similar in stress pattern and syllable structure, phoneme productions tended to be similar, but when syllable structure and/or stress of the pairs differed, monosyllabic words were more likely to be produced correctly than were multisyllabic words. Clinicians should recognize that syllable shape and stress patterns of stimulus words may affect speech sound productions.

Another difficulty with tests that elicit a sample via picture-naming is that they typically elicit only a single production in each of the three word positions. During phonological development, inconsistency in production is common, even in the same stimulus word. Since the production of a sound may fluctuate widely, the client's customary articulatory patterns should not be based on the production of a single stimulus item. The clinician can increase the number of sound samples obtained through a single-word test by transcribing all the sounds in each stimulus (lexical) item, instead of focusing only on a single sound in each stimulus item.

Summary.   Single-word samples, including speech sound tests, provide an efficient and relatively easy method for obtaining a sample of speech sound productions. Although they are frequently a valuable part of the phonological assessment battery, they should not constitute the only sampling procedure. Among their limitations are the small number of phonetic contexts sampled, the failure to fully reflect the effects of coarticulation, the questionable representativeness of single-word naming responses, and the lack of consistency in factors such as syllable shape, prosody, word familiarity, and parts of speech (e.g., nouns, verbs). To increase the number of phonetic contexts sampled through such tests, the clinician is encouraged to transcribe entire stimulus words.

Stimulability Testing

Rationale. Another sample of speech sound productions frequently included in a test battery is obtained through *stimulability testing*—that is, sampling the client's ability to repeat the correct form (adult standard) of error sounds when provided with "stimulation." In essence, this testing examines how well an individual imitates correct models of speech sounds that he or she produced incorrectly in single-word productions or in a connected speech sample. Although definitions of what constitutes stimulability testing have varied in the literature, it is a commonly used procedure in which the examiner asks the respondent to imitate an auditory and/or visual model of a sound, syllable, or word containing the adult form of the segment. The examiner may tell the client to "watch and listen to what I am going to say, and then you say it." It should be recognized, however, that there are no standardized procedures for conducting this type of testing. Some investigators have focused on a single type of response form (e.g., nonsense syllables), but in practice examiners typically seek to elicit imitative productions at three levels: sound in isolation, sound embedded in syllables, and sound embedded in words. The number of models provided by the examiner typically varies from one to five (Diedrich, 1983).

Stimulability testing has been used to predict (1) whether or not a sound is likely to be acquired without intervention, and (2) the level of phonetic production at which instruction might begin (e.g., isolation, syllables, or words). In other words, these data are often used when making decisions regarding case selection and speech sounds targeted for treatment.

Several investigators have reported that the ability of a child (ages 5 through 7 years) to imitate syllables or words containing a specific sound is related to the probability of that child's spontaneously correcting his or her misarticulation of that sound (Carter and Buck, 1958; Farquhar, 1961; Sommers, Leiss, Delp, Gerber, Fundrella, Smith, Revucky, Ellis, and Haley, 1967). Carter and Buck (1958) reported, in a study of first-grade children, that stimulability testing can be used for such prognostic purposes. They inferred that first-grade children who correctly imitated error sounds in nonsense syllables 75 percent of the time were likely to correct those sounds without instruction. Kisatsky (1967) compared the pre- to post-test gains in articulation accuracy over a six-month period of two groups of kindergarten children, one identified as a high stimulability group and the other as a low stimulability group. Although neither group received articulation instruction, results indicated that significantly higher correct scores were obtained by the high stimulability group in the six-month post-test.

Elicitation Procedures. Stimulability assessment is perhaps the least standardized assessment protocol included in phonological evaluation. As stated in the foregoing paragraphs, the examiner typically asks the client to look at the examiner's mouth or watch it in a mirror, listen to what is said, and then imitate the production. The examiner does not point out where teeth, tongue, or lips may be during production; the examinee is simply encouraged to listen and observe a production.

Stimulability testing usually includes imitative testing of those sounds produced in error in word and/or conversational samples. Such sounds are assessed in isolation, nonsense syllables (usually initial, medial, and final positions), and monosyllabic words (again in the three word-positions). The number of productions at each level may vary from one client and/or examiner to the next. Cooperation of the child, number of sounds produced in error, and success with the imitative task are factors the clinician should consider when deciding how extensive the stimulability assessment will be.

It is not uncommon for speech sound tests to include a place on the scoring form to record stimulability results, particularly for sounds in isolation. As suggested, the clinician will usually want to probe imitative skills in syllables and words. The Carter-Buck (1958) procedure discussed earlier included the following format for testing sounds in nonsense syllables for a client who misarticulated /k/:

*k*i	i*k*i	i*k*
*k*æ	æ*k*æ	æ*k*
*k*a	a*k*a	a*k*

Summary.   Stimulability testing is useful in identifying those individuals most likely to need phonological intervention (those with poor stimulability scores), and for determining the level of linguistic production for initiation of instruction. Although stimulability scores have been found to have some prognostic value for identifying those children who will self-correct errors, research data do not indicate that such testing can be totally relied upon to identify clients who will self-correct their errors.

Contextual Testing
Rationale.   As indicated earlier, speech sound errors, especially in children, are often variable and inconsistent. It has been suggested that sounds are often easier to produce in some contexts as opposed to others, thus resulting in inconsistency in production during the phonological acquisition period. Knowledge of the consistency of phonological errors is a factor taken into consideration when deciding on the need for therapy and for making treatment decisions such as choosing a sound to work on in therapy or deciding on a particular phonetic context that may facilitate accurate sound production.

Assessing contextual influences is based on the concept that sound productions influence each other in the ongoing stream of speech. McDonald (1964) suggested that valuable clinical information could be gained by systematically reviewing a sound as it is produced in varying contexts, and coined the term *deep test* to refer to the practice of testing a sound in a variety of phonetic contexts. McDonald was interested in the influence that adjacent sounds have on each other during speech production. For example, /s/ may be produced differently when preceded by /p/ in *capsun* than when it is preceded by 't,' as in *hatsun*. Coarticulatory effects consist of mechanical constraints associated with adjacent sounds and simultaneous preprogramming adjustments for segments later in the speech stream. This overlapping of movements (preprogramming) may extend as far as six phonetic segments away from a given sound (Kent and Minifie, 1977). The result is that segments may be perceived by a listener as being produced correctly in one context but not in another. Such information is of value to the clinician who seeks to establish a particular segment in a client's repertoire.

Elicitation Procedures.   One procedure that has often been used to sample contextual influences is the *Deep Test of Articulation* (McDonald, 1964), a series of phoneme-specific tasks designed to assess individual speech sounds in approximately 50 phonetic contexts.

Deep testing is predicated on the hypothesis that when the consonants preceding or following the sound of interest are systematically altered, the client will usually produce the target sound correctly in at least one phonetic context. In the *Deep Test of Articulation*, each of the stimulus items contains two words, one of which has the target sound. The two words are said together as a single bisyllable unit in order to assess the contextual influence. Phonetic context is varied by systematically changing the segment that immediately precedes or follows the target sound.

A second set of tools sometimes used for consistency-contextual testing are the *Sound Production Tasks* (SPT) developed by Elbert, Shelton, and Arndt (1967). Each imitative task assesses individual consonants in 30 contexts including a sound in isolation, syllables, words, and phrases. For example, items related to the /s/ include the following: /s/, /us/, household, I like soup. It should be pointed out that this measure was designed to facilitate measuring generalization during the course of therapy, and is frequently used for that purpose.

Probably the most comprehensive set of materials that has been developed to assess consistency-contextual influences is the *Clinical Probes of Articulation Consistency* (C-PAC) by Secord (1981). Individual probes elicit responses containing a particular sound in the prevocalic and postvocalic positions, plus clusters, sentences, and storytelling contexts. Probes are developed for all consonant sounds and vocalic /ɝ/. Approximately 100 responses are elicited for each sound.

Another way of doing a contextual analysis is by reviewing a connected speech sample for contexts in which a target sound is produced correctly. Occasionally facilitating contexts can be found in conversation that are not observed in single words or word-pairs.

A final type of contextual assessment, one that clinicians have borrowed from the field of linguistics, is the examination of a phoneme in various morphophonemic alterations (the effect of morpheme structure on phonological production). Such alterations may be examined by having the client produce a sound in differing morphophonemic structures. For example, if word-final obstruent /g/ has been deleted in /dɔg/ (i.e., [dɔ]), the examiner might assess whether or not /g/ is produced in the diminutive /dɔgi/. Likewise, if the child misarticulates /z/ in the word /roz/, the examiner might observe /z/ production in the morphophonemic context of /rozəz/.

Summary. Contextual testing is done primarily to determine phonetic contexts in which a sound error may be produced correctly. These contexts may then be used as a starting point for remediation. Contextual testing is also used as a measure of consistency of misarticulation.

Error Pattern Identification
Rationale. In addition to the traditional speech sound assessments that occur through connected speech sampling and speech sound inventories, many clinicians also employ a phonological process analysis to facilitate error pattern delineation in clients who evidence multiple phonological errors. While the response elicitation procedure is typically identical to that employed in citation testing (i.e., the client names pictures to produce single word responses), the type of scoring and analysis is designed to determine the presence of phonological process/phonological patterns among errors. This type of assessment and analysis

procedure is based on the assumption that children's speech sound errors are not random, but represent systematic variations from the adult standard. Phonologic patterns that describe several individual speech sound errors are identified. These error patterns frequently affect entire sound classes, particular sound sequences, or the syllable structure of words. Clinicians compare the child's productions with the adult standard and then categorize individual errors into phonologic patterns.

The notion of an analysis of error patterns is not a new one. Van Riper (1939), in his book *Speech Correction: Principles and Methods*, talked about substitution analysis and the need to organize speech sound errors into patterns. It was not until the late 1970s and early 1980s, however, that clinicians began to emphasize the identification of phonological patterns, processes, and rules.

One of the reasons pattern analysis procedures have appeal is that they often provide a better description of the child's phonological system than does a traditional categorization of errors as substitutions, distortions, and omissions. Khan (1985) furnished the following illustration of this point. A child who substitutes /wawa/ for *water* might be described in a traditional substitution analysis as substituting [w] for /t/ and substituting [a] for final /ɚ/. On the basis of what we know about phonological acquisition, the [wawa] for *water* substitution is more accurately described as syllable reduplication. The child in this instance is probably repeating the first syllable of the word *water* rather than using sound substitutions for target sounds in the second syllable. A second reason for doing a pattern analysis is the potential for treatment efficacy. When a pattern reflecting several sound errors is targeted for treatment, there is the potential for rapid generalization across sounds related to that pattern.

Systems of pattern analysis, whether based on a place-manner-voicing analysis, distinctive feature analysis, level of phonological knowledge, or more widely employed phonological process analysis procedures, are most appropriate for the client who has multiple errors. The intent of the analysis is to determine if there are patterns or relationships among speech sound error productions which differ from the adult standard. If only a few speech sounds are in error, one need not do a pattern analysis of a child's speech. For example, if a client is misarticulating only two consonants, /s/ and /ʃ/, the clinician would not do a pattern analysis. In this instance, the clinician would develop a remediation plan where both consonants are targeted for instruction.

Phonological patterns identified during analysis become the focus for determining target behaviors for remediation. For example, if a child has eight speech sound substitutions reflecting three error patterns (e.g., stopping of fricatives, gliding of liquids, and fronting), remediation would likely focus on the reduction of one or more of these phonological patterns (processes). The modification of one or more speech sounds (exemplars) reflecting a particular error pattern frequently results in generalization to other speech sounds reflecting the same error pattern. For example, establishment of final /p/ may generalize to all other stops deleted in word-final position. Another example of a remediation strategy would be to target for instruction all speech sounds that reflect a given pattern; that is, all the speech sound errors that appear to be simplified in a similar manner (same phonological pattern). If fricatives were being substituted for stops, the clinician might focus on the contrast between stops and fricatives. By focusing on sounds that reflect a similar error pattern, treatment should be more efficient than if it focuses on individual sounds without regard to phonological patterns.

A phonological *process* or *pattern* is typically defined as a systematic sound change or simplification that affects a class of sounds, or a particular sequence of sounds. This general definition reflects the way the concept has been used by most clinical phonologists. Some authors limit their definition of processes to "natural" phonological processes (Shriberg and Kwiatkowski, 1980; Stampe, 1969, 1973). According to these authors, for a phonologic pattern to be considered a "natural" phonologic process, it cannot be merely a pattern reflecting simplification of a more complex articulatory gesture; it must also occur in sound changes documented in at least some other phonologic phenomenon, such as historical language changes, slips of the tongue, dialectical variation, as well as in normal phonologic acquisition.

Others (Elbert and Gierut, 1986) maintain that only patterns identified through a generative analysis constitute true phonological processes. This type of linguistic analysis examines an individual's phonological system independent of adult standards, in a fashion similar to that used to describe an unknown phonology. Only when patterns are present in a nonrelational description of a child's sound productions are they considered processes.

Elicitation Procedures.   Since the late 1970s, several analysis procedures have been published that are based on the notion of phonologic processes. Phonologic analysis procedures have been published by Compton and Hutton (1978), Weiner (1979), Hodson (1986), Shriberg and Kwiatkowski (1980), Ingram (1981), Khan and Lewis (1986), and Bankson and Bernthal (1990b). In all of these procedures, phonologic patterns are described as phonologic processes. In addition to these published analysis procedures, phonologic productions recorded during connected speech sampling and/or single word testing can be analyzed for the presence of error patterns.

Summary.   Phonologic process instruments, while designed to facilitate a unique type of analysis, are discussed under assessment procedures because they represent a type of testing clinical phonologists often employ. The uniqueness of these kinds of tests is in the type of analysis they facilitate, as opposed to the type of samples obtained. Further discussion of such analyses will be presented later in this chapter under analysis procedures.

Phonologic Assessment in Young Children

Phonologic evaluation of young children (infants and toddlers) must be done within the context of evaluating overall communicative behavior. Since phonologic development is integrally related to development of cognition, language, and motor skills, it does not occur in isolation from these other aspects of a child's development. However, for our purposes, it is useful to isolate phonologic considerations from the overall communication process. The following paragraphs will present information related to this component of communication development that is not covered elsewhere in our discussion of phonologic assessment.

As is characteristic of all aspects of communication development in infants and toddlers, there is much variability among children in terms of the specific phonemes produced at any age. Such variability makes it difficult to formulate strict clinical guidelines for infants and toddlers. Speech sound productions initially emerge within the context of infant vocalizations at the prelinguistic level. One of the first assessments of phonologic development, especially with children at risk for developmental delay, involves determining whether or not the infant is progressing normally through the stages of infant vocalization. Information presented in Chapter 2 regarding the characteristics of these stages is helpful in knowing about sound productions that typically occur during this developmental period, including the gradual shift from prelinguistic to linguistic behavior during the first year.

The point in time and/or development when clinicians frequently become involved in assessing phonology in young children occurs after they have acquired approximately 50 words (completion of the transition stage), or are putting two words together. In normal developing children, first words typically occur about 12 months of age, the transition stage occurs between 12 and 18 months, and words are put together around 24 months. In children with *phonological delay*, obviously these stages may occur at a later chronological age. Phonologic analysis in young children is inextricably bound to development of the child's lexicon. Procedures for eliciting vocalizations from young children depend on the level of the child's development, and can include a range of activities such as stimulating vocalizations during caregiving and feeding activities; informal play with a caregiver, sibling, or clinician; structured play; interactive storytelling; sentence repetition; delayed imitation of a story told by the clinician; narrative generation (about a favorite book); spontaneous conversation.

Stoel-Gammon (1994) indicated that at 24 months children may be categorized into three groups: (1) those who are normal in terms of linguistic development (85 percent of children); (2) those who are slow developing (late talkers), but evidence no major deviations from patterns of normal acquisition; and (3) those whose developmental patterns deviate substantially from the broadest interpretation of norms in terms of order of acquisition or achievement of certain milestones. She indicated that the second and third groups together constitute 15 percent of the population. Children in the second group should be monitored to be certain that they "catch up" with the normal group. Stoel-Gammon indicated that children falling into this category would likely be those who, at 24 months, have a vocabulary smaller than 50 words, who have a phonetic inventory with only 4–5 consonants and a limited variety of vowels, and who, otherwise, are following the normal order of phoneme acquisition and do not have unusual error types. Children in the third group are those who need an early intervention program.

The type of phonological analysis often employed during the early stages of speech sound acquisition is termed an **independent analysis** of **phonological behavior**. An independent analysis identifies the speech sounds produced by a child without reference to appropriateness of usage. This type of analysis is appropriate for the assessment of both normal and delayed phoneme acquisition. For those children who have progressed to the point where they have enough language that intelligibility is a concern (beyond 50 words in their vocabulary), a **relational analysis** may also be employed. In such analyses, the child's phonological productions are compared with the adult standard.

An independent analysis of phonology is typically based on a continuous speech sample and is designed to describe a child's productions without reference to adult usage. Analysis of a child's productions as a self-contained system include the following (Stoel-Gammon and Dunn, 1985):

1. An inventory of sounds (consonants and vowels) classified by word position and articulatory features.

2. An inventory of syllables and word shapes produced (e.g., CVC, CV, VC, CCV).
3. Sequential constraints on particular sound sequences.

These three elements were incorporated by Stoel-Gammon and Dunn (1985) in a framework designed to facilitate organization and analysis of a child's phonological productions. This coding system organizes the sounds and/or words produced by a child and includes a separate coding sheet for different sound classes (e.g., stops, fricatives, vowels). The variables coded include (1) sound class, (2) word position (initial, medial, final), and (3) different word structures (consonants that cross a syllable boundary; multisyllabic words). Figure 6.2 provides an example of a coding sheet for stops. This protocol demonstrates how clinicians can organize sampling data to facilitate the identification of patterns present in the child's phonological system. Data from analyses such as this indicate the segments and syllable structures a child is producing.

A relational analyses of phonological productions is typically used with children in the two year age range evidencing normal language development. Most of the assessment information presented elsewhere in this chapter pertains to relational analyses.

Summary.   Phonological evaluations in infants and toddlers usually are done within the context of an overall communication assessment. Since phonological development is integrally related to other aspects of development such as cognition, motor development, other aspects of linguistic development. Informal assessment involving independent analyses is typically done with very young children and for those with limited verbal repertoires. Usually these include an inventory of sounds, syllables and word shapes produced, and phonological contrasts employed. Once a child has a vocabulary of 50 words, relational analysis may also be employed.

Related Assessment Procedures

The assessment of a child with a phonologic problem includes testing and data gathering procedures supplemental to those focusing directly on phonologic behavior. Some of these procedures are typically administered prior to actual phonologic assessment. Information thus gathered is intended to provide a more comprehensive picture of an individual client and thereby contribute to a better understanding of his or her problem. It may also influence management recommendations that are made regarding a given client.

These additional assessment procedures often include a case history; an oral cavity examination; and hearing, language, fluency, and voice screenings. These procedures can aid the clinician in the identification of factors that may contribute to or be related to the delay or impairment of phonology. Data gathered from these additional measures may lead to referral to other specialists and/or influence remediation decisions. If, for example, a child has a problem with closure of the velopharyngeal port, referral to a cleft palate team may result in pharyngeal flap surgery prior to speech intervention.

Presence of suspected sensory, structural, or neurological deficiencies must be corroborated by appropriate related personnel (e.g., audiological, medical) and recommendations from those sources must be taken into consideration as part of the assessment. Any of these factors may be important in decisions regarding the need for therapy, the point at which

Name: DE   Sampling condition: *The Assessment of Phonological Processes*
Age: 4:6 Date of sampling: 11/24/82

	Initial			Medial		Final		
Stops	1. CV(c)	2. $C^nV(C)$	3. Multisyllabic	4. -C-	5. -C^n-	6. (C)VC	7. (C)VC^n	8. Multisyllabic
P	page [setʃ]	spoon [sũn] spring [swĩn]	paper [ˈfæfɚ]	open [ˈotɛ̃n] paper [ˈfæfɚ] zipper [ˈzɪpə]	airplane [ˈɛɚseˈn]	cup [sʌp] rope [rop] soap [sop]	jump [ʒʌp]	makeup [ˈmetəp]
b	bed [bid] Bo [bo] book [but]	brown [bə̃n]	baseball [ˈbæbʌ] basket [ˈbæsɪt]	cowboy [ˈsoboi]	baseball [ˈbæbʌ] football [ˈfʌtba] toothbrush [ˈtʰusrəʃ]	tub [sʌb]		
t	ten [zɛ̃n] tub [sʌb] two [tsu]	star [saʌ] stick [tʰɪ] string [swĩn] truck [tʰʌt]	TV [sivi] television [ˈtseztĩn] toothbrush [ˈtʰusrəʃ]	glitter [ˈzɪdə] scooter [ˈzʌdə] water [ˈwaə]	football [ˈfʌtba] quarter [ˈtʃwʌdə]	hat [æt]	shirt [ʒɚt]	basket [ˈbæsɪt] minutes [ˈmĩnəz]
d	doll [daʌ]				screwdriver [ˈʃudaɪbɚ] candle [ˈsændl]	bed [bid] sled [sɛd]	and [ʌ] closed [sozd] hand [æ̃n]	
k	couch [tʃaʊtʃ] cup [sʌp]	Claus [sɔz] clothes [soz] closed [sozd] squirrel [swɛl]	candle [ˈsændl] coffee [ˈsɔsi] cowboy [ˈsoboi] colors [ˈsʌzɚz] scooter [ˈzʌdə] screwdriver [ˈʃudaɪbɚ]	makeup [ˈmetəp] wrecker [ˈwɛdə]	basket [ˈbæsɪt]	book [but] like [let] Luke [zʌt] snake [set] stick [tʰɪ] truck [tʰʌt]	fork [sort]	music [ˈmusɪt]
g	gun [zʌ̃n]	glove [sʌz] green [wĩn, sĩn]	Christmas [ˈsɪtmʌs] quarter [ˈtʃwʌdə] glasses [ˈsæzɪz] glitter [ˈzɪdə]		Fall Guy [sʌ daɪ] finger [ˈfĩdə]	rug [wʌd]		

FIGURE 6.2 Data organization for selecting words for analysis.

Source: Stoel-Gammon, C., and C. Dunn, *Normal and Disordered Phonology in Children*, 1985 (Austin, Tex.: PRO-ED), pp. 136–137. Used with permission.

therapy should begin, and the treatment to be prescribed. Although they are routinely screened in phonologic evaluations, language, fluency, and voice screening will not be covered in this text.

Case History

To facilitate an efficient and effective assessment, a case history is obtained from the client or a parent prior to the phonological assessment. This allows the clinician to identify (1) possible etiological factors; (2) the family's or client's perception of the problem; (3) the academic, work, home, and social environment of the client; and (4) medical, developmental, and social information about the client. Case history information is usually obtained through a written form completed by the client or parents. It is frequently supplemented by an oral interview. Specific questions on the phonological status of a young child might include the following: (1) Did your child babble? Can you describe it? (2) When did your child say his or her first words? What were they? When did he or she start putting words together? (3) Describe your child's communication problem, and your concerns about it. (4) How easy is your child to understand? By the family? By strangers? (5) What sounds does your child say? (6) What do you think caused your child's speech difficulty? While case histories obtained from the client or the client's family are products of memory and perception and thus may not reflect total accuracy, parents and clients in general are reliable informants. In spite of its shortcomings, the case history provides the clinician with important background information that frequently influences assessment decisions and subsequent management recommendations.

Oral Cavity Examination

Oral cavity (oral peripheral) examinations are administered to describe the structure and function of the oral mechanism for normal speech purposes. In particular, dentition is observed for bite and missing teeth; hard and soft palates are examined for clefts, submucous clefts, fistulas, and fissures. Size, symmetry, and movement of the lips; size and movement of the tongue; and symmetry, movement, and functional length of the soft palate are also observed.

To examine the intraoral structures, it is recommended that the client be seated immediately in front of the clinician with his or her head in a natural upright position and at a level that allows easy viewing. The examiner should wear surgical gloves. If the client is a child, the examiner may have the child sit on a table or the examiner can kneel on the floor. Although it might seem that the oral cavity would be viewed best when the client extends his or her head backward, such a position can distort normal relationships of the head and neck. The client's mouth usually should be at the examiner's eye level. A flashlight, or other light source, together with a tongue blade will aid in the examination. Observations should start at the front of the oral cavity and progress to the back. Since the oral cavity examination is important in identifying possible etiological factors, a description of how an examination is conducted is presented below. For a more complete presentation of procedures for conducting an oral-mechanism examination, see St. Louis and Ruscello (1981).

Dentition

For the examiner to evaluate the occlusal relationship (i.e., alignment of upper and lower jaws), the client should have the first molars in contact with each other since the occlusal relationship of the upper and lower dental arch are made with reference to these molar contacts. The upper dental arch is normally longer and wider than the lower dental arch; therefore, the upper teeth normally extend horizontally around the lower dental arch; and the maxillary (upper) incisors protrude about one-quarter inch in front of the lower teeth and cover about one-third of the crown of the mandibular incisors. Such dental overjet or overbite is the normal relationship of the dental arches in occlusion.

The teeth are said to be in open bite when the upper teeth do not cover part of the lower teeth at any given point along the dental arch. Mason and Wickwire (1978) recommended that, when evaluating occlusal relationships, the clinician should instruct the client to bite on the back teeth and to separate the lips. They further stated that

> while in occlusion, the client should be asked to produce several speech sounds in isolation, especially /s/, /z/, /f/, and /v/. Although these sounds may not normally be produced by the client with teeth in occlusion, the standardization of airspace dimensions and increases in pressure in the oral cavity can unmask a variety of functional relationships. For example, the child who usually exhibits an interdental lisp may be able to articulate /s/ surprisingly well with teeth together. This occluded position can also unmask and/or counteract habit patterns related to the protrusion of tongue and mandible on selected sounds. (15)

Mason and Wickwire also suggested that an individual with excessive overjet who has difficulty with /s/ should be instructed to rotate the mandible forward as a means of adaptation to the excessive overjet. As pointed out in Chapter 5, however, dental abnormality and speech problems are frequently unrelated, and thus a cause-and-effect relationship between occlusion deviation and articulation problems should not be assumed.

Hard Palate

The hard palate (i.e., the bony portion of the oral cavity roof) is best viewed when the client extends his or her head backward. Normal midline coloration is pink and white. When a blue tint on the midline is observed, further investigation of the integrity of the bony framework is indicated. Such discoloration may be caused by a blood supply close to the surface of the palate and is sometimes associated with a submucous cleft (an opening in the bony palatal shelf). But when a blue tint is seen lateral to the midline of the hard palate, it usually suggests only an extra bony growth, which occurs in approximately 20 percent of the population.

Where a submucous cleft of the hard palate is suspected, palpation (rubbing) of the mucous membrane at the midline of the most posterior portion of the hard palate (nasal spine) is recommended. Although many speech-language pathologists note the height of the hard palatal vault, it probably has little relationship to articulation deviations. The contour or height of the palatal vault may influence certain articulatory contacts, but most individuals with high palatal vaults use compensatory movements that allow for adequate speech sound production.

Soft Palate or Velum

The soft palate should be evaluated with the head in a natural upright position. When the head is not in that position, changes in the structural relationship in the oral cavity area may prevent the viewing of velar function as it occurs during speech.

Mason and Wickwire cautioned that the assessment of velar function, especially velar elevation, should not be done with the tongue protruded or with the mandible positioned for maximum mouth opening. They recommended a mouth opening of about three quarters of the maximum opening since velar elevation may be less than maximum when the mouth is open maximally.

The coloration of the soft palate, like that of the hard palate, should be pink and white. A midline bluish tint should alert the clinician to the possibility of a submucous cleft of the velum, in which case the surface of the velum is covered with mucous membrane, but the underlying layer of periosteum is absent.

The critical factor in velar function is the effective or functional length of the velum and not the velar length per se. Effective velar length is the portion of tissue that fills the space between the posterior border of the hard palate and the pharyngeal closure. Effective velar length is only one factor in adequate velopharyngeal sphincter function and provides little or no information about the function of the sphincter's pharyngeal component, another critical factor for adequate velopharyngeal valving.

The final velar observation typically made is velar symmetry and evaluation. The elevation and posterior movement of the velum is also partially obstructed from view in an intraoral exam. But when the velum does not elevate to the plane of the hard palate during sustained vowel phonation, an inadequately functioning velopharyngeal sphincter should be suspected. It should also be remembered that if the observation is made with the tongue protruded, velar elevation can be restricted.

The posterior-most appendage or extension of the velum is the uvula, which has little or no role in speech production. However, a *bifid* uvula should alert the clinician to other possible anatomical deviations. A bifid uvula appears as two appendages rather than one and is occasionally seen in the presence of submucous clefts and other abnormal anatomical findings.

Fauces

The next area to observe in the oral cavity is the faucial pillars and the tonsillar masses. Only in rare instances are these structures a factor in speech production. The presence or absence of tonsillar masses is noted and, if present, their size and coloration are observed. Redness or inflammation may be evidence of tonsillitis, and large tonsillar masses may displace the faucial pillars and reduce the isthmus.

Pharynx

The oropharyngeal area is difficult to view in an intraoral examination. The pharyngeal contribution to velopharyngeal closure cannot be assessed through intraoral viewing because pharyngeal valving occurs at the level of the nasopharynx, a level superior to that which can be observed through the oral cavity. In some individuals, movement of tissue to form a prominence or ridge (Passavant's Pad) can be seen on the posterior wall of the pharynx; Passavant's Pad is not visible at rest but can usually be seen during sustained phonation.

Passavant's Pad is present in approximately one-third of individuals with cleft palates but is otherwise rare. Since its presence reflects a compensatory mechanism, the examiner should be alert to possible velopharyngeal valving problems. The presence of Passavant's Pad may suggest that adenoidal tissue is needed for velopharyngeal closure, and this factor should be considered in surgical decisions regarding adenoidectomies.

The pharyngeal gag response has been identified as a useful procedure to obtain an idea of the functional potential of the velum. We recommend that the gag response be used only in very rare instances since many clients have a strong aversion to the procedure, and velar function during gagging generally has little relationship to velopharyngeal valving during speech. Elicitation of a gag may provide some useful information in cases where lack of innervation and a paresis of the pharyngeal or palatal function is suspected. Gagging can be induced by pressing firmly on the base of the tongue or by touching the velum with a tongue blade. Gagging usually results in maximum velar excursion and maximum movement of the pharyngeal walls.

Tongue

As pointed out in Chapter 5, the tongue is a primary articulator, and individuals are able to modify tongue movements to compensate for many structural variations in the oral cavity. In terms of tongue size, two problematic conditions are occasionally found. The first, termed *macroglossia*, is an abnormally large tongue. Although this characteristic occurs frequently in certain populations (for example, those with Down's syndrome), the overall incidence is relatively low and research data do not point to the tongue as the cause of speech problems in Down's children. The condition where the tongue is abnormally small in relation to the oral cavity is termed *microglossia*, but this condition rarely, if ever, causes a speech problem.

It has been pointed out that tongue movements for speech activities show little relationship to tongue movements for nonspeech activities. Unless motor problems are suspected, little is gained by having the client perform a series of tongue movements used for nonspeech activities. But protrusion of the tongue or moving the tongue laterally from one corner of the mouth to the other may provide information about possible motor limitations or problems in control of the tongue.

The rapid speech movements observed in diadochokinetic tasks provide limited information with respect to speech function. Winitz (1969) pointed out that the child with a speech problem is at a distinct disadvantage on such tasks because he or she has had less experience producing phonemes correctly than normal developing children. The absolute number of syllables, such as /pʌ/, /tʌ/, /kʌ/, that an individual can produce in a given unit of time usually bears little relationship to articulatory proficiency except when gross motor problems are present. For a discussion of the relationship between diadochokinetic testing and articulation, see Chapter 5. Mason and Wickwire (1978) suggested that the clinician focus on the pattern of tongue movement and the consistency of contacts during diadochokinetic tasks.

A short lingual frenum can restrict movement of the tongue tip. Most individuals, however, acquire normal speech in spite of a short lingual frenum. If the client can touch the alveolar ridge with the tongue tip, the length of the frenum is probably adequate for speech purposes. In the rare instance where this is not possible, surgical intervention may be necessary.

Summary

In an oral cavity examination in which the clinician notes an inadequacy of structure or function that might contribute to the articulation disorders, he or she has several options: (1) refer the client to other professionals (e.g., otolaryngologist, orthodontist) for assessment and possible intervention, (2) engage in further observation and testing to verify the earlier observation and note its impact upon speaking skills, and (3) provide instruction related to compensatory or remedial behaviors.

Audiological Screening

The primary purpose of audiological screening is to determine whether a client exhibits a loss of auditory function, which could be an etiological factor associated with a phonological disorder. Audiological screening is usually conducted with pure tones and/or impedance audiometry prior to phonological assessment.

Pure tone screening typically involves presentation of pure tone stimuli at 500, 1000, 2000, and 4000 Hz at a predetermined intensity level. Usually, a 20 dB HL is used for screening, but this level may be altered to compensate for ambient noise in the room. The pure tone frequencies used in screening are those considered most important for receiving speech stimuli. The loudness of the pure tone stimuli reflects threshold levels needed to function adequately in the classroom.

Impedance screening measures eardrum compliance (movement of the eardrum) and middle-ear pressure as air pressure is altered in the external auditory canal. This screening test yields basic information about the functioning of the tympanic membrane by eliciting the acoustic reflex. The acoustic reflex can be measured by presenting a relatively loud signal to the ear and observing the presence or absence of a change in the compliance of the eardrum. Screening of the acoustic reflex usually involves the presentation of a 1000 Hz signal at 70 dB above a person's threshold. The acoustic reflex is a contraction of the stapedial muscle when the ear is stimulated by a loud sound and serves as a protective device for the inner ear. The client who fails a pure tone for impedance screening test should be referred to an audiologist for a complete audiological assessment.

Summary

As indicated in the discussion of hearing as it relates to speech sound productions in Chapter 5, it is critical to know the status of a client's hearing. There is some indication that even recurrent middle ear problems can contribute to phonological delay. In the case of more severe auditory impairments, there is frequently a correlation between extent of hearing loss and level of speech and language development. Given this relationship, audiological screening must be a routine part of phonological assessment procedures.

Speech Sound Discrimination Testing

A review of the literature on the relationship between speech sound discrimination and articulation is presented in Chapter 5. The information presented there provides background for the assessment of speech sound discrimination.

For many years, clinicians assumed that most children with articulation errors were unable to perceive the difference between the standard adult production and their own error production, and then inferred that many phonological problems were the result of this faulty perception. As a result of this assumption, speech sound discrimination testing became a standard procedure in the assessment battery. Research reported in the last two decades has cast doubt on the cause-and-effect relationship between faulty perception and phonological disorders. Thus, the routine use of speech sound discrimination tests has declined. At the present time, speech sound discrimination testing is typically done only with those clients suspected of having a perceptual problem (e.g., collapsing of two or more adult contrasts into a single sound).

For many years, the most widely used speech sound discrimination tests were general tests of sound discrimination which did not reflect a child's specific speech sound errors. These tests typically involved a paired comparison task of minimal pairs (e.g., coat-boat) produced by the examiner or presented via audio tape. Most of the comparisons did not examine contrasts relevant to a particular child's error productions. An example of a general test of discrimination is the *Goldman-Fristoe-Woodcock Diagnostic Auditory Discrimination Test* (Goldman, Fristoe, and Woodcock, 1970).

Perceptual testing usually involves the client's differentiating the adult standard production from his or her error production, and/or assessment of the child's perception of phonological contrasts. In-depth perceptual testing of an error sound requires numerous phonemic pairings, all focusing on contrasts with the target sound.

Locke's Speech Production Perception Task

One perceptual measure of various phonemic contrasts is the *Speech Production Perception Task* (Locke, 1980), which was designed to assess a child's perception of his or her articulatory errors and involves no preselected stimuli. The stimuli presented are based on the child's error productions. The format for this task, along with an example of the scoring sheet, appear in Table 6.3.

Preliminary to the presentation of Locke's protocol, the child's speech sound errors must be identified. The child's error productions and the corresponding adult (correct) forms are then used to construct the perception task. In this procedure, the adult form is identified as the *production task stimulus*, and the child's substitution or deletion as the *production task response*. A perceptually similar control phoneme is entered as the *production task control phoneme*. For example, if the client substitutes [wek] for /rek/, the stimulus production (SP) would be *rake* /r/, the response production (RP) would be *wake* /w/, and an appropriate control production (CP) would be *lake* /l/.

To administer the task, the examiner presents a picture or an object to the child and names it, using either the correct (SP), incorrect (RP), or control sound (CP) in accord with the test protocol. After the examiner asks "Is this _____?", the child responds yes or no, indicating that he or she accepts or rejects the correct, incorrect, and control phonemes presented. Following administration of the 18 items included in the test, the number of correct responses to the three types of items (SP, RP, CP) are tabulated. A similar procedure would have to be constructed for each sound substitution in which perception is to be examined.

Winitz's Phonological Performance Test

Winitz (1984) suggested that speech sound perception may be adequate on word discrimination tasks but may break down in a conversational context. He described the following

TABLE 6.3   Speech Production Perception Task

Child's Name _____ Sex: M F Birthdate: _____ Age: ____ Yrs. ____ Mos. ____

Date _____		Date _____		Date _____	
Production Task		Production Task		Production Task	
Stimulus	Response*	Stimulus	Response	Stimulus	Response
/θ ʌ m/ →	/f ʌ m/	/r e i k/ →	/w e i k/	/ʃ u/ →	/s u/
SP /θ/ RP /f/	CP /s/	SP /r/ RP /w/	CP /l/	SP /ʃ/ RP /s/	CP /t/
Stimulus-Class	*Response*	*Stimulus-Class*	*Response*	*Stimulus-Class*	*Response*
1 /s/ - CP	yes NO	1 /r/ - SP	YES no	1 /s/ - RP	yes NO
2 /f/ - RP	yes NO	2 /l/ - CP	yes NO	2 /t/ - CP	yes NO
3 /θ/ - SP	YES no	3 /r/ - SP	YES no	3 /t/ - CP	yes NO
4 /θ/ - SP	YES no	4 /l/ - CP	yes NO	4 /ʃ/ - SP	YES no
5 /f/ - RP	yes NO	5 /w/ - RP	yes NO	5 /ʃ/ - SP	YES no
6 /s/ - CP	yes NO	6 /w/ - RP	yes NO	6 /s/ - RP	yes NO
7 /s/ - CP	yes NO	7 /r/ - SP	YES no	7 /s/ - RP	yes NO
8 /θ/ - SP	YES no	8 /w/ - RP	yes NO	8 /ʃ/ - SP	YES no
9 /f/ - RP	yes NO	9 /r/ - SP	YES no	9 /t/ - CP	yes NO
10 /θ/ - SP	YES no	10 /l/ - CP	yes NO	10 /ʃ/ - SP	YES no
11 /f/ - RP	yes NO	11 /l/ - CP	yes NO	11 /t/ - CP	yes NO
12 /s/ - CP	yes NO	12 /w/ - RP	yes NO	12 /s/ - RP	yes NO
13 /f/ - RP	yes NO	13 /t/ - SP	YES no	13 /ʃ/ - SP	YES no
14 /θ/ - SP	YES no	14 /l/ - CP	yes NO	14 /s/ - RP	yes NO
15 /s/ - CP	yes NO	15 /w/ - SP	YES no	15 /ʃ/ - SP	YES no
16 /f/ - RP	yes NO	16 /r/ - SP	YES no	16 /t/ - CP	yes NO
17 /θ/ - SP	YES no	17 /w/ - RP	yes NO	17 /t/ - CP	yes NO
18 /s/ - CP	yes NO	18 /l/ - CP	yes NO	18 /s/ - RP	yes NO
RP ____ CP ____ SP ____		RP ____ CP ____ SP ____		RP ____ CP ____ SP ____	

Source: Adapted by permission from J. Locke, "The Inference of Speech Perception in the Phonologically Disordered Child Part II: Some Clinically Novel Procedures, Their Use, Some Findings." *Journal of Speech and Hearing Disorders*, 45 (1980): 447.

*The correct response is in upper case letters.

procedure for assessing discrimination at what he calls the "phonological level." He devised a mental perceptual measure that is phoneme-specific and designed to assess the contrast between a target sound and a perceptually similar sound in a sentence context. The clinician tells the child to listen to three sentences, each of which contains one example of a given target sound. When they are completed, two pictures will be presented and the child is instructed to select the picture which best represents the meaning of the three sentences. In each sentence the same word (e.g., *rake*) of a minimal pair (e.g., *rake-wake*) is used. At a later point in testing, the contrastive word (e.g., *wake*) is examined within the same three sentences.

In Figure 6.3, items used to assess the /r/-/w/ contrast are presented.

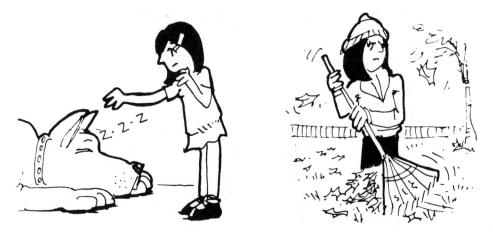

FIGURE 6.3   Phonological Performance Analysis Test.
I was to wake it up.
I didn't want to wake it up.
Finally I was told to wake it up.

I was to rake it up.
I didn't want to rake it up.
Finally I was told to rake it up.

Source: Winitz, H., *Treating Articulation Disorders: For Clinicians by Clinicians.* Austin, Tex.: PRO-ED (1984), p. 35. Used with permission.

Phonological Contrast Testing

An additional type of perceptual testing is the assessment of a child's perception of phonological contrasts. Grunwell (1982) indicated that the child with disordered phonology characteristically lacks perception of the phonological contrasts of the language. It has been hypothesized that one reason for this is the child's small phonetic inventory.

Assessment of a child's awareness of phonological contrasts provides the clinician with data relative to the child's phonemic system at a perceptual level. Most clinicians improvise assessment tasks requiring the child to indicate awareness that certain contrasts are in his or her perceptual repertoire. For example, a child may be shown pictures of the following pairs of words which contrast s/t, s/ʃ, and s/θ, and be asked to pick up one picture from each pair as it is named.

sea	sea	some
tea	she	thumb

Summary.   Once it is determined that perceptual testing is appropriate, the primary concern is the child's ability to differentiate between the adult standard and his or her error productions. External discrimination tests, tests based on the child's specific errors, and tests of phonemic contrasts are used for this purpose. At present, we have only a superficial understanding of the relationship between phonological production and perception. As a result, caution is required when interpreting perceptual test findings relative to performance on production tasks. Further research is necessary if we are to better understand the critical perceptual skills for the clinical management of the child with a phonological disorder.

References

Allen, G., "Some tips on tape recording speech-language samples." *Journal of the National Student Speech-Language-Hearing Association, 12* (1984): 10–17.

Bankson, N., and J. Bernthal, *Quick Screen of Phonology.* Chicago: Riverside Press, 1990a.

Bankson, N. W., and J. E. Bernthal, *Bankson-Bernthal Test of Phonology.* Chicago: Riverside Press, 1990b.

Bush, C. N., M. L. Edwards, J. M. Luckau, C. M. Stoel, M. A. Macken, and J. D. Petersen, On specifying a system for transcribing consonants in child languages: A working paper with examples from American English and Mexican Spanish. Committee on Linguistics, Stanford University, Stanford, Calif., 1973.

Carter, E., and M. Buck, "Prognostic testing for functional articulation disorders among children in the first grade." *Journal of Speech and Hearing Disorders, 23* (1958): 124–133.

Compton, A., and S. Hutton, *Compton-Hutton Phonological Assessment.* San Francisco: Carousel House, 1978.

Curtis, J., and J. Hardy, "A phonetic study of misarticulations of /r/." *Journal of Speech and Hearing Research, 2* (1959): 224–257.

Diedrich, W., "Stimulability and articulation disorders." In J. Locke (Ed.), *Assessing and Treating Phonological Disorders: Current Approaches. Seminars in Speech and Language, 4.* New York: Thieme-Stratton, 1983.

Drumwright, A., *The Denver Articulation Examination.* Denver: Ladoca Project and Publishing Foundation, 1971.

Dubois, E., and J. Bernthal, "A comparison of three methods for obtaining articulatory responses." *Journal of Speech and Hearing Disorders, 43* (1978): 295–305.

Edwards, M. L., *Introduction to Applied Phonetics.* San Diego: College-Hill Press, 1986.

Elbert, M., and J. Gierut, *Handbook of Clinical Phonology Approaches to Assessment and Treatment.* San Diego: College-Hill Press, 1986.

Elbert, M., R. L. Shelton, and W. B. Arndt, "A task for education of articulation change." *Journal of Speech and Hearing Research, 10* (1967): 281–288.

Faircloth, M., and S. Faircloth, "An analysis of the articulatory behavior of a speech-defective child in connected speech and in isolated-word responses." *Journal of Speech and Hearing Disorders, 35* (1970): 51–61.

Farquhar, M. S., "Prognostic value of imitative and auditory discrimination tests." *Journal of Speech and Hearing Disorders, 26* (1961): 342–347.

Fisher, H. B., and J. A. Logemann, *The Fisher-Logemann Test of Articulation Competence.* Boston: Houghton Mifflin, 1971.

Fluharty, N., *Fluharty Preschool Speech and Language Screening Test.* Bingingham, Mass.: Teaching Resources Corporation, 1978.

Gallagher, R., and T. Shriner, "Contextual variables related to inconsistent /s/ and /z/ production in the spontaneous speech of children." *Journal of Speech and Hearing Research, 18* (1975): 623–633.

Goldman, R., and M. Fristoe, *Goldman-Fristoe Test of Articulation.* Circle Pines, Minn.: American Guidance Service, 1969, 1986.

Goldman, R., M. Fristoe, and R. Woodcock, *The Goldman-Fristoe-Woodcock Test of Auditory Discrimination.* Circle Pines, Minn.: American Guidance Service, 1970.

Grunwell, P., *Clinical Phonology*. Rockville, Md.: Aspen, 1982.

Harrington, J., I. Lux, and R. Higgins, "Identification of error types as related to stimuli in articulation tests." Paper presented at the convention of the American Speech-Language-Hearing Association. San Francisco, 1984.

Hodson, B., *The Assessment of Phonological Processes*. Danville, Ill.: Interstate Press, 1986.

Hoffman, P. R., G. Schuckers, and D. Ratusnik, "Contextual-coarticulatory inconsistency of /r/ misarticulations." *Journal of Speech and Hearing Research*, 20 (1977): 631–643.

Ingram, D., *Phonological Disability in Children*. New York: American Elsevier, 1976, 1989.

Ingram, D., *Procedures for the Phonological Analysis of Children's Language*. Baltimore, Md.: University Park Press, 1981.

Jordan, E. P., "Articulation test measures and listener ratings of articulation defectiveness." *Journal of Speech and Hearing Research*, 3 (1960): 303–319.

Kent, R., and F. Minifie, "Coarticulation in recent speech production models." *Journal of Phonetics*, 5 (1977): 115–133.

Khan, L. M., *Basics of Phonological Analysis: A Programmed Learning Test*. San Diego, Calif.: College-Hill Press, 1985.

Khan, L. M., and N. P. Lewis, *Khan-Lewis Phonological Analysis*. Circle Pines, Minn.: American Guidance Service, 1986.

Kisatsky, T., "The prognostic value of Carter-Buck tests in measuring articulation skills in selected kindergarten children." *Exceptional Children*, 34 (1967): 81–85.

Locke, J., "The inference of speech perception in the phonologically disordered child. Part II: Some clinically novel procedures, their use, some findings." *Journal of Speech and Hearing Disorders*, 45 (1980): 445–468.

McDonald, E., *A Deep Test of Articulation*. Pittsburgh: Stanwix House, 1964.

Mason, R., and N. Wickwire, "Examining for orofacial variations." *Communiqué*, 8 (1978): 2–26.

Morrison, J. A., and L. D. Shriberg, "Articulation testing versus conversational speech sampling." *Journal of Speech and Hearing Research*, 35 (1992): 259–273.

Paynter, W., and T. Bumpas, "Imitative and spontaneous articulatory assessment of three-year-old children." *Journal of Speech and Hearing Disorders*, 42 (1977): 119–125.

Pendergast, K., S. Dickey, J. Selmar, and A. L. Soder, *Photo Articulation Test*, Austin, Tex.: PRO-ED, 1984.

Pollack, K., "The identification of vowel errors using transitional articulation or phonological process test stimuli." *Language, Speech, and Hearing Services in Schools*, 22 (1991): 39–50.

The Principles of the International Phonetic Association. London: University College Department of Phonetics, 1978.

Roe, V., and R. Milisen, "The effect of maturation upon defective articulation in elementary grades." *Journal of Speech Disorders*, 7 (1942): 37–50.

Secord, W., *C-PAC: Clinical Probes of Articulation Consistency*. San Antonio, Tex.: Psychological Corporation, 1981.

Shriberg, L. D., and R. D. Kent, *Clinical Phonetics*. New York: John Wiley & Sons, 1982.

Shriberg, L., and J. Kwiatkowski, *Natural Process Analysis*. New York: John Wiley and Sons, 1980.

Shriberg, L. D., J. Kwiatkowski, and K. Hoffman, "A procedure for phonetic transcription by consensus." *Journal of Speech and Hearing Research*, 27 (1984): 456–465.

Shriberg, L. D., and G. L. Lof, "Reliability studies in broad and narrow phonetic transcription." *Clinical Linguistics and Phonetics*, 5 (1991): 225–279.

Siegel, R., H. Winitz, and H. Conkey, "The influence of testing instruments in articulatory responses of children." *Journal of Speech and Hearing Disorders*, 28 (1963): 67–76.

Smith, M. W., and S. Ainsworth, "The effect of three types of stimulation on articulatory responses of speech defective children." *Journal of Speech and Hearing Research*, 10 (1967): 333–338.

Snow, J., and R. Milisen, "The influences of oral versus pictorial representation upon articulation testing results." *Journal of Speech and Hearing Disorders*. Monograph Supplement, 4 (1954): 29–36.

Sommers, R. K., R. Leiss, M. Delp, A. Gerber, D. Fundrella, R. Smith, M. Revucky, D. Ellis, and V. Haley, "Factors related to the effectiveness of articulation therapy for kindergarten, first- and second-grade children." *Journal of Speech and Hearing Research, 10* (1967): 428–437.

St. Louis, K., and D. Ruscello, *The Oral Speech Screening Examination.*" Baltimore, Md.: University Park Press, 1981.

Stampe, D., "The acquisition of phonetic representation." Papers from the Fifth Regional Meeting of the Chicago Linguistic Society, 1969.

Stampe, D., "A dissertation on natural phonology." Ph.D. thesis. University of Chicago, 1973.

Stockman, I., and E. McDonald, "Heterogeneity as a confounding factor when predicting spontaneous improvement of misarticulated consonants." *Language, Speech, and Hearing Services in Schools, 11* (1980): 15–29.

Stoel-Gammon, C., "Normal and disordered phonology in two-year olds." In K. Butler (Ed.), *Early Intervention: Working with Infants and Toddlers.* (pp. 110–121). Rockville, Md.: Aspen Publishers, 1994.

Stoel-Gammon, C., and C. Dunn, *Normal and Disordered Phonology in Children.* Baltimore: University Park Press, 1985.

Templin, M., "Spontaneous vs. imitated verbalization in testing pre-school children." *Journal of Speech and Hearing Disorders, 12* (1947): 293–300.

Templin, M., *Certain Language Skills in Children.* Institute of Child Welfare Monograph Series, 26. Minneapolis: University of Minnesota, 1957.

Templin, M., and F. Darley, *The Templin-Darley Tests of Articulation.* Iowa City, Iowa: Bureau of Educational Research and Service, University of Iowa, 1969.

Van Riper, C., *Speech Correction: Principles and Methods.* Englewood Cliffs, N.J.: Prentice Hall, 1939.

Van Riper, C., and R. Erickson, "A predictive screening test of articulation." *Journal of Speech and Hearing Disorders, 34* (1969): 214–219.

Weiner, F., *Phonological Process Analysis.* Baltimore: University Park Press, 1979.

Winitz, H., *Articulatory Acquisition and Behavior.* Englewood Cliffs, N.J.: Prentice Hall, 1969.

Winitz, H., "Auditory considerations in articulation training." In H. Winitz (Ed.), *Treating Articulation Disorders: For Clinicians by Clinicians.* Austin, Tex.: PRO-ED, 1984.

Wright, V., R. Shelton, and W. Arndt, "A task for evaluation of articulation change: III. Imitative task scores compared with scores for more spontaneous tasks." *Journal of Speech and Hearing Research, 12* (1969): 875–884.

Zimmerman, I., V. Steiner, and R. Pond, *Preschool Language Scale.* Columbus, Ohio: Charles E. Merrill, 1992.

Chapter 7

Analysis and Interpretation of Assessment Data

NICHOLAS W. BANKSON,
James Madison University

JOHN E. BERNTHAL,
University of Nebraska–Lincoln

After the clinician has collected various types of phonological samples, the data gathered during the assessment are analyzed and interpreted to determine (1) whether or not there is a phonological problem; (2) the nature of the problem, if there is one; (3) whether or not the client should be seen for treatment; and (4) if treatment is indicated, a recommended plan of action. The primary goals of *analyses* are to score, sort, or otherwise organize data collected in order to describe phonological performance. The purpose of *interpretation* is to examine the results of the phonological analysis and determine what course of action should be taken. Based on the interpretation of the phonological analysis, the clinician must determine whether or not the client needs instruction, and, if so, select target behaviors for treatment and appropriate intervention strategies. In summary, the clinician reviews responses to the phonological assessment tasks and interprets the analysis of these data in order to make appropriate and efficacious decisions.

Determining the Need for Intervention

Intelligibility

An important consideration for determining the phonological status of an individual is the *intelligibility* or understandability of the client's spontaneous speech. The intelligibility of spontaneous speech is a reflection of the client's verbal communication competence and is a most important factor when determining the need for intervention and for evaluating the effectiveness of intervention strategies. Intelligibility of the speaker is the factor most frequently cited by both speech-language pathologists and naive listeners when judging the severity of a phonological problem (Shriberg and Kwiatkowski, 1982). It should be pointed out that severity, which will be discussed later, and intelligibility are different though related concepts.

Degree of speech intelligibility is a perceptual judgment made by a listener and is based, to a large extent, on the percentage of words in a speech sample that are understood. Intelligibility of speech reflects a continuum of judgments ranging from unintelligible (where the message is not understood) to totally intelligible (where the message is completely understood by the listener). Intermediate points along such a continuum might include the following: speech is usually unintelligible, speech is partially intelligible, speech is intelligible although noticeably in error, or speech sound errors are occasionally noticed in continuous speech.

Factors influencing speech sound intelligibility include the number and types of speech sound errors, consistency of sound errors, frequency of occurrence of error sounds and phonological processes used. In general, the larger the number of a speaker's productions that differ from the adult standard, the more intelligibility is reduced. However, a simple tally of the number of sounds in error is not an adequate index of intelligibility. As Shriberg and Kwiatkowski (1982) reported, there is a low correlation ($r = .42$) between the percentage of consonants correct and the intelligibility of speech sample.

As previously indicated, other factors besides the numbers of errors impact intelligibility. The nature of the clients' errors relative to the target is one such factor. For example, deleting a sound will affect intelligibility more than will a mild distortion of the same sound. Intelligibility is also affected by the consistency of misarticulated sounds and by the frequency with which an error sound occurs in the language. The more consistently a target sound is produced in error, and, likewise, the more frequently target sounds occur in the language, the more likely the listener will perceive the speaker's speech as defective.

Extraneous factors may also influence intelligibility judgments. These factors include listeners' familiarity with the speaker's speech pattern; prosodic factors such as speaker's rate, inflection, stress patterns, pauses, voice quality, loudness, and fluency; the linguistic experience of the listener; the social environment of the communication act; the message content; the communication cues available to the listener; and the characteristics of the transmission media. The complexity of these factors probably accounts for the finding that intelligibility ratings are not highly correlated with the percentage of consonants correct.

There is no standard procedure for quantifying the intelligibility of young children. Gordon-Brannan (1994) identified three general approaches for measuring intelligibility: (1) *open-set word identification*, which calculates the percentage of words understood in a sample where the examiner transcribes a speech sample and determines the percentage of words identifiable; (2) *closed-set word identification*, wherein a listener identifies words read from prescribed word lists; and (3) *rating scale* procedures, which may take the form of either an *interval scaling* procedure, where a listener assigns a rating (number along a continuum of 5–9 points), or a *direct magnitude scale*, where a judgment of a speech sample is made relative to a standard stimulus. In addition, some phonology assessment instruments provide a method of estimating intelligibility based on the frequency of occurrence of misarticulated sounds (Fudala and Reynolds, 1986).

In case selection, a general principle of operation is that the poorer the ratings of intelligibility, the more likely the need for intervention. According to parent reports, normal developing 2-year-old children can be understood by a stranger 50 percent of the time (Coplan and Gleason, 1988). Vihman reported in Chapter 2 a study of normal development wherein her 3-year-old subjects averaged over 70 percent intelligibility in conversation (range of 50–80 percent). Gordon-Brannan (1994) reported a mean intelligibility of 93 percent (range of 73–100 percent) with normal developing 4-year-old children. It is generally recognized that a client 3 years of age or older who is unintelligible is a candidate for treatment and intelligibility expectations increase with age.

Gordon-Brannan (1994), following a review of the literature on the assessment of intelligibility of children, suggested that calculating the actual percentage of words understood in a speech sample may be the most valid way to determine intelligibility. She also suggested that the procedure could be enhanced by including orthographic transcription by a caregiver as a reliability check. Determining percentage of words understood is more time consuming than the common practice of speech-language pathologists to simply make perceptual estimates of intelligibility. She also pointed out that although rating scales for judging speech intelligibility are less time consuming than determining percentage of words understood, such rating scales have not been validated or standardized for children with phonological deficits. For a review of procedures for evaluating the intelligibility of children's speech, see Kent, Miolo, and Bloedel (1994).

Severity

The severity of a phonological disorder frequently needs to be addressed by speech-language clinicians in case selection decisions. Often school systems take severity ratings into consideration in determining caseload size for individual clinicians. Shriberg and Kwiatkowski (1982) developed a metric for quantifying the severity of involvement of children with a developmental phonological disorder which has become widely used. They recommended the calculation of **percentage of consonants correct** (PCC) as an index to quantify severity of involvement based on research that indicated that among several variables studied in relation to listeners' perceptions of severity, the PCC correlated most closely. The percentage of consonants correct requires the examiner to make correct-incorrect judgments of individual sounds produced in a continuous speech sample. Such judgments were found to be a fairly reliable measure for the classification of most children's phonological disorders as mild, mild-moderate, moderate-severe, or severe.

Procedures outlined by Shriberg and Kwiatkowski (1982; 267) for determining PCC are as follows:

> Tape record a continuous speech sample of a child following sampling procedures. Any means that yield continuous speech from the child are acceptable, provided that the clinician can tell the child that his exact words will be repeated onto the "tape machine" so that the clinician is sure to "get things right."

I. Sampling Rules
   A. Consider only intended (target) consonants in words. Intended vowels are not considered.
      1. Addition of a consonant before a vowel, for example, *on* [hon], is not scored because the target sound /ɔ/ is a vowel.
      2. Postvocalic /r/ in fair [feir] is a consonant, but stressed and unstressed vocalics [ɝ] and [ɚ] , as in *furrier* [fɝ·iɚ], are vowels.
   B. Do not score target consonants in the second or successive repetitions of a syllable, for example, *ba-balloon*—score only the first /b/.
   C. Do not score target consonants in words that are completely or partially unintelligible or whose gloss is highly questionable.
   D. Do not score target consonants in the third or successive repetitions of adjacent words unless articulation changes. For example, the consonants in only the first two words of the series [kæt], [kæt], [kæt] are counted. However, the consonants in all three words are counted if the series were [kæt], [kæk], [kæt].

II. Scoring Rules
   A. The following six types of consonant sound changes are scored as incorrect:
      1. Deletions of a target consonant.
      2. Substitutions of another sound for a target consonant, including replacement by a glottal stop or a cognate.
      3. Partial voicing of initial target consonants.
      4. Distortions of a target sound, no matter how subtle.
      5. Addition of a sound to a correct or incorrect target consonant, for example, *cars* said as [karks].
      6. Initial /h/ deletion (*he* [i]) and final n/ŋ substitutions (*ring* [rin]) are counted as errors only when they occur in stressed syllables; in unstressed syllables they are counted as correct, for example, *feed her* [fidɚ]; *running* [rʌnin].
   B. Observe the following:
      1. The response definition for children who obviously have speech errors is "score as incorrect unless heard as correct." This response definition assigns questionable speech behaviors to an "incorrect" category.
      2. Dialectal variants should be glossed as intended in the child's dialect, for example, *picture* "piture," *ask* "aks," and so on.
      3. Fast or casual speech sound changes should be glossed as the child intended, for example, *don't know* "dono," and "n," and the like.
      4. Allophones should be scored as correct, for example, *water* [warɚ], *tail* [teɪ⌐].

III. Calculation of Percentage of Consonants Correct (PCC)

$$PCC = \frac{\text{Number of correct consonants}}{\text{Number of correct plus incorrect consonants}} \times 100$$

Quantitative estimates of severity such as the PCC provide the clinician with an objective means for determining the relative priority of those who may need intervention.

Stimulability

As stated in the discussion of the assessment battery in Chapter 6, stimulability data are often used in making decisions on case selection. Investigators have reported that the ability of a child to imitate syllables and/or words containing a target sound is related to the probability that a child will spontaneously correct his/her misarticulations of that sound.

The use of stimulability for predicting spontaneous improvement or the rate of improvement in remediation has not been documented to the extent that definitive prognostic statements can be made, particularly with reference to an individual client. Diedrich (1983) suggested that a trial period of "diagnostic therapy" provides a stronger basis than do results of stimulability testing for predicting instructional needs.

Stimulability testing is, at best, only a general guide for the identification of clients who may correct their phonological errors without intervention. False positives (i.e., clients identified as needing instruction but who ultimately will outgrow their problems) and false negatives (i.e., clients identified as not needing instruction but who ultimately will require intervention) have been identified in all investigations focusing on stimulability as a prognostic indicator. These findings must be considered when results from stimulability testing are used to make predictive statements in clinical practice. Investigations of imitation as a prognostic indicator have looked at imitation in isolated sounds, syllables, and word productions as predictors of improvement on single-word tests.

In a comprehensive review of literature concerning stimulability, Diedrich (1983) drew the following conclusions regarding stimulability testing as a prognostic measure:

1. Among kindergarten, first, and second graders who received therapy, children with low stimulability scores (less than 25 percent correction) made significantly more improvement than those with high stimulability scores (greater than 60 percent correction) (Carter and Buck, 1958; Sommers, Leiss, Delp, Gerber, Fundrella, Smith, Revucky, Ellis, and Haley, 1967).
2. Among first and second graders who did not receive therapy, children with high stimulability scores (60 percent correction) demonstrated significant improvement in articulation (Snow and Milisen, 1954; Carter and Buck, 1958; Irwin, West, and Trombetta, 1966; Sommers et al., 1967).
3. Among kindergarteners not in therapy, children with high stimulability obtained significant improvement in two studies (Farquhar, 1961; Kisatsky, 1967), but improvement was not significant in a third study (Sommers et al., 1967).

Error Patterns

After the examiner has reviewed a speaker's phonological productions in terms of intelligibility, severity, and stimulability, the next step is to further review for possible patterns of the error productions. Following this, individual sound productions and error patterns are reviewed to determine if a child is using sounds and/or processes at a level appropriate to their age. Procedures designed to review phonological errors for identification of error patterns are particularly appropriate for those clients with multiple errors. In such procedures the clinician reviews the sampling data in an effort to categorize errors according to commonalities, patterns, or phonological processes. Determination of a child's phonological processes may be based on a formal process instrument, a connected speech sample, and/or productions obtained from a single-word articulation test.

Types of Pattern Analysis

Place-Manner-Voicing.   Perhaps the most basic type of pattern analysis involves classifying substitution errors according to place, manner, and voicing characteristics. A **place-manner-voicing analysis** facilitates the identification of patterns such as voiced for voiceless sound substitutions (e.g., voicing errors—/v/→[f] /d/→[t]), replacement of fricatives by stops (e.g., manner errors—/ð/→[d] /s/→/t/), or substitution of lingua-alveolar sounds for lingua-velar sounds (e.g., place errors—/d/→[g]/t/→[k]).

Consider a child with several speech sound errors whose speech patterns reflect correct manner and voicing but produce errors in place of articulation, such as backing of consonants, e.g., /t/→[k] /d/→[g] /b/→[g] /p/→[k]. In this instance, the clinician's strategy might be to teach the client to focus on the place of production. Some clinicians might choose to teach a single sound (for example, /t/) as an exemplar of the correct place of production and then probe for generalization to other sounds, whereas others might choose to teach simultaneously all of the misarticulated stop sounds (same sound class) that reflect the error pattern. When selected exemplars are taught with the assumption that generalization will occur to other untrained sounds, the clinician should not assume that generalization will always occur, especially if the errors occur across sound classes. Generalization from trained to untrained sounds is difficult to predict. In addition, there is a great deal of individual variability in such generalization.

The distinctive feature and phonological process analysis procedures are extensions of analyses based on place, manner, and voicing analyses. These procedures are discussed below.

Distinctive Feature Analysis.   In this second type of pattern analysis, speech sound substitutions are reviewed for presence or absence of particular distinctive features. The idea underlying **distinctive feature analysis** is that a combination of elements or features characterize a given sound segment and that such features can distinguish one sound from other sounds within and across languages. Distinctive features are based on acoustic, perceptual, and/or articulatory characteristics. From a clinical perspective, distinctive features most easily adapted to assessment and treatment of phonological problems are those based primarily on articulatory characteristics. As discussed in Chapter 1, distinctive features typically include between 13 and 16 bipolar characteristics that are used to distinguish speech sound segments. A treatment program based on distinctive features is described in Chapter 8.

Some of the applications that speech-language pathologists have made of distinctive feature analysis have been the subject of criticism. It has been suggested that distinctive features, although helpful in classifying sounds of languages, may not be suited to the analysis of speech sound errors. Since distinctive feature systems were developed to classify the speech sounds of languages, they do not accurately describe many nonstandard (error) productions (e.g., certain sound distortions). The binary (plus or minus feature value) nature of the distinctive features may not reflect the varied productions seen in the speech of children with phonological disorders. A further problem is that the features of a deleted target sound are scored as errors although the sound and, as a result, the features were never attempted. For a critical discussion of the issues regarding the application of distinctive features to clinical analysis and intervention, the reader is referred to the papers by Walsh (1974), Parker (1976), and Foster, Riley, and Parker (1985).

Phonological Process Analysis.   A third type of pattern analysis, often called **phonological process analysis**, was described earlier in terms of case selection. Phonological process analysis is a common method for identifying error patterns, including the influence of sound position within word and syllable shapes. In other words, since speech sound productions are affected by such factors as phonetic context, position in words, and syllable structure of words, these factors are reviewed for any systematic influence they may have. Currently this is the most commonly employed type of pattern analysis, a factor undoubtedly related to the clinical usefulness of the concept. Before discussing interpretation of such analyses, we would like to review again some of the more common processes or patterns observed in the speech of young children. Although the process listings of different authors may vary, most resemble this listing.

Whole Word (and Syllable) Processes.   Whole word and syllable structure processes are changes that affect the syllabic structures of the target word.

1. *Final consonant deletion.* Deletion of the final consonant in a word.

   e.g.   *book*   [bu]
          cap   [ka]
          fish   [fɪ]

2. *Unstressed syllable deletion* (weak syllable deletion). An unstressed syllable is deleted, often at the beginning of a word, sometimes in the middle.

   e.g.   *potato*   [teto]
          telephone   [tɛfon]
          pajamas   [dʒæmiz]

3. *Reduplication.* A syllable or a portion of a syllable is repeated or duplicated, usually becoming CVCV.

   e.g.   *dad*   [dada]
          water   [wawa]
          cat   [kaka]

4. *Consonant cluster simplification.* A consonant cluster is simplified in some manner. The cluster can be reduced to one member of the consonant cluster, another sound can be substituted for the entire cluster, one member of the cluster is retained and a sound substitution is made for the other member of the cluster.

   e.g.   *stop*   [tap]   *brown*   [bwon]   *milk*   [mɪ]
          park   [pak]   *snow*   [ṇou]

5. *Epenthesis.* A segment, usually the unstressed vowel [ə], is inserted.

e.g. *black* [bəlak]
  sweet [səwit]
  sun [sθʌn]
  long [lɔŋg]

6. *Metathesis.* There is a transposition or reversal of two segments (sounds) in a word.

e.g. *basket* [bæksɪt]
  spaghetti [pʌsgɛti]
  elephant [ɛfəlʌnt]

7. *Coalescence.* Characteristics of features from two adjacent sounds are combined so that one sound replaces two other sounds.

e.g. *swim* [fɪm] *tree* [fɪ]

8. *Assimilatory (harmony) processes.* One sound is influenced by another sound where a sound assumes features or becomes similar to a second sound. Thus, the two segments become more alike (hence the term harmony) or, frequently, become identical. These sound changes are sometimes termed **progressive assimilation** if the sound that causes the sound change precedes the affected sound (*gate* [geɪk]) and **regressive assimilation** if the sound that causes the sound change follows the affected sound (*soup* [pup]).

a. *Velar assimilation.* A nonvelar sound is assimilated (changed) to a velar sound because of the influence, or dominance, of the velar.

e.g. *duck* [gʌk] (regressive assimilation)
  take [kek] (regressive assimilation)
  coat [kok] (progressive assimilation)

b. *Nasal assimilation.* A nonnasal sound is assimilated because of the influence, or dominance, of a nasal consonant.

e.g. *candy* [næni] (regressive assimilation)
  lamb [næm] (regressive assimilation)
  fun [nʌn] (regressive assimilation)

c. *Labial assimilation.* A nonlabial sound is assimilated to a labial consonant because of the influence of a labial consonant.

e.g. *bed* [bɛb] (progressive assimilation)
  table [bebu] (regressive assimilation)
  pit [pip] (progressive assimilation)

Segment Change (Substitution) Processes. One sound is substituted for another, with the replacement sound reflecting changes in place of articulation, manner of articulation, or some other change in the way a sound is produced in a standard production.

1. *Velar fronting.* Substitutions are produced anterior, or forward of, the standard production.

   e.g.   *key*   [ti]   (velar replaced by alveolar)
          monkey   [mʌnti]   (velar replaced by alveolar)
          go   [do]   (velar replaced by alveolar)

2. *Backing.* Sounds are substituted or replaced by segments produced posterior to, or further back in the oral cavity than the standard production.

   e.g.   *tan*   [kæn]
          do   [gu]
          sip   [ʃɪp]

3. *Stopping.* Fricatives or affricates are replaced by stops.

   e.g.   *sun*   [tʌn]
          peach   [pit]
          that   [dæt]

4. *Gliding of liquids.* Prevocalic liquids are replaced by glides.

   e.g.   *run*   [wʌn]
          yellow   [jɛwo]
          leaf   [wif]

5. *Affrication.* Fricatives are replaced by affricates.

   e.g.   *saw*   [tʃau]
          shoe   [tʃu]
          sun   [tʃʌn]

6. *Vocalization.* Liquids or nasals are replaced by vowels.

   e.g.   *bird*   [bʌd]
          table   [tebo]
          mother   [mʌðo]

7. *Denasalization.* Nasals are replaced by homorganic stops (place of articulation is similar to target sound).

   e.g.   *moon*   [bud]
          nice   [deis]
          man   [bæn]

8. *Deaffrication.* Affricates are replaced by fricatives.

   e.g.   *chop*   [sap]
          chip   [ʃɪp]
          page   [pez]

9. *Glottal replacement.* Glottal stops replace sounds usually in either intervocalic or final position.

> e.g. *cat* [kæʔ]
> *tooth* [tuʔ]
> *bottle* [baʔl]

10. *Prevocalic voicing.* Voicing of voiceless consonants (obstruents) in prevocalic position.

> e.g. *paper* [bepɚ]
> *Tom* [dam]
> *table* [debi]

11. *Devoicing of final consonants.* Voiced obstruents are devoiced in final position.

> e.g. *dog* [dɔk]
> *nose* [nos]
> *bed* [bɛt]

Multiple Pattern Occurrence.   The examples of phonological patterns given above typically included lexical items in which only a single pattern was used. In reality, the child may produce forms that reflect more than one process, including some that are not reflected in the definitions and descriptions above. A single lexical item may have two or even more processes interacting. When such productions occur, they are more complex and difficult to unravel than words which reflect a single process. For example, in the production of [du] for *shoe*, Edwards (1983) pointed out that the [d] for /ʃ/ replacement reflects the phonological processes of (1) depalatalization, which changes the place of articulation; (2) stopping, which changes the manner of articulation; and (3) prevocalic voicing, which changes a voiceless consonant target to a voiced consonant. In the substitution of [dar] for car, the [d] for /k/ substitution is accounted for by the processes of velar fronting and prevocalic voicing. The identification of the sequence of steps describing how interacting processes account for substitutions is called a **derivation** or **process ordering**. Determining process derivations within a speaker can be difficult and is beyond the scope of this textbook.

Unusual Pattern Occurrence.   As indicated throughout this book, a great deal of individual variation exists in the phonological development of children. Although there are common developmental phonological patterns used by many children, the patterns observed across individuals vary. Unusual phonological patterns (e.g., use of a nasal sound for /s/ and /z/), called *idiosyncratic processes* or patterns, differ from the more common phonological processes and are seen in both children with normal and delayed phonological development. The greatest variation in phonological pattern usage occurs during the early stages of development and is probably influenced, in part, by the lexical items the child uses when acquiring his or her first words. When idiosyncratic patterns persist after age 3;0 to 3;5 years, they likely reflect a phonological disorder.

Sound Preferences.   Another type of sound pattern that some clinicians have reported is called *sound preference*. In these situations, children seem to have a segment or two that they use for a large number of sounds or sound classes. Sometimes a particular sound is substituted for several or even all phonemes in a particular sound class (e.g., fricatives). Other children will substitute a single consonant for a variety of segments, such as [h] for /b, d, s, ʒ, z, d, tʃ, ʃ, l, k, g, r/ (Weiner, 1981). It has been postulated that some children avoid the use of certain sounds in their productions and, instead, use those sounds they find easiest to produce. The phenomenon of sound preference is not viewed as a phonological process by most clinicians.

The list of phonological processes presented above is not exhaustive but represents most of the common patterns seen in normally developing children. These phonological processes have also been used in analyzing the sound errors of phonologically delayed children. Several procedures designed to assist the clinician in the identification of phonological processes in children's speech have been published in monograph or kit form. Included in these procedures are various groupings, as well as additions and deletions to the processes listed above. At first glance, these procedures seem quite similar, but a closer examination reveals differences among them. Table 7.1 reflects a modified version of Edwards's (1983) listing of the characteristics of published phonological assessment procedures.

Theoretical Considerations Regarding Phonological Processes

Description versus Explanation.   Some speech-language clinicians have suggested that the presence of phonological processes is evidence of a cognitive-linguistic deficit, thereby providing an *explanation* of the phonological errors. This is an inappropriate interpretation since phonological process analysis procedures are only *descriptive devices* and do not reveal causes or provide explanations of the error patterns. Smith (1981) warned that in studying phonological development with a linguistic-based pattern analysis, "one must avoid falling into the trap of believing that a child's behavior has been *explained* by having written a series of formal rules or a list of processes relating to particular phonological observations" (11).

An example demonstrating the inherent difficulty in arriving at an explanatory statement for a given phonological process was provided by Hoffman and Schuckers (1984). One explanation for the occurrence of a process might be that the child misperceives the adult word, for example, perceives [dɔg] as [dɔ]. A second explanation might be that the child's underlying lexical representation for *dog* is [dɔ], so the closest match in his storage of lexical items is [dɔ]; thus [dɔg] becomes [dɔ]. A third possible explanation is that the child's perceptual system functions appropriately and the lexical match between what the child perceives and what he or she has stored is consistent with the adult standard, but he or she has a phonological production rule that calls for the deletion of word-final stops. A fourth possibility is that the child has a motor production problem; in this case the child may have the appropriate perception but does not possess the necessary motor skill to make the articulation gesture to produce the sound.

This discussion is not intended to minimize the value of the information provided from a phonological process analysis, but rather to emphasize that when such procedures are used to analyze a child's speech, they serve to describe, not explain, behavior. In other words, in doing an analysis, the clinician cannot assume that because a phonological process (e.g., final consonant deletion) has been identified, that such patterns can be attributed to specific cognitive-linguistic, perceptual, or motor explanations.

TABLE 7.1 Characteristics of the Published Phonological Assessment Procedures

Basis of Comparison	Weiner (1979)	Shriberg and Kwiatkowski (1980)	Hodson (1986)	Khan-Lewis (1986)	Bankson and Bernthal (1990)
Stimuli	"Action" pictures	No specific stimuli	3-dimensional objects	Pictures from the *Goldman-Fristoe Test of Articulation*	Pictures from the *Bankson-Bernthal Test of Phonology*
Elicitation procedures	Delayed imitation and sentence recall	Continuous speech samples	Object-naming; no set order	Picture-naming in citation form	Picture-naming in citation form
Sample size	136 target words, said twice and control items	80–100 different words from 200–250 word sample	50 single words	44 single words	80 single words
Transcription	Live and from recordings	Narrow "on-line" and from tapes	Broad transcriptions are modified; audio taped for reference	Narrow "on-line" and from recordings	Live and from recordings
Number of processes	16	8 "natural" processes	30 processes	12 developmental processes 3 nondevelopmental processes	10 most frequently occurring processes in standardized samples
Target population	Unintelligible children, ages 2–5	Children with severely delayed speech	Children with multiple articulation errors	Normally developing and phonologically disordered children	Normally developing and phonologically disordered children
Time (total)	±45 minutes with a cooperative child	About 1½ hours	±50 minutes	±35 minutes	±30 minutes
Number of processes per word	One test process; others noted	Two processes coded for some words	More than one process per word	All that apply are coded	All that apply are coded
Process descriptions	Conditions of occurrence noted	Organized by sound and position on summary sheet	Number of occurrences tabulated across sounds and positions	Organized by sounds and word-position	Organized by sounds and word-position
Frequency of occurrence	Percent calculated for each test process	Approximate frequency indicated on summary sheet	Calculation for 10 basic processes	Frequency of each of the 15 processes calculated	Frequency of each of the 10 processes calculated
Interacting processes	Not discussed	Only two combinations are coded	Errors coded under all appropriate processes	Errors coded under all appropriate processes	Errors coded under all appropriate processes

Underlying Representation in Phonological Processes.   Shelton (1986) has identified three different theoretical interpretations of phonological processes in the speech-language pathology literature. One view is that phonological processes constitute a taxonomy or listing of speech sound error patterns, a catalog of descriptors that can be used to identify the simplifications or modifications used by children. This view makes no speculations or assumptions regarding the child's underlying representations (mental images or internal knowledge of the lexical items) in relation to the adult standard; it simply describes behavior at the observable or surface level. This atheoretical perspective posits nothing about the operation of processes, the nature of phonological structure, the relationship of surface forms and underlying representations, or even the relationship of production and perception.

A second view of phonological processes assumes that the child has underlying representations of lexical forms that are similar to those of the adult surface forms. This view, which comes from work in normal phonological development, assumes that the child is attempting to produce the adult form of the word and has an adultlike mental image of the lexical item. The surface forms produced by the child, however, reflect an immature development. The child changes the target production in some manner during the production of the word. It is these simplifications that are identified as errors in the individual's speech. The mismatches between the child's productions and his or her underlying representations (which are the same as the adult standard) are expressed as phonological processes.

The third theoretical position acknowledges the existence of underlying representations but makes no assumptions concerning their form. The clinician examines the child's surface forms (the child's articulatory productions) to determine the status or nature of the child's underlying representations. A child who uses a phoneme contrastively is assumed to have the adult underlying form. If the child misarticulates a sound and there is no evidence from phonological testing or acoustical analysis that the sound is in the child's repertoire, it is not assumed the child has the adultlike underlying representation of the sound. For example, if a child says [dɔ] for [dɔg] but uses [g] in the diminutive *doggy* [dɔgi], one can assume that the child has the underlying form for [g] since /g/ is produced in the form [dɔgi]. On the other hand, if /g/ is not observed in any of the child's utterances, no assumption is made about the underlying form for /g/. Thus, this view of underlying structures differs from the second view, described earlier, in that it makes no assumptions concerning the underlying representations; the second assumes the child has the adult form.

Elbert and Gierut (1986) have sought to provide data to support their concept of underlying forms. On the basis of observed phonological productions, they described what they call children's "phonological knowledge" and made inferences from these data about underlying forms. From their perspective, the more knowledge a child has about sounds, the more inferences can be made about the child's underlying forms. Phonological knowledge was determined in a variety of ways, including (1) correct use of the error phoneme in other word positions; (2) correct use of the error phoneme in different contexts; (3) stimulability testing; (4) morphophonemic alternation tasks, for example, [dɔ] for *dog* but [dɔgi] for *doggy*, [pɪ] for *pig* but [pɪgi] for *piggy*; and (5) acoustic analysis, for example, evidence of a glottal gesture in the word-final position on a spectrogram when the examiner transcribed the final consonant as a deletion. When a child demonstrated phonological knowledge on one of the tasks, the investigators inferred that the child's underlying representation was similar to the adult.

Developmental Appropriateness

A fifth factor to consider in deciding if a client is a candidate for intervention is the age appropriateness of his or her phonological productions. If a child misarticulates sounds that are ordinarily produced by children at that age, or if a child's total number of correct speech sounds produced is below the age norm, or if a child evidences phonological processes that typically are eliminated by other children of his/her age, the child is identified as having a developmental delay. How much delay is necessary before a child is considered a candidate for intervention is a judgment the clinician must make.

The number of correct speech sound productions in relation to age is a metric frequently used to qualify children for speech services in the public schools. For example, if a 4-year-old child produces 32 target items correctly on a particular measure and the mean number of correct responses for children of the same age is 49, with a standard deviation of 12, the child's speech would usually be identified as phonologically delayed. Likewise, a 5-year-old child who uses final consonant deletions, stopping, and backing would be identified as phonologically delayed since these phonological patterns are no longer operating in normally developing children of that age.

Two methods traditionally have been employed to compare articulation performance and chronological age: (1) The number of correct responses on a speech sound articulation test are tabulated and then compared with normative data for a given age level on the same test (e.g., *Bankson-Bernthal Test of Phonology*, Bankson and Bernthal, 1990); and (2) a comparison is made of the child's individual segmental productions with developmental norms for individual sounds (e.g., Prather, Hedrick, and Kern, 1975; Iowa-Nebraska norms, Smit, Hand, Freilinger, Bernthal, and Bird, 1990).

The comparison of a child's segmental productions with developmental norms for individual sounds is one way norms are frequently used. Although this appears to be a simple task, one must be cautious in assigning an age norm to a particular sound. Normative data are typically statistical averages that reflect overall patterns of mastery. One must remember that children learn sounds at different rates and in different sequences. Thus caution is required in the application of these normative data for individual sounds produced by a child.

As discussed earlier, investigators have attached an age expectation to specific speech sounds by listing the age levels at which 75 percent and 90 percent of the children in a normative group have mastered each sound tested. Sander (1972) pointed out that such normative data are group standards that reflect upper age limits rather than average performance and suggested instead that the concept of customary production be used. He defined customary production as the point at which 51 percent of the children correctly produced a sound in two of the three word positions. Sander (1972) also argued that "variability among children in the ages at which they successfully produce specific sounds is so great as to discourage pinpoint statistics" (58).

Prather and colleagues (1975) reported speech sound acquisition norms for children from age 2 through 4 years on a test designed to elicit consonants in the prevocalic and postvocalic positions. With respect to the age levels at which 75 percent of the children had mastered specific sounds, these investigators reported earlier age levels than Templin (1957) although the sequence of acquisition was similar in both studies. They pointed out that the differences in findings could be due to their use of two-position versus Templin's three-position testing. A useful set of normative data for individual sound acquisition, which reflects an age range for sound development, is shown in Figure 7.1.

Smit (1986) reanalyzed the data from Prather and colleagues (1975) and Templin (1957) and found that methodological differences could account for the apparent downward shift in ages of acquisition reported by Prather and colleagues. She reported that when two-position data sets from Prather and colleagues were compared with two-position results from Templin, the findings were similar; and in fact, in a few instances the ages of acquisition for specific sounds reported by Prather and colleagues were later than those reported by Templin.

Smit and colleagues (1990) gathered three-position data from children in two Midwestern states. Using a 75 percent criterion level, they reported that children acquire sounds at ages equal to or younger than ages reported by Templin. They found that /ŋ/ and /r/ reached the 75 percent criterion later than reported by Templin. They also found that clusters tended to reach the 75 percent criterion at the same age or later than singletons contained in the cluster. It is interesting to note the overall similarity between the data gathered by Smit and colleagues and those of Templin collected 33 years earlier.

The clinician should keep in mind that in using the data from any large group study, individual subject data are obscured. Although the precise sequence and nature of phonological development varies from one person to another, in general certain segments are mastered earlier than others, and this information is used in determining presence of phonological delay and the direction of treatment. For example, if 6-year-old Kirsten says all sounds usually produced by 75 percent of 3-year-old children, but is not yet using sounds commonly associated with 4-, 5-, and 6-year-olds, her phonological productions would be considered delayed. This developmental aspect of phonological acquisition makes age a useful factor in determining whether a child has a phonological delay.

A second commonly employed way of comparing phonology and chronological age is to compare a child's phonological performance with norms for a specific phonological measure (as opposed to individual segmental norms). In this procedure, the number of speech sound productions produced correctly on a specific test are compared with normative data for that instrument. In other words, the number of sounds that the child produces correctly are compared with normative data to determine whether a child's articulatory performance is typical for the child's age. This analysis is appropriate for children 8 years old and younger since correct production of speech sound segments is usually expected by age 8 in normal children. This procedure is the basis by which many states and school districts determine if children with phonological delay and disorders qualify for services. Tests such as the *Goldman-Fristoe Test of Articulation* (Goldman and Fristoe, 1986), the *Arizona Articulation Proficiency Scale* (Fudala and Reynolds, 1986), and the *Bankson-Bernthal Test of Phonology* (1990) are examples of tests that contain overall test norms.

The age appropriateness of certain processes that may be present in a young child's speech is an additional normative factor taken into consideration in case selection. Several

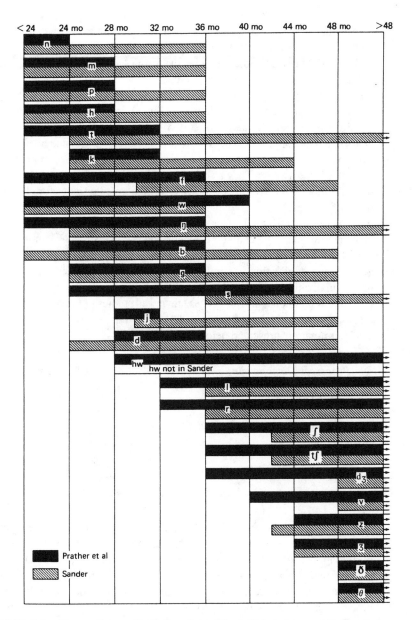

FIGURE 7.1   Normative articulation data. The left-hand margin of each bar represents the age at which 50 percent of the children in a normative study used the specified sound correctly. The right-hand margin shows the age at which 90 percent of the children used the sound correctly.

Data reported in the lower bars are from Sander (1972). Data in the black bars are from the work of Hedrick, Prather, and Tobin (1975). Adapted by permission from E. M. Prather, D. L. Hedrick, and C. A. Kern, "Articulation Development in Children Aged Two to Four Years," *Journal of Speech and Hearing Disorders*, *40* (1975): 179–191 (p. 186).

investigators have provided information that is relevant to this matter. Preisser, Hodson, and Paden (1988), in a cross-sectional study, examined phonological process usage in young children. Between 24 and 29 months, the most commonly observed processes were cluster reduction, liquid deviation (which included deletions of a liquid in a consonant cluster, e.g., *black* → [bæk]), vowelization (e.g., *zipper* → [zɪpo]), and gliding of liquids (e.g., *red* → [wɛd]). Next most common were patterns involving the strident feature.

Roberts, Burchinal, and Footo (1990) observed a group of children between 2;5 and 8 years in a quasilongitudinal study—that is, children were tested a varying number of times over the course of the study. They reported a marked decrease in process use between the ages of 2;5 and 4 years. They also reported percentage of occurrence (i.e., dividing the total number of occurrences for each process of 20 percent or more for cluster reductions, deletion of final consonants, syllable reductions, liquid gliding, fronting, stopping, deletion of medial consonants, and deaffrication. By age 4, only cluster reduction, liquid gliding, and deaffrication had a percentage of occurrence of 20 percent or more. They also reported that at 2;5 years the percentage of occurrence was less than 20 percent for the following processes: reduplication, assimilation, deletion of initial consonants, addition of a consonant, labialization shifts, methathesis, and backing.

Stoel-Gammon and Dunn (1985) reviewed studies of process occurrence and identified those processes which typically are deleted by age 3 and those that persist after 3 years. Their summary is presented below:

Processes Disappearing by 3 Years	*Processes Persisting after 3 Years*
Unstressed syllable deletion	Cluster reduction
Final consonant deletion	Epenthesis
Consonant assimilation	Gliding
Reduplication	Vocalization
Velar fronting	Stopping
Prevocalic voicing	Depalatalization
	Final devoicing

Table 7.2 from Grunwell (1981) reflects "simplifying processes" used by young children in normal phonological development. The table is derived largely from data reported by Ingram (1976) and Anthony, Bogle, Ingram, and McIssac (1971) and is based on a relatively small number of subjects. The solid lines reflect typical ages at which particular processes are evidenced, and the broken lines reflect the approximate age at which the processes are modified or begin to disappear.

Bankson and Bernthal (1990) reported data on the processes most frequently observed in a sample of over 1,000 children, 3 to 9 years of age, tested during the standardization of the *Bankson-Bernthal Test of Phonology* (BBTOP). The BBTOP ultimately included the 10 processes that appeared most frequently in children's productions during standardization testing. The processes that persisted the longest in children's speech were gliding of liquids, stopping, cluster simplification, vocalization, and final consonant deletion. These data are almost identical to those reported by Khan and Lewis (1986). They also reported velar fronting as a process persisting in young children's speech.

TABLE 7.2   Chronology of Phonological Processes

	2;0–2;6	2;6–3;0	3;0–3;6	3;6–4;0	4;0–4;6	4;6–5;0	5;0→
Unstressed Syllable Deletion	████	████	████	─ ─			
Final Consonant Deletion	████	████	─ ─				
Reduplication	─ ─						
Consonant Harmony	████	─ ─ ─					
Cluster Reduction (Initial)							
Obstruent—Approximant	████	─ ─	─ ─	─ ─			
/s/ + Consonant	████			─ ─			
Stopping							
/f/	████	─ ─	─ ─				
/v/	████	─ ─	─ ─				
/θ/ θ → [f]	████	─ ─	─ ─	─ ─	─ ─	─ ─	─ ─
/ð/ /ð/ → [d] or [v]					─ ─	─ ─	─ ─
/s/	████	─ ─					
/z/			─ ─	─ ─			
/ʃ/ Fronting '[s] type'		─ ─		─ ─	─ ─		
/tʃ, dʒ/ Fronting [ts, dz]		─ ─	─ ─		─ ─	─ ─	
Fronting/k, g, ŋ/	████	─ ─	─ ─				
Gliding r → [w]	████	─ ─	─ ─	─ ─	─ ─	─ ─	─ ─
Context-Sensitive Voicing	████	─ ─					

Source: Adapted by permission from P. Grunwell, "The Development of Phonology: A Descriptive Profile." *First Language,* 3 (1981): 161–191. Used with permission.

Some investigators have called for quantitative criteria to be used in determining whether certain phonological processes are significant in terms of case selection or target behavior selection. McReynolds and Elbert (1981) suggested that some percentage of occurrence of a process be applied in determining if a given error pattern constitutes a phonological process. As a guideline for identifying error patterns as phonological processes, they recommended that an error pattern occur in at least four instances and in at least 20 percent of the items that could be affected by the process. McReynolds and Elbert (1981) also urged that certain qualitative conditions be met before a pattern is considered a process. For example, they recommended that the error sound be produced correctly and used contrastively in some context but not necessarily in the context in which the process appeared to be operating. For example, if /k/ is deleted in the word-final position but is used appropriately in word-initial position, this observation would indicate that the client can make the /k/ and a process is operating in the word-final position.

Comparison of age and phonological development is widely practiced and certainly such data must be taken into consideration in recommending intervention. Justifiable criticism has been made of using such data as the single criterion for case selection (Turton, 1980; Sander, 1972; Winitz, 1969). Criticism is based on the following factors: (1) Speech sound developmental norms typically reflect upper age limits of customary consonant production (between 75 and 100 percent of children produce the sounds correctly) rather than average age estimates; (2) the norms are based on production in the initial, medial, and final positions of single words rather than spontaneous speech; (3) there is a great deal of variability across children; (4) norms frequently are based on a single production of a particular sound in one or two contexts; (5) norms represent a statement of average performance by age, but the resulting sequence of acquisition may not be applicable to a given individual; (6) although sounds generally appear to be acquired in a sequence, prior acquisition of certain sounds is not necessarily required for the learning of other sounds; and (7) the nature of the error may be a critical factor. For example, Stephens, Hoffman, and Daniloff (1986) reported that unlike most errors, lateralization of /s/ did not spontaneously improve with age. As a result of this finding, together with our clinical experience, we do not consider such errors developmental. We would concur with the suggestion of Smit and colleagues (1990) that lateralized /s/ errors be treated earlier than other /s/ errors because unlike most speech sound errors they do not generally spontaneously correct with age. This lack of improvement in lateralization with age has led Smit (1993) to suggest that lateralization of /s/ is not a developmental error.

The use of process norms in helping to determine caseload is relatively new. In this case, one is looking for processes or simplifications to have disappeared by a particular age. If processes persist beyond the expected age level, their presence is one of the factors that should be taken into consideration in case selection.

Case Selection Guidelines and Summary

The first question that must be answered through analysis of phonological sampling procedures is whether or not there is a phonological problem that warrants intervention. By reviewing the intelligibility of the speaker, the severity of the phonological differences that may be present, and the developmental appropriateness of the child's phonological productions as well as error patterns, such a question can be answered.

As a general guideline for initiating intervention, the child should be at least one standard deviation (some guidelines call for 1.5 to 2 standard deviations) below his or her age norm in the number of sounds produced correctly or in the use of phonological processes. The clinician should recognize, however, that this is only a general guideline and that other considerations, such as intelligibility, speaker's perception of his or her problem, nature of the errors and error patterns, consistency of errors, and other speech characteristics may also be important. In the case of an unintelligible child, the use of normative data may be of minimal value because the concern is not to determine whether the child has a problem, but rather to understand the nature of the problem and to delineate the error patterns.

Clients age 3 years or older who evidence pronounced intelligibility and/or severity problems or who evidence idiosyncratic phonological problems are priority candidates for intervention; children younger than 2;5 years and candidates for intervention are usually recommended for early intervention programs which include parent programs. Children, age 8 and below, whose phonological performance is at least 1 standard deviation below the mean for their age are candidates for intervention. Most children 9 years or older are candidates for intervention if they have consistently produced speech sound errors. Teenagers and adults who perceive that their phonological errors constitute a handicap should be considered for instruction. Likewise, children should be considered for intervention when they or their parents are very concerned about their speech sound productions.

Target Behavior Selection

Once the need for intervention is established, sampling data are further reviewed to determine recommended goals for intervention. The following paragraphs will delineate how the various components of the assessment battery are utilized to establish target behaviors for remediation.

Stimulability

As you will recall, stimulability testing consists of assessing client performance when the client is asked to imitate the adult form of speech sound errors in isolation, syllables, and words. Clinicians have postulated that error sounds that can be produced through imitation are more rapidly corrected through intervention than sounds that cannot be imitated. In terms of target behavior selection, stimulable sounds have often been viewed as sounds to be taught early (Secord, 1989) so that clients may more readily achieve success in their therapy and so that these sounds can provide a foundation for the acquisition of sounds not in the client's repertoire ("harder sounds"). McReynolds and Elbert (1978) reported that once a child could imitate a sound, generalization occurred to other contexts. Thus, imitation served as a predictor of generalization. Powell, Elbert, and Dinnsen (1991) reported that stimulability explained the generalization patterns observed during treatment. They found that sounds that were stimulable were most likely to be added to the phonetic repertoire regardless of the sounds selected for treatment. Miccio and Elbert (1996) suggested that "teaching stimulability" may be a way to facilitate phonological acquisition and generalization by increasing the client's phonetic repertoire.

Intervention is usually initiated at the level of the most complex linguistic unit the client can imitate (i.e., isolation, syllable, word, phrase). Diedrich (1983) stated that even if stimulability would fail as a predictor for self-correction, it can serve to indicate whether treatment should begin at the isolated, syllable, word, or phrase level. For children with error patterns, choosing an *exemplar* (target sound) on which the child is stimulable will hopefully facilitate generalization. Sounds from different sound classes are often chosen as exemplars, with stimulability data aiding in their selection. For example, if word-final stops, fricatives, and nasals are all deleted, the clinician might target one stimulable stop, fricative, and nasal as exemplars. Hodson (1989), in her cycles approach to remediation, suggested finding target sounds on which the child is stimulable when targeting processes.

Although there seems to be general agreement that sounds children can produce or are stimulable on take less time to treat, some clinicians assign such sounds a lower priority for remediation than sounds on which the child is not stimulable. It is postulated that the establishment of sounds where the child demonstrates the "least knowledge" are the sounds that have the best potential to positively affect the child's overall phonological system although such sounds may be more difficult to teach (Elbert and Gierut, 1986). This recommendation is in contrast to the notion that target selections should include sounds on which the client is stimulable since therapy will move rapidly and the child will enjoy faster success (Secord, 1989; Diedrich, 1983).

It has been postulated (Dinnsen and Elbert, 1984) that imitation of words by the child may also reflect correct underlying representations (storage of the adult form). One might speculate, then, that if a child is able to imitate a word, this performance may indicate that the child has acquired at a cognitive level the linguistic contrasts of the language necessary to produce a sound in at least some appropriate contrastive contexts. From this perspective, correct imitation is a reflection not only of phonetic or motor skill but also of the child's possession of the adult's (correct) underlying form of the error word. In a study of this issue, Lof (1994) concluded that stimulability testing reflects phonetic behavior only.

Frequency of Occurrence

A factor used in target behavior selection is the frequency with which the sounds produced in error occur in the language. Obviously, the greater the frequency of a sound in a language, the greater its potential effect on intelligibility. Thus, treatment will have the greatest impact on a client's overall intelligibility if frequently occurring segments produced in error are selected for treatment.

Table 7.3 lists the rank order and frequency of occurrence of the 24 most frequently used consonants in conversational American English (Shriberg and Kwiatkowski, 1983). These statistics are based on a collection of natural speech data from a variety of sources. Mines, Hanson, and Shoup (1978) noted a relatively high correlation among all frequency counts, based on both spoken and written expression. Seven consonants /n, t, s, r, d, m, z/ account for over half of all consonant occurrences in our language. However, consonants /n, t, s, r, l, d, ð, k, m, w, z/ occur very frequently in connected speech and errors on these sounds will adversely affect intelligibility. Other data reported in the table showed that almost two thirds of the consonants used are voiced, 29 percent are stops, 19 percent are sonorants, and 18 percent are nasals. Moreover, three of the six stops /t, d, k/, three of four sonorants /r, l, w/, and two of three nasals /n, m/ are among the 11 most frequently occurring consonants. Dental and alveolar consonants accounted for 61 percent of the produc-

TABLE 7.3 Percentage of Occurrence of (Intended) English Consonants in Continuous Speech

Sound	Rank	Mean %	Hoffman (1982)	Irwin and Wong (1983)[a]	Carterette and Jones (1974)	Mader (1954)	Shriberg and Kwiatkowski (1982)	Shriberg and Kwiatkowski (1983)	Mines et al. (1978)
n	1	12.01	11.22	9.84	13.63	13.14	11.7	13.04	11.49
t	2	11.83	12.43	14.05	7.91	11.74	13.7	13.08	9.88
s	3	6.90	6.78	6.66	6.94	6.50	7.1	6.43	7.88
r	4	6.68	7.06	5.99	8.20	7.83	5.2	5.84	6.61
d	5	6.41	4.26	6.89	6.31	10.25	5.8	5.33	5.70
m	6	5.93	5.20	5.52	7.49	4.63	5.6	7.97	5.11
z	7	5.36	8.69	4.88	4.58	3.70	3.0	3.97	4.70
ð	8	5.32	6.90	6.04	4.42	6.40	4.1	4.04	5.37
l	9	5.25	3.42	5.41	4.96	5.55	5.6	5.59	6.21
k	10	5.13	4.60	5.20	4.96	4.25	6.0	5.57	5.30
w	11	4.88	4.19	4.70	5.57	5.33	4.8	4.79	4.81
h	12	4.38	7.47	5.17	3.37	3.33	4.2	4.97	2.23
b	13	3.28	2.84	3.40	3.18	2.97	3.5	3.92	3.24
p	14	3.12	2.98	3.12	2.12	2.73	3.9	3.90	3.07
g	15	3.08	3.93	3.29	2.90	2.38	4.1	2.93	2.02
f	16	2.07	2.38	1.64	2.21	1.83	2.4	1.37	2.65
ŋ	17	1.58	.94	1.86	1.05	1.61	2.5	1.24	1.85
j	18	1.56	1.22	1.49	1.41	0.77	2.2	1.94	1.87
v	19	1.52	1.03	1.46	1.64	1.91	1.2	0.42	2.97
ʃ	20	0.93	0.87	1.14	0.84	0.84	1.5	0.38	0.95
θ	21	0.89	0.59	0.84	1.03	0.93	0.9	0.76	1.19
dʒ	22	0.58	0.62	0.50	0.53	0.69	0.6	0.19	0.95
tʃ	23	0.55	0.34	0.31	0.51	0.55	0.7	0.56	0.85
ʒ	24	0.03	0.01	0.01	0	0.01	0	0	0.15

Source: L. Shriberg and F. Kwiatkowski, "Computer-Assisted Natural Process Analysis (NPA): Recent Issues and Data." In *Assessing and Treating Phonological Disorders: Current Approaches.* J. Locke (Ed.), *Seminars in Speech and Language, 4* (1983): 397. Used by permission.

[a]Data calculated from page 156, Table 8.4 to reflect only children aged 3, 4, and 6 years.

tions and labial and labiodental sounds, 21 percent. In other words, over four-fifths of consonant occurrences are produced at the anterior area of the mouth.

Developmental Appropriateness

Earlier in this chapter we discussed, at length, the role of normative data in case selection. That discussion is also relevant to target behavior selection. Traditionally, clinicians have tended to select sounds for intervention that should already be in a client's repertoire (i.e., are developmentally appropriate) or process should no longer be present. While age appropriateness is one to take into consideration, it should be pointed out that the other variables discussed in this section may override a selection solely based on developmental norms.

Contextual Analysis

As stated earlier, contextual testing is concerned with the influence of surrounding sounds on a particular sound that is not produced correctly. Contextual testing may identify facilitating phonetic contexts in which surrounding sounds have a positive influence on the production of error sounds. Contextual testing provides data on phonetic contexts in which an error sound may be produced correctly and be helpful in determining a treatment program. Through the identification of such contexts, the clinician may find that a specific sound doesn't have to be taught because it is already in the client's repertoire. Both the client and clinician may save time and frustration that often accompany initial attempts to produce a speech sound by focusing first on a certain context in which a sound is produced correctly and then gradually shifting to other contexts. In general, when contexts can be found where target sounds are produced correctly, such sounds take less time to correct in remediation. The number of contexts in which a child can produce a sound correctly on a deep test may provide some indication of the stability of the error. It seems logical that the less stable the error, the easier it may be to correct. However, some clinicians find that a stable error pattern is easier to focus on than a more "elusive error." The clinician can utilize those contexts in which a segment is produced correctly to reinforce correct production and facilitate generalization to other contexts. If a client's error tends to be inconsistent across different phonetic contexts, one might assume that the chances for improvement are better than if the error tends to persist across different phonetic contexts or situations. This assumption, however, has yet to be demonstrated.

Phonological Process Analysis

The comparison of a client's use of phonological processes with normative data can be used in target selection. The processes used by a phonologically delayed child can be compared with those that might be expected in the speech of normally developing children. Those processes that usually are not present in normal children are targeted for intervention. One caution about this procedure should be pointed out. Few, if any, data would suggest that reduction in the use of phonological processes occurs in a prescribed order, although some processes tend to persist in older children and others tend to occur only in younger children. Moreover, no data suggest that the elimination of one process in a child's speech should occur before another process is targeted for treatment. There are some general trends that may be helpful in targeting processes for treatment, but a universally prescribed development order for the deletion of processes has not been established.

Hodson (1989) suggested that clinicians focus on teaching appropriate phonological patterns (rather than eliminate inappropriate patterns) and that stimulable patterns be those given priority for intervention. She further indicated that priority target patterns often include early developing patterns, posterior-anterior contrasts, and *s* clusters.

Phonological Knowledge Analysis

Elbert and Gierut (1986) suggested that phonological assessment and target selection should include a determination of a client's "productive phonological knowledge" (child's cognitive awareness of a particular sound at a linguistic level). These authors have postulated that the consistency with which a phoneme is used across morphemes and word positions is a reflection of the child's phonological knowledge of that phoneme. Gierut (1986) identified a continuum of knowledge types, with 1 representing "most knowledge" about a sound and 6 representing "least knowledge" of a sound. As can be seen in Table 7.4, a child displaying Type 2 knowledge of [s] would produce the sound correctly for all morphemes and word-positions, with the occasional substitution of /t/ for /s/ in word-final position. By contrast, a child displaying Type 5 knowledge of [s] would inconsistently produce this sound correctly in the initial position, while [s] morphemes in word-final positions would always be produced incorrectly.

Gierut, Elbert, and Dinnsen (1987) reported that when phonological intervention was directed toward those error sounds that evidenced "least knowledge" (as opposed to "most knowledge"), the greatest changes in a child's phonology occurred. In the continuum of knowledge, as reflected in Table 7.4, it is assumed that the extent of misarticulation is a reflection of the degree of an individual's phonological knowledge. In terms of making the most efficacious decisions relative to target behavior selection, Elbert and Gierut (1986) suggested selecting those sounds for treatment that reflect the least phonological knowledge. They observed greater generalization to untrained sounds when they targeted sounds reflecting least phonological knowledge than when they targeted those with most phonological knowledge. They hypothesized that focusing on least knowledge resulted in greater overall reorganization of a child's phonological system, and thus greater generalization.

Gierut (1986) outlined several steps involved in determining a person's phonological knowledge at a productive level. Included among these steps are the following:

1. Obtain a representative sample of speech. Ideally this would include both connected speech and spontaneous single-word utterances in order that a sample of all English sounds in at least three word-positions can be obtained. Sounds should be sampled more than once in each position.
2. Determine the type of knowledge that a child displays for each target sound (Table 7.4).
3. Establish what the child has yet to learn. This is done by ranking a child's phonological knowledge on a continuum ranging from "most" to "least" phonological knowledge for each target phoneme.
4. Select treatment sounds and goals based on the least phonological knowledge on the treatment continuum.

TABLE 7.4 Phonological Knowledge Continuum

Knowledge Type	Description	Example		
1	A child displaying Type 1 knowledge of target [s] would produce this sound correctly in all word-positions and for all morphemes; [s] would never be produced incorrectly.	[sʌn] [sup] [mɛsi] [mɪsɪŋ] [mɪs]	*sun* *soup* *messy* *missing* *miss*	
2	A child displaying Type 2 knowledge of target [s] would produce this sound correctly for all morphemes and positions. However, a phonological rule would apply to account for observed alternations between, for example, [s] and [t] in morpheme-final position.	[sʌn] [sup] [mɛsi] [aɪs] BUT: [mɪs]–[mɪt] [kɪs]–[kɪt]	*sun* *soup* *messy* *ice* *miss* *kiss*	
3	A child displaying Type 3 knowledge of target [s] would produce this sound correctly in all positions. However, certain morphemes that were presumably acquired early and acquired incorrecly (i.e., "fossilized") would always be produced in error.	[sʌn] [mɛsi] [mɪs] BUT: [nænə] [wu]	*sun* *messy* *miss* *Santa* *juice*	
4	A child displaying Type 4 knowledge of target [s] would produce this sound correctly for all morphemes in, for example, initial position. However, production of [s] would be incorrect for all morphemes in medial and final positions.	[sʌn] [sup] BUT: [mɛti] [mɪtɪŋ] [mɪt] [kɪt]	*sun* *soup* *messy* *missing* *miss* *kiss*	
5	A child displaying Type 5 knowledge of target [s] would produce this sound correctly in, for example, initial position. However, only some morphemes in this position would be produced correctly. All [s] morphemes in postvocalic positions would be produced incorrectly.	[sʌn] [sup] BUT: [top] [tak] [mɛti] [kɪt]	*sun* *soup* *soap* *sock* *messy* *kiss*	
6	A child displaying Type 6 knowledge of target [s] would produce this sound incorrectly in all word-positions and for all morphemes; [s] would never be produced correctly.	[tʌn] [tup] [mɪtɪŋ] [mɪt] [kɪt]	*sun* *soup* *missing* *miss* *kiss*	

Source: Description and examples of six types of productive knowledge. From J. Gierut, "On the Assessment of Productive Phonological Knowledge." *NSSLHA Journal, 14* (1986), p. 88.

Target Behavior Selection Guidelines

When selecting target behaviors, consideration should be given to the following: (1) sounds that are stimulable; (2) sounds produced correctly in particular contextual environments; (3) sounds that have a high frequency of occurrence in the language; (4) sounds that are likely to diminish phonological error patterns; (5) sounds in patterns that are inappropriate or unusual; and (6) sounds selected on the basis of a productive phonological knowledge continuum. Of these factors, the impact that the target selected may have on the child's overall phonological system, especially intelligibility, is of utmost importance.

Other Factors to Consider in Case Selection— Intervention Decisions

Dialectal Considerations

The linguistic culture of the speaker is a factor that must be considered when deciding on the need for speech-language intervention, particularly for those clients from ethnic or minority populations, where standard English may not be the norm. *Dialect* refers to a consistent variation of a language, reflected in pronunciation, grammar, or vocabulary, that is used by a particular subgroup of the general population. Although many dialects are identified with a geographical area, those of greatest concern to clinicians are dialects related to sociocultural or ethnic identification.

The phonological patterns of a particular dialect will differ to some degree from the general cultural norm, but these variations reflect only *differences* and not delays or deficiencies in comparison to the so-called standard version of the language. To view the phonological or syntactic patterns used by members of such subcultures as delayed, deviant, or substandard is totally inappropriate. As Williams (1972) put it years ago, "The relatively simple yet important point here is that language variation is a logical and expected phenomenon, hence, we should not look upon nonstandard dialects as *deficient* versions of a language" (111). This perspective has obvious clinical implications, since persons whose speech and language patterns reflect a cultural dialect should not be considered for remediation unless their phonological patterns are outside the cultural norm for the region or ethnic group, or the individual wishes to learn a standard dialect.

Phonological differences may also occur in the speech of individuals within subcultures. The language patterns of inner-city African Americans in New York City, for example, may be quite different from those in New Orleans. The point, then, is that (1) one cannot use normative data based on general American English to judge the phonological status of individuals of some subcultures, and (2) one should not assume that members of certain subcultures have homogeneous linguistic patterns, especially when geographic or ethnic factors are considered. The phonological characteristics of selected dialects with implications for treatment are discussed in Chapter 4. The reader should refer to this chapter for further information on this topic.

Social-Vocational Expectations

Another factor to consider in the analysis and interpretation of a phonological sample is the attitude of the client or the client's parents toward the individual's phonological status. In borderline cases (those for whom a treatment recommendation is debatable), attitude may be a factor in decisions for or against intervention. Extreme concern over a relatively minor articulatory difference by the client or the client's parents may convince the clinician to enroll an individual for instruction. For example, the child who has a frontal lisp and also has a name that begins with /s/ may feel very strongly that the error is a source of embarrass-ment. Crowe Hall (1991) and Kleffner (1952) found that fourth- and sixth-grade children reacted unfavorably to children who had mild articulation disorders. There are many reports in the literature wherein elementary children have recounted negative experiences in speak-ing or reading situations when they produced only a few speech sounds in error. Even "minor distortions" can influence how one is perceived. Silverman (1976) reported that when a female speaker simulated a lateral lisp, listeners judged her more negatively on a personality characteristics inventory than when she spoke without a lisp.

The standard for acceptance of communication depends, to a large extent, on the speak-ing situation. People in public speaking situations may find that even minor distortions de-tract from their message. Some vocations, for example, radio and television broadcasters, may call for very precise pronunciations, and thus, some individuals may feel the need for intervention for what may be relatively minor phonetic distortions. We suggest that if an in-dividual, regardless of age, feels handicapped by speech errors, treatment should usually be provided.

References

Anthony, A., D. Bogle, T. Ingram, and M. McIsaac, *Edinburgh Articulation Test*. Edinburgh: Churchill Livingston, 1971.

Bankson, N. W., and J. E. Bernthal, *Bankson-Bernthal Test of Phonology*. Chicago: Riverside Press, 1990.

Carter, E., and M. Buck, "Prognostic testing for func-tional articulation disorders among children in the first grade." *Journal of Speech and Hearing Disor-ders*, 23 (1958): 124–133.

Carterette, E., and M. Jones, *Informed Speech: Alpha-betic and Phonemic Texts with Statistics Analysis and Tables*. Berkeley: University of California Press, 1974.

Coplan, J., and J. Gleason, "Unclear speech: Recogni-tion and significance of unintelligible speech in pre-school children." *Pediatrics*, 82 (1988): 447–452.

Crowe Hall, B. J., "Attitudes of fourth and sixth graders toward peers with mild articulation disorders." *Lan-guage, Speech, and Hearing Services in Schools, 22* (1991): 334–340.

Diedrich, W., "Stimulability and articulation disorders." In J. Locke (Ed.), *Assessing and Treating Phono-logical Disorders: Current Approaches. Seminars in Speech and Language, 4.* New York: Thieme-Stratton, 1983.

Dinnsen, D., and M. Elbert, "On the relationship be-tween phonology and learning." In M. Elbert, D. Dinnsen, and G. Weismer (Eds.), *Phonological Theory and the Misarticulating Child, ASHA Monographs*, 22. Rockville, Md.: ASHA, 1984.

Edwards, M., "Issues in phonological assessment." In J. Locke (Ed.), *Assessing and Treating Phonological Disorders: Current Approaches. Seminars in Speech and Language, 4*. New York: Thieme-Stratton, 1983.

Elbert, M., and J. Gierut, *Handbook of Clinical Phonology Approaches to Assessment and Treat-ment*. San Diego: College-Hill Press, 1986.

Farquhar, M. S., "Prognostic value of imitative and au-ditory discrimination tests." *Journal of Speech and Hearing Disorders*, 26 (1961): 342–347.

Foster, D., K. Riley, and F. Parker, "Some problems in the clinical applications of phonological theory." *Journal of Speech and Hearing Disorders, 50* (1985): 294–297.

Fudala, J. B., and W. M. Reynolds, *Arizona Articula-tion Proficiency Scale* (2nd ed.). Los Angeles: Western Psychological Services, 1986.

Gierut, J. A., "On the assessment of productive phono-logical knowledge." *Journal of the National Stu-dent Speech-Language-Hearing Association, 14* (1986): 83–100.

Gierut, J. A., M. Elbert, and D. A. Dinnsen, "A functional analysis of phonological knowledge and generalization learning in misarticulating children." *Journal of Speech and Hearing Research, 30* (1987): 462–479.

Goldman, R., and M. Fristoe, *Goldman-Fristoe Test of Articulation.* Circle Pines, Minn.: American Guidance Service, 1969, 1986.

Gordon-Brannan, M., "Assessing intelligibility: Children's expressive phonologies." In K. Butler, and B. Hodson (Eds.), *Topics in Language Disorders, 14* (1994): 17–25.

Grunwell, P., "The development of phonology: A descriptive profile." *First Language, 3* (1981): 161–191.

Hedrick, D. L., E. M. Prather, and A. R. Tobin, *Sequenced Inventory of Communication Development.* Seattle: University of Washington Press, 1975

Hodson, B., *The Assessment of Phonological Processes.* Danville, Ill.: Interstate Press, 1986.

Hodson, B., "Phonological remediation: A cycles approach." In N. Creaghead, P. Newman, and W. Secord (Eds.), *Assessment and Remediation of Articulatory and Phonological Disorders.* Columbus, Ohio: Charles E. Merrill, 1989.

Hoffman, K., "Speech sound acquisition and natural process occurance in the continuous speech of three-to-six year old children." Unpublished master's thesis, University of Wisconsin, Madison. 1982.

Hoffman, P. R., and G. H. Schuckers, "Articulation remediation treatment models." In R. G. Daniloff (Ed.), *Articulation Assessment and Treatment Issues.* San Diego: College-Hill Press, 1984.

Ingram, D., *Phonological Disability in Children.* New York: American Elsevier, 1976, 1989.

Irwin, J., and S. Wong, *Phonological Development in Children 18–72 Months.* Carbondale, Ill.: Southern Illinois University Press, 1983.

Irwin, R., J. West, and M. Trombetta, "Effectiveness of speech therapy for second grade children with misarticulations: Predictive factors." *Exceptional Children, 32* (1966): 471–479.

Kent, R. D., G. Miolo, and S. Bloedel, "Intelligibility of children's speech: A review of evaluation procedures." *American Journal of Speech-Language Pathology,* May (1994): 81–95.

Khan, L. M., and N. P. Lewis, *Khan-Lewis Phonological Analysis.* Circle Pines, Minn.: American Guidance Service, 1986.

Kisatsky, T., "The prognostic value of Carter-Buck tests in measuring articulation skills in selected kindergarten children." *Exceptional Children, 34* (1967): 81–85.

Kleffner, F., "A comparison of the reactions of a group of fourth grade children to recorded examples of defective and nondefective articulation." Ph.D. thesis, University of Wisconsin, 1952.

Lof, G. L., "A study of phoneme perception and speech stimulability." Ph.D. thesis, University of Wisconsin–Madison, 1994.

Mader, J., "The relative frequency of occurrence of English consonant sounds in words in the speech of children in grades one, two and three." *Speech Monographs, 21* (1954): 294–300.

McReynolds, L. V., and M. Elbert, "An experimental analysis of misarticulating children's generalization." *Journal of Speech and Hearing Research, 21* (1978): 136–150.

McReynolds, L. V., and M. Elbert, "Criteria for phonological process analysis." *Journal of Speech and Hearing Disorders, 46* (1981): 197–204.

Miccio, A., and M. Elbert, "Enhancing stimulability: A treatment program." *Journal of Communication Disorders, 29* (1996): 335–363.

Mines, M., B. Hanson, and J. Shoup, "Frequency of occurrence of phonemes in conversational English." *Language and Speech, 21* (1978): 221–241.

Parker, F., "Distinctive features in speech pathology: Phonology of phonemics?" *Journal of Speech and Hearing Disorders, 41* (1976): 23–39.

Powel, T. W., M. Elbert, and D. A. Dinnsen, "Stimulability as a factor in the phonological generalization of misarticulating preschool children." *Journal of Speech and Hearing Research, 34* (1991): 1318–1328.

Prather, E., D. Hedrick, and C. Kern, "Articulation development in children aged two to four years." *Journal of Speech and Hearing Disorders, 40* (1975): 179–191.

Preisser, D. A., B. W. Hodson, and E. P. Paden, "Developmental phonology: 18-29 months." *Journal of Speech and Hearing Disorders, 53* (1988): 125–130.

Roberts, J. E., M. Burchinal, and M. M. Footo, "Phonological process decline from 2½ to 8 years." *Journal of Communication Disorders, 23* (1990): 205–217.

Sander, E., "When are speech sounds learned?" *Journal of Speech and Hearing Disorders, 37* (1972): 55–63.

Secord, W., "The traditional approach to treatment." In N. Creaghead, P. Newman, and W. Secord (Eds.), *Assessment and Remediation of Articulatory and Phonological Disorders.* Columbus, Ohio: Charles E. Merrill, 1989.

Shelton, R., personal communication, 1986.

Shriberg, L. D., and J. Kwiatkowski, "Phonological disorders III: A procedure for assessing severity of involvement." *Journal of Speech and Hearing Disorders, 47* (1982): 256-270.

Shriberg, L., and J. Kwiatkowski, *Natural Process Analysis.* New York: John Wiley & Sons, 1980.

Shriberg, L., and J. Kwiatkowski, "Computer-assisted natural process analysis (NPA): Recent issues and data." In J. Locke (Ed.), *Assessing and Treating Phonological Disorders: Current Approaches, Seminars in Speech and Language, 4.* New York: Thieme-Stratton, 1983.

Silverman, E., "Listeners' impressions of speakers with lateral lisps." *Journal of Speech and Hearing Disorders, 41* (1976): 547–552.

Smit, A. B., "Ages of speech sound acquisition: Comparisons and critiques of several normative studies." *Language, Speech, and Hearing Services in Schools, 17* (1986): 175–186.

Smit, A. B., "Phonological error distributions in the Iowa-Nebraska articulation norms project: Consonant singletons." *Journal of Speech and Hearing Research, 36* (1993): 533–547.

Smit, A. B., L. Hand, J. J. Freilinger, J. E. Bernthal, and A. Bird, "The Iowa articulation norms project and its Nebraska replication." *Journal of Speech and Hearing Disorders, 55* (1990): 779–798.

Smith, B. L., "Explaining the development of speech production skills in young children." *Journal of the National Student Speech-Language-Hearing Association, 9* (1981): 9–19.

Snow, J., and R. Milisen, "The influences of oral versus pictorial representation upon articulation testing results." *Journal of Speech and Hearing Disorders.* Monograph Supplement, 4 (1954): 29–36.

Sommers, R. K., R. Leiss, M. Delp, A. Gerber, D. Fundrella, R. Smith, M. Revucky, D. Ellis, and V. Haley, "Factors related to the effectiveness of articulation therapy for kindergarten, first- and second-grade children." *Journal of Speech and Hearing Research, 10* (1967): 428–437.

Stephens, M. I., P. Hoffman, and R. Daniloff, "Phonetic characteristics of delayed /s/ development." *Journal of Phonetics, 14* (1986): 247–256.

Stoel-Gammon, C., and C. Dunn, *Normal and Disordered Phonology in Children.* Baltimore: University Park Press, 1985.

Templin, M., *Certain Language Skills in Children.* Institute of Child Welfare Monograph Series, 26. Minneapolis: University of Minnesota, 1957.

Turton, L. J., "Development bases of articulation assessment" (pp. 129–155). In W. D. Wolfe and D. J. Goulding (Eds.), *Articulation and Learning* (2nd ed.) Springfield, Ill.: Charles C Thomas, 1980.

Walsh, H., "On certain practical inadequacies of distinctive feature systems." *Journal of Speech and Hearing Disorders, 39* (1974): 32–43.

Weiner, F., *Phonological Process Analysis.* Baltimore, Md.: University Park Press, 1979.

Weiner, F. F., "Systematic sound preference as a characteristic of phonological disability." *Journal of Speech and Hearing Disorders, 46* (1981): 281–286.

Williams, F., *Language and Speech: Introductory Perspectives.* Englewood Cliffs, N.J.: Prentice Hall, 1972.

Winitz, H., *Articulatory Acquisition and Behavior.* Englewood Cliffs, N.J.: Prentice Hall, 1969.

C h a p t e r **8**

Remediation Concepts, Principles, and Methodologies

NICHOLAS W. BANKSON,
James Madison University

JOHN E. BERNTHAL,
University of Nebraska–Lincoln

Basic Considerations

Introduction

In most instances, the long-range objective of remediation for phonologic disorders is the client's spontaneous use of speech sounds that reflect the adult standard of his or her linguistic community. Once a speech-language clinician has determined that an individual's phonology is disordered or otherwise warrants intervention, assessment data are used in the planning of management strategies to accomplish this objective. As described in Chapter 7, phonologic analyses are designed to assist the clinician in identifying appropriate target behaviors for instruction. Once specific goals and objectives for intervention have been determined, the clinician is then faced with the task of determining the type of treatment approaches that are best suited for an individual client. The factors described in this chapter are those clinicians will want to take into consideration in planning, organizing, and ultimately carrying out their instructional program for given clients.

Principles of Instruction

Clinical speech instruction, regardless of the disorder area being treated or the use of a motor or linguistic approach to intervention, typically employs certain principles of instruction in order to ensure that instructional time is well spent and that optimal progress is made toward both short- and long-term goals. Included under these principles of instruction are two categories of recommendations and guidelines for successful interventions.

Temporal Sequencing of Instructional Components

Once instruction objectives have been determined, the clinician formulates an instructional plan that spells out the temporal sequence of instructional components. The typical sequence of clinical speech instruction components is:

Antecedent events (AE)	A delineation of stimulus events designed to elicit particular responses
Responses (R)	The behavior elicited
Consequent events (CE)	The reinforcement, punishment, or neutral consequences that may follow the response

Antecedent events are the stimulus events present during or just prior to a response. Such events typically consist of a verbal model, a picture, printed material, or verbal instructions designed to elicit particular verbal responses.

Responses, the behaviors the clinician wants the client to produce, may range from approximations of the desired behavior (e.g., movement of the tongue backward) to production of the correct behavior (e.g., production of /k/ in connected speech). The clinician is concerned with the functional relationship between an antecedent event and a response or, in other words, the likelihood that a given stimulus will elicit the desired response. Movement to the next level of instruction is often contingent upon a certain number of correct responses. It is important in phonologic training that clients have the opportunity to produce many utterances in the course of a therapy session. A high rate of utterances provides the opportunity for both the clinician's external monitoring as well as the client's automatization of the response. It is typically important that responses are stabilized on one level of complexity before proceeding onto the next level.

The third aspect of the temporal sequence for instruction is **consequent events** (CE). Consequent events are events that occur following a particular response, and usually are labeled reinforcement or punishment. Whether or not a response is learned (and how quickly it is learned) is closely related to the nature and frequency of the consequent events. The most frequently used consequent event is *reinforcement*. Tangible reinforcers such as tokens, points, chips, and informal reinforcers such as a smile or verbal feedback are used equally. Consequent events should immediately follow the correct or desired behavior and should only be used when the desired or correct response is produced. Reinforcement is defined by an increase in a behavior following the presentation of consequent events. Using consequent events after an incorrect behavior sends the "wrong message" to the speaker and does not facilitate learning of correct responses.

Instructional steps are organized so that a sequential series of AE-R-CE steps are followed as one moves through therapy, such as Step 1, AE-R-CE; Step 2, AE-R-CE; Step 3, AE-R-CE.

Modeling

Modeling is an instructional technique in which the clinician provides a verbal model for the client. Sometimes the goal of modeling is that the client will immediately imitate the clinician's production, and sometimes it is that the client will hear and/or see utterances produced in accord with the adult standard. Modeling is a treatment technique frequently employed in speech therapy.

Strategies for Attacking Treatment Goals

An early treatment decision relates to the number of treatment goals targeted in a given session. Fey (1986) outlined two "goal attack strategies" applicable to children with phonologic disorders. The first strategy is called a *vertically structured treatment program*, in which one or two goals (targets) are trained to some performance criterion before proceeding to another target. The traditional treatment of phonologic disorders, to be described in detail later in this chapter, is an example of a vertically structured program. In this approach, one or two phonemes are targeted for treatment and are worked on until they are produced in sentences before training is initiated on other target sounds. Likewise, for a client who exhibits five different phonologic processes, the clinician would target one process and focus treatment on that process until some criterion level is reached before proceeding to the next target process. If the target is final consonant deletions, only one or two exemplars would be the focus of the training. Elbert and Gierut (1986) termed this vertical type of strategy *training deep*. The assumption behind the vertical strategy is that mass practice on a restricted number of target sounds with a limited number of training items will facilitate generalization to other non-trained items. For examples of this type of training, see Elbert and McReynolds (1975, 1978) and McReynolds and Bennett (1972).

A second instructional strategy is a *horizontally structured treatment program* (Fey, 1986), or what Elbert and Gierut (1986) have called *training broad*. Using this strategy, the clinician works on several targets at the same time. Obviously, the time needed to reach a specific performance level will vary across targets. One example, also described later in the approach, is the multiphonemic approach, in which the clinician selects several sounds for treatment in the same session. By working on several sounds simultaneously, the client will presumably learn commonalities or relationships among target sound productions and treatment will be more efficient. In other words, the client receives less training about more aspects of the sound system than in the vertical approach. Several target sounds are taught in many treatment items. The concept behind training broad is that limited practice, with a wide range of exemplars, is an efficient way to modify a child's phonologic system. The goal is to expose the child to a wide range of target sound productions so that this broad-based training will facilitate simultaneous acquisition of several treatment targets.

A third strategy, which combines aspects of the vertical and horizontal approaches, is a *cyclically structured treatment program* (Hodson and Paden, 1991). In this approach, the clinician works with the child on selected goals in a cyclical schedule (two to four days per week, two to four weeks per cycle). Hodson and Paden (1991) recommended structuring treatment so that each cycle included instruction on several error patterns (processes). Within each pattern, instruction is focused on two to five exemplars (phoneme targets) that the child can produce in which a process is not operating. Regardless of the progress at the end of a particular cycle, the next cycle focuses on a second set of processes. It may be necessary, however, to return to certain targets in subsequent cycles. The important difference between this strategy and the previously discussed vertical and horizontal strategies is that treatment proceeds to other target processes regardless of the progress at the end of the cycle. Hodson (1989) suggested that such an approach reflects the manner in which children learn phonology—that is, sounds are not acquired in a straight line progression from initial appearance to adult usage; rather, sounds emerge in young children, and may or may not always progress toward the adult (ambient) norm in an even fashion. Some children regress in usage of particular sounds. In other words, children seem to acquire phonemes in a start-and-stop manner, as reflected in a cyclical approach.

Historically, the most common strategy employed in remediation was the vertical approach, but the horizontal and the related cyclical approaches are now favored by many clinicians and more typically used. Our preference is for the horizontal and cyclical approaches, although all three approaches have been shown to improve phonologic productions.

Scheduling of Treatment

Another basic consideration in planning for phonologic intervention relates to the scheduling of treatment sessions. Relatively little is known about the influence that scheduling of instruction has upon remediation efficacy and sufficient research has not been reported to determine which scheduling arrangements are most desirable. In addition, it is often not practical to schedule treatment sessions on an "ideal" basis. Scheduling of treatment is obviously connected to the treatment methodology employed, the type of client treated, and practical realities such as availability of instructional services.

Investigators who have studied scheduling have generally been concerned with the efficacy of intermittent scheduling versus block scheduling of treatment sessions. *Intermittent scheduling* usually refers to twice weekly scheduling over an extended period of time (such as eight months); *block scheduling* refers to daily sessions for a shorter temporal span (such as two eight-week blocks) separated by time between the blocks.

Several investigators during the 1960s compared dismissal rates associated with traditional (intermittent) and block scheduling, primarily for public school students with articulation disorders (Van Hattum, 1969). A typical study compared dismissal rates for two groups of clients, one of which received treatment twice weekly for eight months, and the other four times per week for eight consecutive weeks in two separate eight-week cycles during an eight-month period. Unfortunately, variables such as articulation severity, phonologic knowledge, stimulability, and treatment methodology employed were not well controlled. In commenting on these studies, Van Hattum (1969) stated: "Research reports relating to scheduling are usually confusing and seldom conclusive. Further, research methodology, due to the complexity of the problem and the number of variables involved, is open to question" (171). Within the limitations of such experimental procedures, however, the following observations on scheduling of articulation intervention can be made:

1. Scheduling of intervention four to five times per week for eight to ten weeks would appear to result in slightly higher dismissal rates than intermittent scheduling for a longer period of time, the greater gains being made early in the treatment process.

2. Intensive scheduling on a short-term basis does not appear to be as successful with clients who have articulation disorders associated with organic impairment when compared to clients without known organic impairment.

Other aspects of scheduling have received even less attention in the literature than session frequency. Powers (1971) suggested that for children under age 8, treatment sessions should probably not exceed one half hour, and if they do, the type of activity should be varied considerably after the first half hour. Older children may be able to work effectively for 40 minutes or more; however, even most adults cannot be expected to maintain sustained attention or effort for longer than one hour at a time.

Group Versus Individual Treatment

Another basic consideration prior to launching phonologic intervention is the matter of deciding if therapy is to be individual, provided in a small group (2–4 people) format, or in a combination of the two. This decision is based on the assumption that clients are being served by the "pull-out" model of treatment (i.e., children are taken from the classroom and provided speech instruction in a separate room) or are receiving services in a speech and hearing center not part of a school system. Later in this section we will discuss speech and language instruction that is classroom based.

Although group instruction is sometimes conducted because of large caseloads, reports have indicated that group instruction may well be as effective as individual instruction in remediating articulation disorders (Sommers, Furlong, Rhodes, Fichter, Bowser, Copetas, and Saunders, 1964; Sommers, Schaeffer, Leiss, Gerber, Bray, Fundrella, Olson, and Tomkins, 1966).

Sommers and colleagues (1964) reported that 50-minute group instruction resulted in as much articulatory change as 30-minute individual instruction when both group and individual sessions were conducted four times per week for four weeks. In a subsequent study (Sommers et al., 1966), similar results were obtained from group sessions held 45 minutes each week and individual instruction sessions held 30 minutes each week over a period of eight and a half months. These investigators concluded that group and individual sessions were equally effective and that the results were not influenced by the grade level (fourth to sixth grade versus second grade) or the severity of the phonologic disorder. Phonologic groups usually contain three or four clients of about the same age who work on similar target behaviors. Van Hattum (1969) pointed out that, unfortunately, such sessions may become so regimented that all individuals work on the same activity, the same target behavior, and the same level of behavior; they are even given the same homework assignments. We have found success working with small groups in which clients reflect different target behaviors and different training levels.

It should be pointed out that *group instruction* should be different from *individual instruction in a group*. Often the beginning clinician has had experience primarily in treating individual clients. When assigned a group of clients, the clinician may simply work with each client individually while remaining group members observe. Group instruction can and should be structured so that individuals in the group can benefit from interaction with other members and from activities that involve the entire group. For example, individuals can monitor and reinforce each other's productions and can serve both as correct models for each other and as listeners to see if the communication intent of the message was met. Powers (1971) stated that a combination of group and individual sessions would be most advantageous for individuals with phonologic problems. She also recommended that instructional groups be limited to three or four individuals whose ages do not exceed a three-year range.

The trend for speech-language pathologists working in the schools to function in a collaborative/consultative role with the classroom teacher, in contrast to the "pull-out" model mentioned above, has added new emphasis and direction to the concept of group instruction. Masterson (1993) has suggested that classroom-based approaches for school-age children allow the clinician to draw on textbooks, homework, and classroom discourse to establish instructional goals and procedures. For preschoolers, classroom activities such as crafts, snacks, and toileting are similarly helpful activities for language and phonologic instruction. Masterson further indicates that classroom-based approaches may be most useful for treating conceptual or linguistic rule type errors, as opposed to errors that require more motor based habilitation. Instruction in the context of the classroom setting is typically less direct than that involved in a pull-out model and requires careful planning from the clinician. This setting is particularly appropriate when a client is in the generalization, or "carryover," phase of instruction, in which academic material and other classroom activities allow for an emphasis on communication skills and intent. It is likely that both of these models (i.e., pull-out; classroom) may be appropriate for a given client during the course of intervention.

Intervention Style

A final consideration before we begin our discussion of specific therapy approaches is *intervention style*. In addition to selecting target behaviors and training stimuli to be used in treatment, the clinician must also consider the management mode or style most appropriate for a given client. A key issue here is the amount of structure that may be prescribed for or tolerated by a given client.

Shriberg and Kwiatkowski (1982) described the structure of treatment as a continuum ranging from drill (highly structured therapy) to play (little structure to therapy), with combinations of these *two end points as in-between stages* on the continuum. These authors described the following four modes of management:

1. *Drill.* This type of therapy relies heavily on clinician presentation or some form of antecedent instructional events, followed by client responses. The client has little control over the rate and presentation of training stimuli.
2. *Drill play.* This type of therapy is distinguished from drill by the inclusion of an antecedent motivational event (e.g., activity involving a spinner; card games).
3. *Structured play.* This type of instruction is structurally similar to drill play. However, training stimuli are presented as play activities. In this mode, the clinician moves from formal instructional antecedent events to playlike activities when the child becomes unresponsive to more formal stimuli presentations.
4. *Play.* The child perceives what he or she is doing as play. However, the clinician arranges activities so that target responses will occur as a natural component of the activity. Clinicians may also use modeling, self-talk, and other techniques to elicit responses from a child.

Shriberg and Kwiatkowski (1982) conducted several studies with young children to compare the relative effects of these four treatment modes. Their data indicated that drill and drill play modes were more effective and efficient than structured play and play modes. In addition, drill play was as effective and efficient as drill.

Clinicians' evaluation of the four modes indicated that they felt drill play was most effective and efficient for their clients, and they personally preferred it. They also urged that three factors be considered when making a choice of management mode: (1) a general knowledge of the child's personality, (2) the intended target response, and (3) the stage of therapy (Shriberg and Kwiatkowski, 1982).

Summary

Before deciding on a specific treatment methodology, the clinician must make several administrative decisions that interact significantly with treatment approaches and, potentially, clients' progress. These include the following:

1. How many targets will I work on in a given session, and how long will I stay with a target before I move on to another?
2. How frequently will therapy sessions be held, and how long will each session last?
3. Will instruction be individual or in a small group? If it is conducted in a school environment, will it be pull-out, classroom based, or a combination of the two?
4. How much structure is most effective with a given client? Is drill and practice the best approach, or play, or a combination of the two?

Treatment Approaches

Introduction

Historically, speech-language pathologists have approached the correction of speech sound productions from the standpoint of teaching a motor behavior, since speech sound errors were thought to reflect an individual's inability to produce the complex motor skills required for the correct articulation of speech sounds. In recent years, clinicians have come to view many developmental phonologic disorders from a linguistic perspective rather than a motor perspective. The linguistic perspective is based on the notion that some individuals produce phonologic errors because they have not learned to use certain phonologic rules, such as sound contrasts, in accord with the adult norm. In other words, error productions reflect the fact that some clients have not acquired the rules for appropriate sound usage rather than an inability to produce the adult sounds.

Although it is convenient to dichotomize the **motor** and **linguistic** aspects of phonology for organization purposes, normal phonologic use obviously involves both the production of sounds at a motor level and their use in accordance with the rules of the language. Thus, the two skills are intertwined and may be described as two sides of the same coin. At a clinical level, it is often difficult or impossible to determine whether a client's errors reflect a lack of motor skills to produce a sound, a lack of linguistic knowledge, or deficiencies in both. It may be that, in a given client, some errors relate to one factor, some to another, and some to both.

Even though a disorder may be related primarily to either the motor or linguistic aspects of phonology, instructional programs typically involve elements of both. It should be recognized that although it is often difficult to determine whether a given instructional procedure is primarily a motor-based or a linguistic-based technique, some activities undoubtedly assist the client in both the development of linguistic knowledge and the development of appropriate motor skills. We recommend that both motor and linguistic aspects of phonology be a part of most therapy programs. One notable exception is the case of a phonetic distortion (e.g., lateral /s/), where a motor approach is the treatment of choice since the "higher level" linguistic aspects of the sound can be assumed (i.e., the child uses lateral /ṣ/ in situations where /s/ is to be used). By careful observation of a client and the nature of his or her problem, the clinician may be able to determine when one approach should be emphasized to a greater degree.

Although we have categorized the treatment approaches presented in this chapter as motor or linguistic, that does not mean that the approaches were necessarily developed from a particular theoretical perspective. In fact, many phonologic treatment approaches have emerged from pragmatic origins and continue to be used simply because "they work." In the pages that follow, several approaches to remediation are described. Some of these can be related to theory, some are atheoretical, and others lie somewhere in between. In the summary of each approach we have presented a "Background Statement" that reflects our perception of the theoretical perspective from which the approach has emerged. A challenge for the future is to develop, refine, and revise theories that provide rationale, support, explanations, and direction for intervention procedures. Ingram (1986) and Schwartz (1992) have strongly indicated that language and phonologic intervention should be based on theory.

Motor-Based Approaches to Intervention

Motor Learning Principles

The remediation approaches we are about to describe were designed to focus primarily on the motor skills involved in producing target sounds and frequently include perceptual tasks as part of the treatment procedures. Most of them represent variations of the traditional approach to remediation. Remediation based on a motor perspective views phonologic errors as motor based, with treatment focused on the placement and movement of the articulators so that segmental productions are consistent with adult standard pronunciations. The usual remediation approach involves the selection of a to-be-corrected target speech sound or sounds, with instruction proceeding through a sequence of increasingly complex linguistic units (e.g., isolation, syllables, words, phrases) until target sounds are used appropriately in spontaneous conversation. Thus, speech production is viewed as a learned motor skill, with remediation requiring repetitive practice at increasingly complex motor and linguistic levels until the targeted articulatory gesture becomes automatic.

Ruscello (1984) has indicated that phonological errors may be modified in two ways when viewed from a motor perspective: (1) movements may be taught to replace incorrect movements, or (2) movements may be taught where they were formerly absent. On the basis of the literature related to motor skill learning, Ruscello has outlined the following critical features in motor skill development:

1. *Cognitive analysis.* A mental or cognitive analysis is important in the early phase of movement formation. In this process, the learner evaluates his or her anticipated performance mentally and then incorporates those adjustments necessary for appropriate execution of the movement. Once stabilization of the movement occurs, such cognitive planning is minimized. This internalization of a skilled movement is thought to contribute to the generalization of skilled movement across a variety of contexts. Based on experimental data, Ruscello and Shelton (1979) reported that mental planning was helpful in the acquisition of articulatory skills in a treatment paradigm.

2. *Practice.* Practice is the key variable thought necessary for mastery of any skilled motor behavior. As the learner practices a particular motor skill, modifications based on internal and/or external feedback are made so that accuracy of performance is increased. A motor skill is best practiced in limited contexts until correct execution of the movement is achieved. Early treatment sessions involve discrete productions, such as isolated sound or word practice, while later sessions introduce more advanced tasks in the context of continuous discourse.

3. *Stages of motor skill development.* Initially there is a sluggishness in the execution of motor skills because the learner is acquiring the movement. With practice, the motor skill is perfected and stabilized. Ultimately, the skill becomes a part of the learner's repertoire of skilled movements and becomes automatic for the speaker.

4. *Feedback.* Sensory feedback processes (internal and external) are described in the motor learning literature as being of great importance in the early development of a skill. When the individual perfects a skill pattern through practice, the error response is diminished and feedback becomes less important.

The treatment approaches described here are based on a motor perspective of phonologic disorders, and some of the attributes outlined by Ruscello are incorporated in these treatment approaches, albeit in a rather nonsystematic fashion.

From a motor-based perspective, the treatment process can be viewed as a continuum comprising three stages—establishment, facilitation of generalization, and maintenance. Such a temporal continuum may also be viewed as an ordered sequence of short-range goals that ultimately lead to the terminal objective for remediation. This continuum, applicable to most types of speech and language disorders, constitutes a framework for a wide variety of specific teaching techniques and procedures. Although the concepts of establishment and maintenance come from the motor literature, the concept of a treatment continuum fits disorders that would be considered linguistic in nature.

The goal of the first phase of instruction, called *establishment*, is to elicit target behaviors from a client and then stabilize such behaviors at a voluntary level, and/or establish phonologic contrasts. Establishment procedures are often based on production tasks, as in the example of a clinician teaching a child who does not produce /l/ where to place his tongue to say /l/. In addition, for a child who can say /l/ but deletes it in the final position (e.g., *bow* for *bowl*), the contrast between word-pairs, such as *bow* and *bowl*, may need to be taught during the establishment phase. Once the client is able to produce the correct form of an error sound and is aware of how it is used contrastively, he or she is ready to move into the generalization phase of instruction.

The second phase of instruction, called *generalization*, is designed to facilitate transfer or carryover of behavior at several levels—positional generalization, contextual generalization, linguistic unit generalization, sound and feature generalization, and situational generalization. The treatment process includes instructional activities or strategies designed to facilitate generalization of correct sound productions to sound contrasts, words, and speaking situations that have not been specifically trained. An example of a context generalization activity would be practicing /s/ in a few key words with high vowels (e.g., *see*, *sit*, *seek*) and then determining whether /s/ is produced correctly in words where /s/ is followed by low vowels (e.g., *soft*, *sock*, *sat*). An example of a situational generalization activity would be practicing /l/ in sentences in the treatment setting and then observing whether the child uses /l/ in sentences produced in his or her classroom or home.

The third phase of remediation, *maintenance*, is designed to stabilize and facilitate retention of those behaviors acquired during the establishment and generalization phases. Instructional activities related to the generalization and maintenance phases of treatment generally overlap. Frequency and duration of instruction are often reduced during maintenance, and the client assumes increased responsibility for "maintaining" correct speech patterns. The client may also engage in specific activities designed to habituate or automatize particular speech patterns. A maintenance activity may consist of a client's keeping track of his or her /s/ productions at mealtime or use of r-clusters during 5-minute phone conversations every evening for a week or longer.

A traditional approach to remediation has been to focus on correcting a single sound, move it through the treatment continuum to later in the generalization phase or to the maintenance phase, and then initiate the correction of another sound. As indicated earlier, many clinicians prefer to focus on several error sounds or phonologic patterns simultaneously, proceeding along the treatment continuum with several segments or processes.

Clients may enter the treatment continuum at different points, the exact point being determined by the individual's current articulatory skills and phonological rules. Consider these two examples: Mark is able to produce a sound correctly in certain words and is able to perceive the target contrastively. Mark therefore begins instruction at the generalization stage. Kristy is able to produce a sound imitatively in syllables, perceives the sound contrast in word-pairs, but fails to incorporate the target production of the sound into words. She also enters the treatment continuum at the generalization stage, but at an earlier point than Mark. The clinician must identify not only the appropriate phase of the treatment continuum but also the appropriate level within a phase at which to begin instruction. In the cases of Mark and Kristy, the clinician determined from assessment data that instruction for Kristy might start at the syllable level to reinforce correct target sound production at that level, while Mark would start on words that contained facilitating contexts.

Teaching Sounds: Establishment of Target Behaviors

As stated earlier, the first phase of remediation for clients who do not produce target behaviors upon request, or who have perceptual and/or production difficulty with particular adult phonologic contrasts, is called *establishment*. During this phase of instruction, the clinician seeks to teach target behaviors and/or establish phonologic contrasts. Thus, the focus in this treatment phase is usually the production of a sound in "isolation," syllables, words, and/or the perception of sound contrasts in words. Clients who enter the treatment continuum at the establishment phase are those who (1) do not have a specific sound in their repertoire and are not stimulable on it, (2) produce a sound in their repertoire (produced only in a limited number of phonetic contexts or occasionally in conversation) but are not able to produce the segment on demand, (3) are unable to perceive the sound in minimal pairs, (4) do not use the segment in a particular context or position (positional, sequential, or contextual constraints), and (5) produce a sound on demand but do not easily incorporate the sound into syllabic units.

Two basic teaching strategies are used to establish target behaviors. The first involves perceptual training prior to production training. The second focuses almost exclusively on production tasks. *Perceptual training* may be described as including conceptualization or phonologic contrast training (e.g., sorting word-pairs such as *two* and *tooth* into two categories that reflect the presence of the final consonant and the deletion of the consonant) as well as traditional discrimination tasks (e.g., discrimination of [s] from [θ]).

Perceptual Training

The type of perceptual training that historically was used most commonly is called *ear training* or *speech sound discrimination training*. Instructional tasks designed to teach discrimination stem from the traditional motor approach to articulation treatment and typically involve making same-different judgments about what is heard (e.g., "Tell me if these are the same or different—*rake–wake*").

Van Riper and Emerick (1984), Winitz (1975, 1984), Powers (1971), and Weber (1970) recommended that discrimination training occurs prior to production training during the establishment phase of the treatment continuum. Winitz (1975) stated, "A child who does not hear differences between sounds hardly can be expected to produce sounds precisely" (48). Only sounds produced in error should be included in speech sound discrimination training since little, if any, relationship is reported between an individual's misarticulation of speech sounds and his or her performance on general speech sound discrimination tasks (Aungst and Frick, 1964; Monnin and Huntington, 1974; Locke, 1980).

Traditionally, speech sound (auditory) discrimination training has focused on judgments of external (clinician produced) speech sound stimuli, sometimes referred to as interpersonal discrimination. Speech sound discrimination training procedures are often sequenced so that the client goes from judgments of another speaker's productions to delayed external self-discrimination (judgments of one's own tape-recorded productions) to simultaneous productions and monitoring of sounds (judgments of one's own sounds as they are produced).

Winitz (1984) suggested that auditory discrimination training precede articulation production training and also be concurrent with production training at each stage of production (e.g., isolation, syllable, word, sentence, conversation) until the client can make the appropriate speech sound discrimination easily at that level. The idea that discrimination training should precede production training is based on the assumption that certain perceptual distinctions are prerequisites for establishing the production of a speech sound in the child's phonologic system. This assumption is not universally accepted, either in terms of developmental theory or in intervention models. A critical question that remains to be answered is whether or not speech sound discrimination training has an impact on the establishment or production of a target sound.

The extent to which perceptual instruction is an inherent aspect of production training is not clear. For example, when a client is asked to say *house* and he or she says *hout*, the clinician may say "no, not *hout* but *house*." In this instance, instruction is production oriented, but perceptual training becomes an inherent part of the task. Williams and McReynolds (1975) reported that production training generalized to speech sound discrimination tasks. They also found that sound discrimination training had little initial effect on production of sounds. Shelton, Johnson, and Arndt (1977) reported that production training did not significantly affect speech discrimination scores and discrimination training did not affect production scores. Rvachew (1994) reported that an interpersonal [external monitoring] speech perception training program involving a computer-driven word-pair training program facilitated sound production learning. This study varied from earlier studies, however, in that subjects received both production and perceptual training simultaneously. Rvachew also reported that perceptual training was most effective for subjects who learned to produce the correct form of their error sound (i.e., became stimulable) during the course of instruction. Although there is a lack of evidence about the precise nature of the relationship between sound discrimination and the establishment of correct productions, it has frequently been assumed that perceptual training is an inherent part of teaching articulatory productions.

The reported failure, in some investigations, of discrimination training to positively influence phonologic productions may be related to the nature of the training task. Savin (1972) questioned children's ability to analyze syllables into phone-size units (individual segments) before 5 or 6 years. Based on that assumption, Shelton (1978) inferred that speech sound discrimination training focused on segmentation of phones from "larger units" may be of questionable value in children younger than 6 years. Likewise, Bernthal, Greenlee, Eblen, and Marking (1987) found that 4- to 6-year-old normal children with age-appropriate phonology had difficulty identifying certain speech sound errors in sentences. Tasks such as these require a metalinguistic (phonemic) awareness that is often difficult for children with phonologic errors. As will be discussed later, such skills may be as beneficial for learning to read and spell as for speech production itself.

A second type of perceptual training that has gained increased acceptance in recent years is conceptualization or contrast training. The idea of conceptualization training was proposed by La Riviere, Winitz, Reeds, and Herriman (1974) as a strategy for the treatment of certain phonologic problems. For example, they recommended that when consonant clusters are reduced, the child be taught to sort contrasting word-pairs (e.g., *led–sled*) into categories that reflect simplification of a consonant cluster and those that reflect appropriate production of the target consonant cluster.

Winitz (1975) pointed out that some children with phonologic errors may not have a true speech sound discrimination problem, but rather are simply not able to conceptualize and use sound contrasts ranging from word-pair contrasts to running speech. For example, the client may be lacking the phonologic concept of word-final consonant usage (i.e., the client evidences final consonant deletion—*so* and *soul*; *tea* and *teeth*). To facilitate the reduction of the final consonant deletion process, Winitz (1975) suggested that the child be trained to contrast and compare speech sounds and syllable structures at the word level and in sentence contexts. Other clinicians (Weiner, 1981; Elbert, Rockman, and Saltzman, 1980) have labeled treatment of this nature **contrast training**. In contrast to conceptualization training, the client is taught to sort contrasting words or syllables into two classes or categories. As suggested, such training might include a task in which the client picks up pictures of "tea" and "teeth" as they are randomly named by the clinician. The intent of this training is to develop a perceptual awareness of differences between minimal pairs and serve to establish and produce the appropriate phonologic contrasts.

In summary, many speech clinicians teach their clients to perceive the distinction between the target and error sounds or to identify phonemic contrasts as part of the establishment process. Such activities may precede and/or accompany production training. Traditional discrimination training has been questioned because many individuals with phonologic disorders do not reflect discrimination problems. In addition, production training, unaccompanied by direct discrimination training, has been shown to modify phonologic errors. The type of perceptual training that appears most useful during the establishment phase is that of conceptualization or phonemic contrast training (for those clients who have not established phonemic contrasts).

Production Training

Many clinicians begin phonologic intervention by focusing on production in establishing a sound production. Whether or not perceptual training precedes or is interwoven with production training, the goal during the establishment phase of production training is to elicit a target sound from a client, stabilize it at a voluntary level, and make certain that the target segment (speech sound) is perceived in minimal pair contrasts.

When a sound is not in a person's repertoire, it is sometimes taught in isolation or syllables rather than words. It should be remembered that some speech sounds, such as stops in isolation, are nearly impossible to teach since stops by their physical nature are produced in combination with vowels or vowel approximations. Glides, likewise, involve production of more than the glide when they are produced.

Whether sounds should be taught initially in isolation, syllables, or words is a matter of some controversy. McDonald (1964) urged that syllables be used in production training since he assumed that the syllable is the basic unit of motor speech production. Some clinicians (e.g., Van Riper and Emerick, 1984) argue that since isolated sounds or syllables are the least complex units of production and afford the least interference between the client's habitual speech sound error and the learning of a correct (adult) production, they should be taught first. Words sometimes elicit interference from old error patterns and in such cases are not a good place to initiate instruction. Others advocate words (lexical items) as the best place to begin instruction because the client can benefit from contextual influences in meaningful productions, and because of the communicative benefits that accrue from the use of "real words."

Four methods are commonly employed by speech-language clinicians to establish the motoric production of a target sound: imitation, contextual utilization, phonetic placement, and successive approximation. Each of these approaches is discussed below.

1. *Imitation.* We recommend that the clinician attempt to elicit responses through imitation as an initial instructional method for production training. Usually the clinician presents several auditory models of the desired behavior (typically a sound in isolation, syllables, or words), instructs the client to watch his or her mouth and listen to the sound that is being said, and then asks the client to repeat the target behavior. Sometimes, the clinician may wish to amplify the model through an auditory trainer. Following this auditory stimulation, the client is asked to produce the sound, syllable, or word. Often, imitation is used in conjunction with phonetic placement (described below) to establish a sound. Correct productions are sometimes tape recorded by the clinician so that the client may play back and evaluate his or her own productions. Clients may also be asked to focus on how a sound feels during correct production and to modify their productions to maintain this kinesthetic awareness.

When an individual can imitate a target sound, the goal during establishment is to stabilize target productions. Subsequent instruction should begin at the most complex linguistic level at which the client is able to imitate, whether it be isolation, syllables, words, phrases, or sentences. This should have been determined during stimulability testing but should also be rechecked periodically during the instructional sequence. Even if the client was not stimulable on a sound during assessment, it is recommended that the clinician begin remediation by asking the client to imitate target productions using auditory, visual, and tactile cues.

2. *Contextual utilization.* As a second approach to establishment, especially when the client does not imitate the target behavior, we recommend that the clinician look for contexts in which the target sound can be produced correctly. As indicated earlier, correct sound productions can frequently be elicited through contextual testing since segments are affected by phonetic and positional context. In Chapter 6, contextual or deep testing was recommended for many clients selected for remediation. The intent of such testing is to identify environments and instances where correct production of target behaviors occurs. It is also recommended that a clinician who is listening to the client's spontaneous speech note any words in which misarticulated sounds are produced correctly. Production training would then begin on such "key" words.

As previously pointed out, although consonants are less likely to be in error when they appear as singletons, correct consonant productions are occasionally elicited in clusters even when absent in singletons. Therefore, clusters should also be included in contextual testing. Curtis and Hardy (1959) reported that more correct responses of /r/ were elicited in consonant clusters than in consonant singletons.

Usually, less than 30 minutes are needed to do a systematic search for correct productions through contextual testing of an individual sound. If a particular context can be found in which the target behavior is produced correctly, it can be used to facilitate correct production in other contexts. For example, if /s/ is produced correctly in the context of the word-pair *bright sun*, the /t/ preceding the /s/ may be viewed as a facilitating context. As a treatment methodology, the client can be instructed to say these two words and prolong the /s/. Later, surrounding sounds may be changed to represent other contexts (e.g., *watch–sun*, *weep–sun*). By modifying the context, correct productions may become stabilized in the client's repertoire.

The rationale for using phonetic context is similar for the use of imitation as an instructional method. Because contextual utilization allows the clinician to capitalize on a behavior already in the client's repertoire, it can be an efficient means of establishing the target behavior.

3. *Phonetic placement.* When the client is unable to imitate a target sound and no contexts are identified in which the target is produced appropriately, the clinician can instruct the client about how to produce a particular sound. This type of instruction is called phonetic placement. In teaching phonetic placement, the clinician

    a. Instructs the client where to place the articulators to produce a specific speech sound
    b. Provides verbal descriptions of how to make the sound
    c. Provides visual and tactile cues to supplement verbal description
    d. Analyzes and describes differences between the error production and the target production

The phonetic placement method has probably been used for as long as clinicians have attempted to modify speech patterns. Over a half century ago, Scripture and Jackson (1927) published *A Manual of Exercises for the Correction of Speech Disorders* that included phonetic placement techniques for speech instruction. These authors suggested

    a. Mirror work
    b. Drawings designed to show the position of the articulators for the production of specific sounds
    c. "Mouth gymnastics"; that is, movements of the articulators (lips and tongue) in response to models and verbal cues and instructions
    d. The use of tongue blades in order to teach placement of sounds

The phonetic placement approach involves explanations and descriptions of idealized phoneme productions. The verbal explanations provided to the client include descriptions of motor gestures or movements and the appropriate points of articulatory contact (tongue, jaw, lip, and velum) involved in producing the target segments. This approach to teaching sounds frequently is used alone or in combination with imitation and context utilization. The Appendix describes techniques for teaching various consonants, some of which utilize phonetic placement cues. The following description is an example of a phonetic placement approach to teaching [s]:

    a. Instruct the client to raise the tongue so that its sides are firmly in contact with the inner surface of the upper back teeth.
    b. Instruct the client to slightly groove the tongue along the midline. Insert a tongue depressor along the midline of the tongue to provide the client a tactile cue as to the place to form the groove.
    c. Instruct the client to place the tip of the tongue immediately behind the upper or lower teeth. Show the client in a mirror where to place the tongue tip.
    d. Instruct the client to bring the front teeth (central incisors) into alignment (as much as possible) so that a narrow small space between the rows of teeth is formed.

  e. Instruct the client to direct the airstream along the groove of the tongue toward the cutting edges of the teeth.

4. *Successive approximation.* Complex behavioral responses such as speech sound productions often need to be broken down into a series of successive steps or approximations that lead to the production of the target behavior(s). A teaching method that utilizes successive approximation is termed **shaping**. The shaping process begins with the elicitation or imitation of a response that the client can emit and proceeds through a series of graded steps or approximations, each progressively closer to the target behavior. Shaping has been found to be an efficient method for teaching complex behavioral tasks but requires careful planning in the sequencing of events to be used for treatment.

The first step in shaping is to identify an initial response that the client can produce and one that is related to the terminal goal. One common way that this method can be initiated is by the modification of other speech sounds already in the repertoire. Instructional steps move successfully from the initial response to the desired behavior. For example, a client who is unable to produce /s/ could be instructed to:

  a. Make [t] (the place of constriction is similar for both sounds)
  b. Make [t] with a strong aspiration on the release, prior to the onset of the vowel
  c. Prolong the strongly aspirated release
  d. Remove the tip of the tongue slowly during the release from the alveolar ridge to make a [ts] cluster
  e. Prolong the [s] portion of the [ts] cluster in a word like oats
  f. Practice prolonging the last portion of the [ts] production, and finally
  g. Produce [s]

Likewise, for a child who produces [ɝ] in error, the clinician might shape the child's production according to the evocation program reported by Shriberg (1975):

  a. Stick your tongue out (model provided).
  b. Stick your tongue out and touch the tip of your finger (model provided).
  c. Put your finger on the bumpy place right behind your top teeth (model provided).
  d. Now put the tip of your tongue "lightly" on that bumpy place (model provided).
  e. Now put your tongue tip there again, and say [l] (model provided).
  f. Say [l] each time I hold up my finger (clinician holds up finger).
  g. Now say [l] for as long as I hold my finger up, like this: (model provided for 5 seconds). Ready. Go.
  h. Say a long [l] but this time as you're saying it, drag the tip of your tongue slowly back along the roof of your mouth—so far back that you have to drop it. (Accompany instructions with hand gestures of moving fingertips back slowly, palm up.) (104)

These two examples reflect ways that clinicians capitalize on successive approximations: by shaping behaviors from a sound in the client's repertoire (e.g., /t/), and by shaping from a nonphonetic behavior in the client's repertoire (e.g., protruded tongue). Once the client produces a sound that is close to the target, the clinician can use other techniques, such as auditory stimulation, imitation, and phonetic placement cues to reach the target production. Descriptions of the other possible ways to elicit various sounds are provided in the Appendix.

Establishment Guidelines

Although we have attempted to formulate the following guidelines on the basis of available literature, more often than not they reflect our own clinical biases. Recognizing that individual variations among clients preclude a detailed set of specific instructions applicable to all clients, these guidelines are general.

1. Perceptual training, particularly contrast training employing minimal pairs, is suggested as part of establishment when there is evidence that the client is unable to perceive appropriate phonologic contrasts or that the error pattern is based on a phonologic rule.
2. When teaching the motor production of a target sound,

   a. Look for the target sound in the client's response repertoire through stimulability (imitation) testing, contextual testing (including consonant clusters and other word-positions), and connected speech samples. The recommended sequence for eliciting sounds which cannot be produced on demand is (1) imitation (verbal stimulation), (2) contextual utilization, (3) phonetic placement, and (4) successive approximation (shaping). Stabilize correct productions and use them as a starting point for production training.

   b. When correct productions of the target patterns are not located via stimulability, contextual testing, or in the speech corpus, such productions may have to be taught.

   c. When several sounds are in error and such errors reflect underlying patterns, the clinician should look for correct production of at least one sound (exemplar) within each sound class during stimulability testing, contextual testing, or in a spontaneous speech corpus. The exemplar(s) should then be stabilized and used to facilitate generalization.

In summary, imitation, phonetic placement, contextual utilization, and successive approximation are all methods that can be used to establish speech sound productions. Perceptual training should be utilized when appropriate phonologic contrasts are not made. If the target behavior can be elicited via imitation, instruction should then proceed to the generalization and maintenance phases of the treatment continuum. For the client who is unable to imitate target sounds correctly, context utilization, phonetic placement, and successive approximation should be used.

Beyond Teaching Sounds: Overall Treatment Approaches

Traditional Approach

While teaching a sound may be the first step in intervention, correction of phonologic errors involves phases of instruction that go beyond establishment. Several treatment approaches are designed to move a client through a multi-step process of habilitation. The **traditional approach** to articulation therapy was formulated during the early decades of the 1900s by the pioneering clinicians of the field. By the late 1930s, Charles Van Riper had assimilated these treatment techniques into a theory of articulation disorders and published them in his text entitled *Speech Correction: Principles and Methods* (originally published in 1939 and modified in subsequent editions). As an outgrowth of his writings, the traditional approach is sometimes referred to as the "Van Riper method."

The traditional or motor approach was developed at a time when the treatment clientele was primarily school-age and adult clients whose errors were primarily substitutions and distortion (residual errors). Years later, unintelligible preschoolers came into focus and at that point linguistic approaches designed to address error patterns came into use. This traditional approach is still used and appropriate for individuals with few phonologic errors whose speech sound errors do not reflect an error pattern that cuts across a group of sounds or class of sounds.

The traditional approach progresses from the identification of error productions to the establishment of correct productions and moves on to transfer and finally to maintenance. As Van Riper and Emerick (1984) stated:

> The hallmark of traditional articulation therapy lies in its sequencing of activities for (1) sensory-perceptual training, which concentrates on identifying the standard sound and discriminating it from its error through scanning and comparing; (2) varying and correcting the various productions of the sound until it is produced correctly; (3) strengthening and stabilizing the correct production; and finally (4) transferring the new speech skill to everyday communication situations. This process is usually carried out first for the standard sound in isolation, then in the syllable, then in a word, and finally in sentences (206).

A characteristic of the traditional approach is its emphasis on perceptual training (i.e., speech sound discrimination or ear training). During this part of therapy, the client is not required to produce the sound, but rather, instruction is designed to provide a perceptual standard by which the client can contrast his or her own productions. Thus, perceptual training becomes a precursor to production training. Van Riper and Emerick's (1984) perceptual, or ear, training is outlined as follows.

Perceptual Training/Ear Training

The goal of this phase of instruction is for the client to develop an auditory model that will serve as an internal standard against which comparisons of his or her own productions can be made. Several suggested phases of ear training precede production training. While initially the phases usually proceed in the order listed here, the clinician may wish to reinforce these skills at any point in therapy by going back to earlier ear training activities.

Phases of Ear Training (Perceptual Training)

1. Identification

    a. The clinician demonstrates the sight, sound, and feel of a target sound.

    b. For young children, the sound is often labeled (e.g., /t/ is the ticking sound; /f/ the angry cat sound).

    c. The client recognizes the target sound in isolation from among dissimilar and similar sounds.

2. Isolation

    a. The client is able to indicate when he or she hears (e.g., raise hand, show happy face) or does not hear (e.g., keeps hand down, shows sad face) the target behavior and is able to do so in increasingly complex environments (i.e., words, phrases, sentences).

    b. The client is able to identify the position of a target sound in a word (initial, medial, final).

3. Stimulation

    a. The clinician "bombards" the client with productions of the target sound. This may be accomplished by repetitions of the target sound (e.g., tongue twisters) or variations in the loudness or duration at which target sounds are presented by the clinician.

4. Discrimination

    a. The client makes external discriminations (judgments) of correct and incorrect productions (produced by the clinician) in increasingly complex contexts (i.e., words, phrases, sentences). In this instance the client is comparing someone else's production with his or her own internal image of the correct form of a sound. A clinical narrative that reflects the clinician teaching the client to make an external judgment related to a θ/s substitution is as follows: "Here is a picture of a 'thun.' 'Thun.' Did I say that word right? Did you see my tongue peeking out at the beginning of the word? Did you hear /θ/ instead of /s/? Can you help me remember to keep my tongue in and say the /s/ right?"

Additional suggestions for perceptual training including error detection and error correction have been presented by Winitz (1975), who stated that when the client is unable to imitate the correct form of the target sound or segment, speech sound discrimination is an important prerequisite to motor production. Winitz (1975) also speculated that discrimination training can affect changes in production and outlined the following principles for discrimination training:

1. The acoustic contrast in discrimination training should be large at first, then the phonemic distance should gradually be narrowed. It is suggested that the sound error or sound substitution should be contrasted with other sounds before it is contrasted with standard productions of the target sound. Thus, if /θ/ → /s/, the /θ/ should be contrasted with other sounds and only later in the instructional sequence should /s/ be contrasted with /θ/.

2. It could be hypothesized that ultimately the most important perceptual contrast the client must learn is the distinction between error and standard productions. The client should learn to discriminate between the clinician's imitation (external monitoring) of the client's speech sound error and the standard pronunciation before judging his or her own productions (internal monitoring).

3. Instruction should involve active participation by the client. For example, when the child misarticulates, wait a few seconds, imitate the child's production, and then respond by repeating the target words correctly several times before handing the object to the child. As training continues, wait for the child to correct him- or herself.
4. Once the client can discriminate correct-incorrect productions at the word level, discrimination of sounds in running speech should be trained.

In summary, many of the comments made in this section on traditional perceptual training derive from the perspective that speech sound errors are motor based. Later in this chapter we will talk about perceptual training that derives from a linguistic orientation. One should keep in mind that at a practical level the clinician may wish to incorporate instructional procedures from both perspectives in clinical instruction that focus on speech sound perception.

Production Training

The second but primary ingredient of traditional instruction is production training. Production training usually includes four sequential instructional phases wherein a target sound is (1) produced in isolation (the target sound is elicited in isolation or, in the case of stops and certain glides, in a CV context such as /pa/); (2) produced in syllables (the sound is produced in CV, VC, and VCV syllables); (3) produced in words (the target sound is produced in a word or lexical context in initial, final, and medial positions); and (4) produced in a meaningful connected speech context. Secord (1989) outlined the following instructional steps for traditional production training:

1. *Isolation.* An explanation for beginning with production of the target sound in isolation is the assumption that the articulatory gestures of a sound are most easily learned when the sound is highly identifiable and in the least complex context. The goal at this level is to develop a consistently correct response. Specific techniques for teaching sounds are included in the Appendix. It should be pointed out, however, that when a client is able to produce a sound at a more complex level (such as syllables or words), production training should begin at that level.

2. *Nonsense syllables.* The goal at this step is consistently correct productions in a variety of nonsense syllable contexts. A suggested sequence for syllable practice is CV, VC, VCV, and CVC. It is also suggested that the transition from the consonant to the vowel should be accomplished with sounds that are similar in place of articulation. For example, an alveolar consonant such as /s/ should be facilitated in a high front vowel context, as in [si]. The clinician might also wish to use the target sound in nonsense clusters.

3. *Words.* Once the client can consistently produce the target sound in nonsense syllables, instruction proceeds to word level productions. Instructions at this level should begin with monosyllabic words with the target consonant (assuming instruction is focusing on consonants as opposed to vowels) in the prevocalic position (CV). Instruction then moves to VC, CVC, CVCV, monosyllabic words with clusters, followed by more complex word forms. Table 8.1 reflects a hierarchy of phoneme production complexity at the word levels identified by Secord (1989).

TABLE 8.1   Substages of Word Level Stabilization Training (Secord, 1989)

Substage	Syllables	Examples for /s/
1. Initial prevocalic words	1	*sun, sign, say*
2. Final postvocalic words	1	*glass, miss, pass*
3. Medial intervocalic words	2	*kissing, lassie, racer*
4. Initial blends/clusters	1	*star, spoon, skate*
5. Final blends/clusters	1	*lost, lips, rocks*
6. Medial blends/clusters	2	*whisper, outside, ice-skate*
7. All word positions	1–2	*(any of above)*
8. All word positions	any	*signaling, eraser, therapist*
9. All word positions; multiple targets	any	*necessary, successful*

Once a core group of words is established in which the client is readily able to produce the target sound, the clinician seeks to expand the small set of core words to a somewhat larger set of training words. Usually target words are selected on the basis of meaningfulness to the client (e.g., family names, places, social expressions, academic curriculum, and so forth), but other factors such as phonetic context and syllable complexity should also be taken into consideration, just as they were for the initial set of core words.

4. *Phrases.* At this point instruction shifts from single-word productions to practicing a target sound in two- to four-word phrases. This level of production represents a complexity level in between single words and sentence level productions. This is especially true if carrier phrases are employed. *Carrier phrases* are phrases where only a single word is added with each repetition (e.g., I see the *car*; I see the *cup*; I see the *cane*). In phrase level productions, only the target word should initially contain the target sound.

5. *Sentences.* An extension of phrase level productions is sentence level practice. Just as practice at other levels has involved careful sequencing of task complexity, that principle also holds at this level. This includes factors such as phonetic context, syllable structure of words, and number of words in the sentence. Secord (1989) suggested the following sequence of sentence level complexity:

1. Simple short sentence with one instance of the target sound
2. Sentences of various lengths with one instance of the target sound
3. Simple short sentences with two or more instances of the target sound
4. Sentences of various lengths with two or more instances of the target sound

6. *Conversation.* The final step in production involves using a target sound in everyday speech. At this point the clinician is seeking to facilitate generalization of productions that have already proceeded through more structured production tasks. Initially, generalization situations are structured so that the client produces his or her sound correctly in situations where his speech is monitored. Activities such as role playing, talking about future plans, attempting to get information, interviewing, and oral reading can be used at this level. Following such structured generalized conversations, subsequent conversations are more spontaneous and free and sometimes characterized as "off-guard" type conversations. The intent is to provide activities to facilitate transfer that approximate real-life situations. Activities should include speaking situations where the client focuses not on self-monitoring skills but on what he or she says. Telling personal experiences, talking about topics that evoke strong feelings, and taking part in group discussions are appropriate activities. Van Riper (1978) suggested that at this final stage of instruction negative practice helps to stabilize a new response. In negative practice, a client deliberately produces a target sound incorrectly; Van Riper and Erickson (1996) stated that such deliberate error productions increase the rate of learning.

At this point, the clinician also seeks to facilitate the carryover of conversational usage to situations beyond the therapy environment. It is also suggested that such situational generalization be encouraged once the client can produce a target sound at the word level. By encouraging transfer in earlier stages of instruction, it is assumed that generalization beyond the word level will be significantly enhanced and will perhaps decrease the amount of time needed at the phrase, sentence, and conversational levels.

Van Riper and Erickson (1996) recommended that sensory-perceptual training should be included as production training moves forward from word level productions so that internal perceptions of phonological productions will accompany external perceptions. It is assumed that when the client is able to perceive correct and incorrect productions in another person's speech, such discrimination will facilitate an internal concept of such phonological contrasts. This latter awareness is necessary for clients to make judgments about their own error productions.

Facilitating internal or "intra-auditory" discrimination involves helping the client learn how to recall, perceive, and predict errors. Detecting one's own phonological errors after they occur and being able to predict where they may occur are part of what becomes self-monitoring. Unfortunately, techniques for facilitating these skills are not as easy to devise as for external monitoring. Recommended techniques for this type of instruction have been short loop tape recordings, amplification of one's speech, and shadowing of speech by clinician and client.

Summary of the Traditional Approach

Background Statement.   The underlying assumptions of the traditional approach to remediation include the following: (1) Faulty perception of speech sounds is often related to phonological errors, and (2) phonological errors may be viewed as inadequate development of oral motor skills. Thus, the traditional approach relies heavily on motor production combined with activities related to discrimination training (ear training).

Unique Features.   The traditional approach to articulation remediation has for many years constituted the basic framework for articulation instruction and focuses on motor learning of individual speech sounds. The approach provides general instructional guidelines and a sequence for correcting articulatory errors from the establishment phase through the maintenance phase, but it does not provide step-by-step detail. Although some suggested teaching activities are included, no criterion levels are suggested, no reinforcement schedule is recommended, and no data collection system is presented. The approach can be modified to fit the needs of clients of all ages. The perceptual training (ear training) suggested in this approach includes discrimination, identification, auditory stimulation with verbal models, and self-monitoring.

Strengths and Limitations.   It may be said that from a historical perspective this is the most widely employed approach to phonological remediation, and one that forms the basis of several treatment approaches. This fact, no doubt, is related to the logical sequence of training tasks, the success that accrues through motor practice, and the adaptability and applicability of the approach. It may not, however, be the most efficacious approach for clients whose phonological problems are not motor based or when client's phonological patterns affect entire sound classes.

Research Support.   This approach has stood the test of time because it has "worked" for many clinicians, with many clients. Many investigators have reported phonological change in association with intervention that has been based on this approach; however, comparative studies between the "traditional approach" and others are limited. The emphasis on external discrimination training as part of the treatment process for all children has been questioned because of the difficulty involved in separating discrimination training and production training, as well as the lack of data to support its effectiveness. This approach is still appropriate for the treatment of clients who have a limited number of errors. Elements of this approach are also utilized in linguistic approaches to remediation.

Multiple Phoneme Approach

The **multiple phoneme approach** was designed by McCabe and Bradley (1975) to facilitate instruction on several error sounds during each treatment session and is characterized by a traditional treatment sequence combined with a method for collecting data on articulatory responses. In addition, the approach calls for the application of behavioral principles to treatment and the analysis of sound productions in conversation (Bradley, 1989). The multiple phoneme approach is divided into establishment, transfer, and maintenance phases.

Phase I, called *establishment*, is designed to elicit correct target sound productions in isolation in response to a grapheme (printed letter) or phonetic symbol. Production is initiated first under conditions of auditory-visual-tactile stimulation (the client hears the model, sees the associated grapheme, and receives phonetic placement cues); then follows auditory-visual stimulation (pairing of the grapheme and clinician's model), and finally visual stimulation (the grapheme alone is presented). The goal of establishment is correct production of the target in isolation via visual stimulation on four out of five attempts.

Step 2 of Phase I is called a *holding procedure*, and it is designed as a branching step to maintain correct target productions in isolation. It is to be used if time limitations in a particular training session preclude additional training on all target segments. For example, consider the client who produces /s, z, ʃ, t, f, v, r, l/ in error in connected speech but has met the criterion for establishment of these sounds in isolation. The clinician may choose for the client to work on generalization of /s/, /z/, and /ʃ/ at the word level and /t/, /f/, and /v/ at the syllable level during a particular session. Since time may not allow generalization activities with the /r/ and /l/ in the session, /r/ and /l/ are elicited through a holding procedure, which involves using one or more of the activities in Step 1 of this phase.

Phase II, **transfer**, is designed to facilitate production of sounds along the treatment continuum from isolation to correct production in conversational speech. The transfer phase contains five steps or activities, and clients can be producing different sounds at any of these levels during a single session.

In Step 1 of the transfer phase, an *imitative word probe* is administered to determine whether or not the subject should receive instruction at the syllable or word level. If the client does not produce a target sound in 6 to 10 monosyllabic words, instruction begins at the syllable level. In this step the consonant is produced in combination with all commonly occurring vowels in CV and VC combinations, along with multisyllable sequences in response to presentation of grapheme and auditory stimuli.

In Step 2 of transfer, target productions are elicited in initial, medial, and final *word-positions* in response to printed words (picture stimuli are used with nonreaders). Care is taken to ensure that verbs, adjectives, prepositions, articles, and nouns are utilized as training words, with no more than 25 to 30 total target words. Criterion for moving to the next step is 90 percent accuracy for one session or 80 percent accuracy for two sessions.

Step 3 of transfer involves *phrase and sentence* practice with the goal of having all sounds in words produced correctly. Control of vocabulary and phrase-sentence length is important initially. If a client has established only a limited number of phonemes, the clinician may have to calculate accuracy on the basis of words that actually contain target sounds. At this stage clients are also encouraged to monitor their own productions. Criterion for advancement is the same as that at the word level.

Step 4 of transfer, *reading–storytelling*, has as its goal accurate production of target sounds in connected speech in utterances of four to six word-units. Reading and storytelling are the suggested ways to elicit responses.

Step 5 of transfer, *conversation*, is the final stage of instruction. The criterion level for termination of this stage is 90 percent whole-word accuracy (all sounds articulated correctly within every word) for one entire session or 80 percent for two sessions.

Phase III, called **maintenance**, focuses on whole-word accuracy in various speaking situations. At this stage, accuracy of productions is monitored in various speaking situations by the clinician, the client, and others in the environment.

A primary emphasis in the multiple phoneme approach is placed on counting and charting correct and incorrect responses during a treatment session, with all responses of the client tabulated. Throughout each session the clinician records responses on an Articulation Data Sheet shown in Figure 8.1. The sheet is arranged to record the level and accuracy of production for each sound.

The multiple phoneme approach may be viewed as a structured outline for (1) sequencing training steps and (2) data collection. Specific instructional techniques are left to the judgment and preferences of the clinician.

Summary of the Multiple Phoneme Approach
Background Statement.   This approach was originally developed with clients evidencing severe phonological disorders associated with cleft palate. Reliance on the traditional treat-

Client _____   Date _____

Clinician _____   Transfer _____

Maintenance _____

Step _____

Date	Session	Activity	Isolation	Syllables	Words	Sentences	Reading	Conversation	Time	Total Response	Total Error	Total Correct	% Correct	Comments

FIGURE 8.1   Articulation data sheet.

Source: Used with permission of R. McCabe and D. Bradley.

ment sequence and the fact that all error sounds are targeted for remediation suggests that this approach views articulation errors from a motor perspective.

Unique Features.   Unique features of this approach include the following: the structured format for collecting response data; the procedures employed during the establishment phase; the use of graphemes in association with target sounds and words; the use of several parts of speech (e.g., nouns, verbs, adjectives) as training words; and the teaching of several target sounds in each session.

Strengths and Limitations.   This approach provides an organized way to teach several sounds simultaneously and to collect data on client performance. Because of the complexity of the data collection system, the approach lends itself to individual rather than group instruction. Preschool children may find simultaneous instruction on all sounds in error to be somewhat confusing and may also find the use of written symbols to be difficult. Even though the approach is designed to focus on the motor production of several error sounds, clinicians can use the data collection system with more linguistically oriented approaches. For example, a clinician may still follow the traditional teaching sequence and utilize this data collection system when teaching exemplars of phonological error patterns. In those instances where a clinician has a need to work on several sounds simultaneously because of a limited number of treatment sessions (e.g., the child's insurance will cover no more than 12 sessions) and no error patterns, this approach is appropriate. In such instances, the clinician may wish to provide some instruction on all error sounds rather than relying on across-phoneme generalization for sound acquisition.

Research Support.   McCabe and Bradley (1975) reported data from 44 clients, ages 5 to 14, who were exposed to the multiple phoneme approach to instruction. They found statistically significant gains on both the *Arizona Articulation Proficiency Scale* and a specially designed articulation protocol. It should be pointed out, however, that no control group was used in this study. Black (1972) reported an 80 percent dismissal rate of a public school caseload during the first year the multiple phoneme approach was used. Only 20 percent of the caseload had been dismissed the previous year, when a different remediation approach was used. Such data, while supportive, lack scientific rigor because of the lack of control procedures.

Programmed Conditioning for Articulation

The **Programmed Conditioning for Articulation: Monterey Articulation Program** is a behaviorally oriented program authored by Baker and Ryan (1971), based on the traditional approach to articulation remediation. Developed from the principles of programmed instruction, this program can be adapted to focus on any sound segment the clinician may wish to teach. It consists of an establishment phase, which includes a basic program of 18 steps, 91 branching steps, and several sound evocation programs; a transfer phase of 15 steps; and a maintenance phase of five steps.

   Sound evocation programs are intended to teach target productions when such behaviors are not in the client's response repertoire. These programs are available for /s/, /r/, /l/,

/θ/, /ʃ/, and /tʃ/. General instructional suggestions and guidelines for teaching other phonemes are presented. Testing is prescribed prior to the initiation of the establishment phase
to allow the clinician to select the target sound(s) and determine the appropriate entrance
step in the program.

The same basic instructional pattern is followed for all phases of the program: The
client responds to a stimulus and is given reinforcement. Verbal modeling, or imitation,
is the most frequently used method of stimulus presentation in the program. Pictures,
graphemes, and storytelling are also used to elicit responses. The authors recommend that
instruction be conducted so that clients produce an average of 300 responses per hour of
instruction. Reinforcement for correct responses is presented according to a schedule that
begins with continuous reinforcement and shifts to a fixed ratio of 10 to 1 as the student
progresses.

The criterion level for advancing from one step to the next in the program is 10 correct
responses in a row. If errors are consistently produced, then branching activities are initiated. Criteria for shifting to branching is ten consecutive errors or three consecutive sessions with a correct response rate of less than 80 percent.

The establishment phase in this program progresses from sound evocation through
production in conversational speech in the instructional setting. Thus, the definition of establishment is broader than the definition used throughout this book. Table 8.2 presents the
program outline for the establishment phase. The instructional sequence proceeds from
Step A (imitation of the sound in isolation) to Step B (imitation of the sound in syllables)
and continues with stimulus and response complexity increasing through the steps. The program delineation includes specific instructions regarding the nature of the stimulus, the expected response, and the schedule of reinforcement.

The transfer phase of the program is designed to facilitate situational transfer. Series A
(Table 8.3) of the transfer program is initiated during the establishment phase of the program. When the student reaches certain criterion levels on the establishment program, the
instructor gives the client word lists, phrases, and sentences to take home for practice with
a parent. The parent is instructed to work with the child during a 5-minute period and
record his or her responses.

During Series B and subsequent series (see Table 8.3) of the transfer phase, the clinician monitors the client during speaking situations, culminating with the client giving a
speech or participating in show-and-tell with his or her peers. During such speaking situations, the clinician must record at least 10 target responses, and the client must produce
90 percent correct responses to proceed to the next step.

The maintenance phase of the program covers a two-month period following completion of the transfer phase. It includes periodic rechecks to help the student maintain the
newly acquired sounds. During the first month, the client is seen weekly; during the second
month, only once. Criterion for each step in this phase is 10 consecutively produced correct
responses in conversation.

Summary of the Programmed Conditioning for Articulation

Background Statement.   This behavioral program views remediation from the perspective that speech sounds are learned motor behaviors. Instruction involves a progression
of motor skills and employs behavioral principles that are used in modifying behaviors.

TABLE 8.2 Establishment Phase: Programmed Conditioning for Articulation

Step		Stimulus	Response	Schedule of Reinforcement
Series A		Take Criterion Test Placement Start		
	1	Sound in isolation	Sound	
Series B	1	Sound in nonsense syllable, random presentation of short vowels (a, e, i, o, u) with X* in initial position (Xa)	Syllable	
	2	Sound in nonsense syllable, random presentation of short vowels (a, e, i, o, u) with X in final position (aX)	Syllable	
	3	Sound in nonsense syllable, random presentation of short vowels (a, e, i, o, u) with X in medial position (aXa)	Syllable	100% (continuous)
Series C	1	Word with X in initial position	Word	50%
	2	Word with X in final position	Word	50%
	3	Word with X in medial position	Word	50%
Series D	1	Word with X in initial position appearing randomly in 2- or 3-word phrase	Phrase	50%
	2	Word with X in final position appearing randomly in 2- or 3-word phrase	Phrase	50%
	3	Word with X in medial position appearing randomly in 2- or 3-word phrase	Phrase	50%
Series E	1	Word with X in initial position appearing randomly in 4- to 6-word sentence	Sentence	50%
	2	Word with X in final position appearing randomly in 4- to 6-word sentence	Sentence	50%
	3	Word with X in medial position appearing randomly in 4- to 6-word sentence	Sentence	50%
Series F	1	Contextual reading material (If nonreader, go to series G-2.)	Reads a sentence	100%
Series G	1	Story: Instruct to read silently and then tell a story about it.	Reads story silently Tells what he/she reads in phrases and sentences Phrases	100%
	2	Pictures: (Instructor models first picture by telling short story about the picture.)	Tells story about picture in sentences	100%
Series H	1	Conversation	Conversation	100%
	2	Conversation End of Program Stop Take Criterion Test Go to Transfer Program Series B. Begin Program again with New Sound(s).	Conversation	10%

Source: Used with permission of Monterey Learning Systems, 900 Welch Road, Palo Alto, Calif.

*X = target sound

TABLE 8.3 Transfer Phase: Programmed Conditioning for Articulation

Step	Stimulus	Response	Schedule of Reinforcement
Series A	Child working with parent at home:		
1	Says word containing X	Repeats word	100%
2	Says phrase containing word with X	Repeats phrase	100%
3	Says sentence containing word with X	Repeats sentence	100%
4	Reading material or pictures	Reads or tells about pictures	100%
5	Conversation	Conversation	100%
Series B	Take Transfer Criterion Test Different physical settings with the clinician:		
1	Outside clinic (outside the door)	Conversation	100%
2	Outside clinic (down the hall)	Conversation	100%
3	Outside clinic (outside the building or in another room)	Conversation	100%
4	Playground or cafeteria or off school or clinic grounds	Conversation	100%
5	Outside classroom	Conversation	100%
Series C	In the classroom:		
1	With clinician in classroom	Conversation	100%
2	With clinician and teacher in classroom	Conversation	100%
3	Small-group activity	Conversation	100%
4	Large-group activity	Conversation	100%
5	"Speech" or "Show and Tell" in front of class Take Transfer Criterion Test End of Program Stop Go to Maintenance	Conversation or monologue	100%

Source: Used with permission of Monterey Learning Systems.

Instruction consists of several series of small, sequential steps associated with contingent reinforcement. Thus, this program represents a formal programmed approach to instruction that is based on behavioral conditioning.

Unique Features. The detailed, step-by-step instructions for correcting misarticulations provide the clinician with what some might call a "recipe" for sequencing therapy. The scope of the program, which moves from establishment to transfer to maintenance, including a home program, is more comprehensive than most. As with all programmed instruction, the course of treatment is based on data that accrue from tabulation of responses made by the client.

Strengths and Limitations.   The reason this program is included in this text is that it provides clinicians or instructional aides with a systematic, step-by-step instructional procedure that takes a client from establishment to dismissal for a given sound. The emphasis on numerous responses per session ensures much repetition and motor practice. Program methodology relies heavily on imitation, which may become tedious for some clients and clinicians. The inclusion of branching steps allows some individualization of the program, but the basic assumption is that the program is particularly suitable for school-age children and adults with residual errors.

Research Support.   Data to support the program have been reported by Baker and Ryan (1971) and Gray (1974). These investigators reported that significant gains can be achieved by subjects when comparing pretest and posttest scores for all phases of the program. However, experiments that have included control groups or other controls have not been reported.

Sensory-Motor Approaches

Perhaps the most widely recognized **sensory-motor approach** to articulation remediation was developed by McDonald (1964) and focused on motor productions in various phonetic contexts. This system, while motor based, is quite different from the traditional approaches presented earlier. It is based on the assumption that phonetic contexts can be used to facilitate generalization of target sounds from simple to more complex productions. When first introduced, this system was unique in rejecting notions that (1) perceptual training should precede production training, and that (2) the initial step in production training should be production of sounds in isolation. Rather, McDonald pointed out that sounds in conversational speech do not occur in isolation but instead are organized into syllables. Thus, it would follow that if the syllable is assumed to be the basic unit of speech production, instruction should begin at and focus upon production at the syllabic level.

The initial objective of treatment is to heighten the client's awareness of kinesthetic and auditory sensations associated with connected speech. At this point, the client imitates combinations of bisyllables and trisyllables following the presentation of verbal models by the clinician. The stimuli are arranged to follow a hierarchy from simple movements to more complex movements with a variety of stress patterns. The intent of such practice is to enable the client to "listen and then to hear and feel his or her reproductions of the stimulus."

Practice begins with sounds that the child can produce correctly (nonerror sounds) in bisyllable (CVCV) productions. The second CV of the bisyllable is a duplication of the first CV syllable, and each syllable is produced with equal stress. The consonant is then combined with each of the commonly used vowels; as in the example: [titi], [tɪtɪ], [tete], [tætæ], [tʌtʌ], [tutu], [tʊtʊ], [toto], [tata]. Next the client imitates syllables with primary stress on the first syllable followed by practice with primary stress on the second syllable. Following this, the vowels used in each syllable are changed, as in /titɪ/, and then other consonants that the client can produce correctly are substituted in a variety of vowel contexts and stress patterns. Combinations that will produce a variety of movement patterns (i.e., changes in place of consonant-vowel articulation) should be included.

Following practice with bisyllables, imitation of trisyllables, such as [lalala], is initiated. Practice with trisyllables follows the same general pattern presented for bisyllables, including a variety of movement sequences and stress patterns. As a part of bisyllable and trisyllable practice, clients are instructed to describe the placement of the articulators and describe the articulatory movements. Some of the error sounds should be included in bisyllabic and trisyllabic contexts, but no effort should be made to remediate these sounds if they are produced incorrectly.

Instruction for articulatory errors is initiated in a context where the error sound can be produced correctly. McDonald provided an example of a child with a defective /s/ who produced [s] correctly on a deep test in the context of *watchsun*. He suggested the following sequence of instructions after *watchsun* was identified as a context where /s/ was correctly produced: (1) Say *watchsun* with "slow-motion" speed; (2) say *watchsun* with equal stress on both syllables, then with primary stress on the first syllable, and then with primary stress on the second syllable; (3) say *watchs* and prolong [s] until a signal is given to complete the bisyllable with [ʌn]; (4) say short sentences with the same facilitating context such as "Watch, sun will burn you." The sequence is repeated with other sentences and stress patterns. The meaningfulness of the sentence is not important since the primary focus of the activity is the movement sequences.

The third objective is "to facilitate the correct articulation of the sound in systematically varied phonetic contexts." The client is instructed to alter slightly the movement patterns associated with the correct /s/ by changing the vowel following the segment. For example, when /s/ was correct in *watchsun*, McDonald suggested a sequence such as:

watch-sum	*watch-sat*
watch-sea	*watch-soon*
watch-sit	*watch-sew*
watch-send	*watch-saw*

The next step is to practice words that include a second contextual modification. Using the previous example, segments preceding and following /tʃ/ would be altered. Words like *teach*, *reach*, *pitch*, *catch*, and *beach* would be used in combination with one-syllable words beginning with /s/ and followed by a variety of vowels (such as *sand*, *sun*, *said*, and *soon*). Practice is then conducted with various combinations of the words that terminate with /tʃ/ in combination with words that begin with /s/ (for example, *teachsun*). Various sound combinations are practiced with different rates and stress patterns and should also be practiced in sentence contexts.

The next phase of instruction is directed toward a phonetic context other than [tʃ] in which the /s/ is correct, and then vary the phonetic context, rate of speech, and syllable stress in alternative contexts. Situational transfer procedures and activities are similar to those used with other treatment systems.

Hoffman, Schuckers, and Daniloff (1989) described a variation of the sensory motor approach that involves a sequenced set of production-based training tasks designed to facilitate the motoric automatization of articulatory performance. The basic assumption behind their suggestions is that "revision of over learned, highly automatic behavior is possible through carefully planned and executed performance rehearsal" (248). They also indicated that once *inappropriate* patterns of a behavior are automatized or habituated the process of revising those behaviors may differ from development of the original behavior.

Intervention is seen as involving instruction and extensive practice of motor articulatory adjustments to replace previously learned (incorrect) production. The paragraphs that follow present the sequence of tasks and instructional activities these authors suggest.

Prior to working directly on error targets, the clinician elicits, via imitation, sound segments that the client can produce correctly. Such "stimulability tasks" provide the client with an opportunity to experience success in a speech task as well as the opportunity to observe and imitate the clinician's productions. It is suggested that the clinician not only model the correct form of sounds in the child's repertoire but also distort such productions through excessive movements (e.g., lip rounding for /m, p, f/) for the purpose of giving the client the opportunity to practice manipulation of the articulators in response to the clinician's model. Such activity will hopefully facilitate the client's skill at identifying, comparing, and discriminating the clinician's and his/her own sound productions.

Following stimulability tasks, the clinician and client work together to employ the articulatory adjustments necessary for correct target sound production. It is suggested that the clinician be able to repeat sentences using error productions similar to those of the client in order to be aware of the motoric acts involved in the client's misarticulations. Instead of focusing instruction on "correct" or "better" target sound productions, the emphasis is on doing interesting things with the speech mechanism, with the ultimate goal the production of a target sound. Activities designed to provide information about the anatomy and physiology of the speech mechanism are suggested at this stage, and children are encouraged to view their productions in the mirror and listen to themselves on audio/video tapes.

Rehearsal involves four levels of complexity: nonsymbolic units, words and word pairs, sounds in sentences, and narratives. Once the narrative level is reached, rehearsal can include a mixture of the four levels.

Practice with nonsymbolic units (the authors use the term *nonsymbolic* rather than *nonsense syllables*) provides for manipulation of articulatory gestures that were begun during pretraining. Nonsymbolic instruction focuses on target productions in VC, CV, VCV, and VCCV syllables. It is asserted that production of nonsymbolic units imposes minimal constraints on the speaker by allowing him or her to focus on the speech task rather than also including morphologic, syntactic, and semantic concerns. Table 8.4 reflects nonsymbolic sound unit rehearsal matrices. The authors suggest that motoric success at this rudimentary level facilitates success at more linguistically and socially complex levels.

Word and word-pair practice is the next step in the program. Initial targets should reflect a transition from nonsymbolic units to meaningful units that encompass the nonsymbolic syllables already practiced. Practice activities at this level may require memory and speed but should be designed to encourage the client to assume responsibility for recognizing and judging the adequacy of his/her performance. Table 8.5 reflects a list of words and word-pairs by word-position that might be used at this level.

The next step in the program involves *sound in context rehearsal sentences*. At this stage the client repeats the clinician's model of sentences that includes words practiced at the word level. As in target word selection, it is important that sentences selected for imitation are appropriate for the client's age, abilities, and interests.

A second phase of this level consists of presenting a stimulus word containing the target segment to the client, then requiring the client to repeat the word, and then embed it in a spontaneously generated sentence.

TABLE 8.4 Nonsymbolic Sound Unit Rehearsal Matrices

V	C		V	C	V		C	V		V	C	C	V
i	s		i	s	i		s	i		i	t	s	i
a	s		i	s	a		s	a		i	t	s	a
u	s		i	s	u		s	u		i	t	s	u
æ	s		i	s	æ		s	æ		i	t	s	æ
			a	s	i					a	t	s	i
			a	s	a					a	t	s	a
			a	s	u					a	t	s	u
			a	s	æ					a	t	s	æ
			u	s	i					u	t	s	i
			u	s	a					u	t	s	a
			u	s	u					u	t	s	u
			u	s	æ					u	t	s	æ
			æ	s	i					æ	t	s	i
			æ	s	a					æ	t	s	a
			æ	s	u					æ	t	s	u
			æ	s	a					æ	t	s	a

The final step in this program involves using a target sound in narratives. This activity employs stories that can be illustrated, acted out, or read. Felt boards and figures are particularly recommended. A series of clinician-generated narratives are employed; for example, "This is Poky the turtle. Today is his birthday. He is 6 years old. He says, 'It's my birthday." What does he say?' This is followed by the client saying "It's my birthday." Through such narratives, practice of the target sound is embedded in communicative tasks. The clinician may have a client practice individual sentences from these narratives for additional practice at the sentence level.

While this program has been presented as a series of steps or levels, the authors point out that these steps should overlap. Throughout the program the client is the primary judge

TABLE 8.5 Word and Word-Pair List for [s]

Prevocalic		*Intervocalic*	*Postvocalic*	
Initial	Cluster	Medial	Final	Word-Pair
Sam	*scat*	*passing*	*pass*	*Jack sat*
seed	*ski*	*receive*	*niece*	*jeep seat*
soup	*scooter*	*loosen*	*loose*	*room soon*
saw	*scar*	*bossy*	*toss*	*cop saw*
sit	*skit*	*kissing*	*miss*	*lip sip*
sign	*sky*	*nicer*	*mice*	*right side*

of productions, describing the movement patterns, articulatory contacts, and adequacy of production of each target sound. For children misarticulating more than a single phoneme, once training on one target has moved from stimulability through rehearsal, a second target can be introduced while continuing to work on the first.

Summary of Sensory-Motor Approaches

Background Statement.   The theoretical concept underlying sensory-motor approaches is that articulatory errors can be corrected by extensive practice of articulatory behaviors, with syllabic units as a basic building block for later motor practice at more complex levels. To employ this approach, a sound must be in the client's repertoire.

Unique Features.   The emphasis on imitated, repetitive productions is a unique aspect of this approach. The systematic variation of phonetic contexts in productions of both sounds produced correctly and error sounds targeted for remediation sets this approach apart from others.

Strengths and Limitations.   A major strength of this approach is that it builds on behaviors (segmental productions in particular phonetic contexts) that are in a client's repertoire and capitalizes on syllabic units plus auditory, tactile, and kinesthetic awareness of motor movements. It may be particularly useful to clients who use a sound inconsistently and need methodology to facilitate consistent production in other contexts. The concept of syllable practice and systematic variation of phonetic contexts and stress may be useful to any training method that includes syllable productions. It has not been shown, however, that bisyllable and trisyllable practice with nonerror productions will aid in the elicitation of correct productions for those that are in error. This methodology would not typically be used with clients exhibiting multiple and/or linguistically based errors.

Research Support.   Although a deep test to facilitate the location of facilitating contexts has been widely used, published clinical investigations that provide support for the efficacy of this intervention approach are lacking.

Summary of Motor Approaches to Remediation

The treatment approaches described on the previous pages focus on the development and habituation of the motor skills necessary for target sound productions, with the traditional approach to remediation largely forming the basis of these approaches. An underlying assumption is that motor practice leads to generalization of correct productions to untrained contexts and to automatization of behaviors. Motor approaches to remediation are especially appropriate for phonetically based errors but are also employed by some clinicians with disorders which reflect a linguistic basis.

Remediation Guidelines for Motor Approaches

1. A motor approach to remediation is recommended as a teaching procedure for clients who evidence motor production problems with individual segments such as lisping for

/s/ and /z/ and other residual errors. It can also be incorporated into treatment programs for clients reflecting linguistic or pattern-based errors, especially if the patterns reflect motor constraints (e.g., prevocalic voicing or certain cluster simplifications). Instruction should be initiated at the linguistic unit level (isolation, syllable, word) at which a client can produce target sounds.

2. Perceptual training is recommended as part of a motor remediation program for those clients who evidence perceptual problems related to their error sounds.

3. A horizontal and/or cyclical approach is recommended for clients with multiple errors.

4. For clinicians who wish to follow a detailed treatment protocol based on a traditional treatment approach, the Programmed Conditioning for Articulation provides such a model.

5. Since motor practice is necessary even with linguistically oriented approaches, the steps and procedures of this approach are often used in linguistic-based approaches.

Linguistic-Based Approaches to Intervention

The primary focus of linguistic approaches to remediation is the establishment of phonological rules in a client's repertoire. Instruction is oriented toward relationships among sounds (contrasts and other rules), as opposed to the focus on individual sounds of motor-oriented approaches to remediation.

Treatment programs designed to facilitate acquisition of linguistic rules are not associated with a single unified method; however, two primary characteristics are frequently associated with linguistic oriented treatment approaches. The first characteristic relates to the process whereby behaviors are targeted for treatment, the second to the instructional procedures themselves.

Selection of target behaviors is based on an analysis of phonological errors to determine patterns or rules that may account for the errors. Following pattern or phonological process identification, individual sound(s), called **exemplars**, are chosen that are likely to facilitate generalization to an entire class of sounds or sound positions (e.g., other sounds containing a certain feature; other sounds in the same word position). Treatment is then designed to facilitate the acquisition of appropriate sound contrasts and/or sequences, with the expectation that generalization will occur to other sounds that are part of the same pattern (e.g., teaching one final consonant will generalize to other final consonants).

Most treatment protocols that are based on a linguistic model employ minimal contrast word-pairs, which involve minimal or maximal feature contrasts (Weiner, 1981; Gierut, 1989; Fey, 1992). For example, minimal pairs such as bu*s*-buc*k* and bu*s*-bu*t* represent minimal pairs with greater and lesser contrasts, respectively, because of the differences in place of articulation between /s/ and /k/ (greater contrast because of the alveolar-velar contrast), and /s/ and /t/ (lesser contrast because both /s/ and /t/ are alveolar consonants).

The remainder of this chapter will focus on treatment approaches that derive from a linguistic perspective. The primary focus of these approaches has been to (1) establish feature contrasts, and (2) eliminate or reduce phonological processes (simplifications). Linguistic approaches have also been concerned with other aspects of the phonological system. Included among these are elimination of homonyms and the establishment of new syllable shapes and new sound classes. In addition, language-based approaches have been recommended for those who have linguistically based phonological disorders as well as other types of language disorders (i.e., syntax, semantics, pragmatics).

The reader will note that remediation approaches associated with distinctive features and phonological processes stem from a similar theoretical base, and treatment procedures associated with each resemble one another. Since the treatment approaches for distinctive features and phonological processes are similar, a single critique will be presented for these approaches.

Distinctive Feature Approaches

Distinctive features may be considered subphonemic elements of phonemes that determine the linguistic contrasts between sounds and sound classes. In other words, unique bundles of distinctive features underlie the distinctions among phonemes in a language. For a review of information concerning distinctive features, refer back to Chapters 1 and 7.

The intent of instructional programs based on distinctive features is to establish feature contrasts that are lacking in a client's repertoire, thus accounting for one or more error patterns. Distinctive feature programs usually focus on the establishment of a feature through teaching a sound containing that feature. It is then assumed that the newly established feature will generalize from the exemplar to other members of the sound class in which the feature may be absent (e.g., + continuant generalizes from target /f/ to /θ/, /s/, and /ʃ/).

Stoel-Gammon and Dunn (1985) identified the following remediation concepts and treatment strategies that evolved from distinctive feature treatment programs:

1. Selection of target phonemes shifted from isolated phonemes to sound classes. The clinician focuses on features common to several phonemes and thus learns a feature common to a class of sounds rather than learning unrelated sounds one at a time.
2. Emphasis on facilitating generalization as a treatment goal requires the clinician to look at the influence that treatment may have on a sound class rather than isolated sounds.
3. Emphasis is placed on phonological contrasts as the basis for correcting errors and acquiring the adult sound system.

McReynolds and Bennett (1972) reported data indicating that features established in one sound (exemplar) will generalize to other sound segments in which the target feature is absent. They inferred from this finding that remediation based on distinctive features should be an efficient treatment approach. As in other types of generalization, the nature and extent of feature generalization that takes place is highly variable. Generalization seems to be significantly influenced by the similarity between the segment selected for training and other segments in which the generalization occurs (e.g., segments in the same sound class). In general, the more features two sound segments share, the more potential there is for generalization to occur from one sound to the second sound.

In the paragraphs that follow, we describe several distinctive feature treatment approaches that have appeared in the literature. The reader will note that distinctive feature approaches to remediation frequently incorporate methodologies that were described earlier in the motor approaches to therapy. Since the establishment of distinctive feature contrasts often involves production of individual sound segments, remediation frequently follows a similar sequence to that seen in motor approaches.

McReynolds and Bennett (1972) described instructional procedures used in a distinctive feature training study that investigated the nature of feature generalization. Their approach was designed to teach a feature contrast that was absent in a child's productive repertoire and included two overall teaching phases.

In Phase 1, production focused on nonsense syllables which contained the target feature (e.g., + continuant) in the initial position (e.g., *f*a). In Phase 2, the child was taught to produce a sound containing the target feature in the final position of a nonsense syllable (e.g., a*f*). Within each phase there were several steps. In Step 1, the child was instructed to produce a consonant in which this feature was lacking. In Step 2, the child was taught to contrastively produce two consonant sounds in syllables, the segment learned in Step 1, and a second consonant selected to contrast with the first. For example, if [+ continuant] was the feature contained in the first sound taught, [− continuant] was the feature selected for the second or contrast sound ([fi] vs. [pi]). Subsequent steps in Phase 1 consisted of producing the two phonemes, each in the initial position, and in combination with four vowels (e.g., [fi] vs. [pi], [fa] vs. [pa], [fʌ] vs. [pʌ], and [fo] vs. [po]). Phase 2 was identical except for position of the target sound. In the example above, the child used stops instead of fricatives/ continuants (e.g., *fun* was said *tun*; *show* was said *toe*, etc.). In Phase 1, the client was taught the continuant /f/ and then was taught to produce it in the initial position of a nonsense syllable (e.g., fi, fæ, fa, fo). Step 2 focused on having the child produce pairs of nonsense syllables that reflected the + continuant/− continuant contrast (e.g., *fa–pa*; *fi–pi*). In Phase 2, the two steps were repeated except /f/ was taught in the final position (e.g., af; af–if).

In a subsequent monograph, McReynolds and Engmann (1975) recommended that whenever possible, distinctive feature training should be initially restricted to sound units that reflect a single contrast, such as voicing in [p] versus [b]. They also recommend that when sound contrasts involve two or more feature differences, training should focus on segments with the least number of feature differences. For example, if a child uses /g/ for /s/ (e.g., /gʌn/ for /sʌn/) and also uses /g/ for /d/ (/gæd/ for dæd/), the clinician may wish to focus initially on the /g/–/d/ contrast rather than the /g/–/s/ contrast because of fewer feature differences (i.e., /g/ and /d/ have the same manner and voicing features but differ only in place of articulation, whereas /g/ and /s/ differ in place, manner, and voicing features).

Weiner and Bankson (1978) published an exploratory program that attempted to teach a feature (i.e., [+ frication]) in specific segments where the feature was not used correctly. Rather than relying on feature generalization from trained sounds to nontrained sounds, as did McReynolds and Bennett (1972), they attempted to establish a feature in segments that reflected the feature deletion without focusing on the correct production of a particular sound segment, but rather on the presence of the feature only (e.g., [+ frication]). Their client was a child who substituted stops (plosives) for fricatives. The first task in the training program consisted of an identification procedure that directed attention to developing awareness of [+ frication] in a number of contexts. The client was then required to contrast production of fricatives and stops. The client imitated fricative sounds and was reinforced for the production of [+ frication] regardless of the correctness of the remaining features in the segments. In other words, the sound imitatively produced might have been in error, but if [+ frication] was present, the response was reinforced. More specifically, [+ frication] was taught in the following instructional sequence:

1. Introduction of the concept of "dripping" sounds (stops) and "flowing" sounds (fricatives).
2. Identification of words that begin with dripping as compared to flowing sounds.
3. Imitation of words containing fricatives in the initial position, with such fricatives emphasized through duration of initial sound (e.g., *f-f-f-f*ish). Following his or her production, the client was required to judge whether the word began with a dripping or flowing sound. Feedback was provided for both production and identification.
4. Repetition of Step 3 without exaggeration of the word-initial fricative.
5. Presentation of a 20-item picture-naming task in which each item began with a fricative.

These investigators reported that as a result of this instructional sequence their client was able to produce [+ frication] successfully on a 20-item picture-naming task.

Blache (1989) published a distinctive feature approach to remediation of phonological delay. The approach is organized into four basic steps:

Step 1. *Discussion of words.* Determine whether or not the child knows the concept of the lexical items to be used in therapy. Once a minimal pair contrast has been selected to teach a distinctive feature, it is important to determine if the child understands both lexical items in the word-pair. For example, if the word-pair selected is the letter *T* and *key*, the child might be asked: "Which one opens the door? Which one is a letter of the alphabet? Which one goes into a lock? Which one do you write?" (See Figure 8.2.)

Step 2. *Discrimination testing and training.* The child is tested to determine if he or she can perceive the feature contrast. The clinician presents one word of a minimal pair, for example, *fan–pan* or *bear–pear*. The child is instructed to point to the picture that the clinician has named. A criterion of seven consecutive correct responses is used to establish perception of the contrasting word-pairs.

Step 3. *Production training.* After the client has demonstrated that he or she perceives the minimal contrast, the next step is to demonstrate the feature in a production task. In this step, the child is instructed to say the word and the clinician points to the picture of the word the client pronounced. The client should always be able to correctly pronounce one word of the pair but may not be able to pronounce the other member of the word-pair; thus, a correct production of an error sound may not be required at this stage.

Step 4. *Carryover training.* Once the child is able to pronounce the target word, the word is placed in longer and more complex linguistic environments. The word is used with the indefinite article *a* in varied phonetic contexts, two-word expressions, three-word carrier phrases, and the like, until the word is used in meaningful situations, social situations, and in the school and home.

Blache (1989) pointed out that this distinctive feature approach serves as a program that "provides a context in which learning can occur but does not teach the child how to pro-

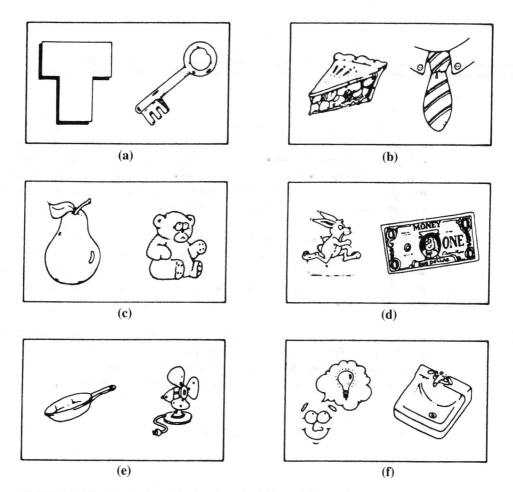

**FIGURE 8.2   Exemplars illustrating six different distinctive feature contrasts
(a = front–back lingual; b = labial–lingual; c = voiced–voiceless; d = nasal–nonnasal;
e = continued–interrupted; f = strident–mellow).**

Source: "Minimal Word-Pairs and Distinctive Feature Training" by S. E. Blache, in *Phonological Intervention:
Concepts and Procedures* (p. 65), M. Crary (Ed.), San Diego: College-Hill Press, Inc., 1982. Copyright 1982 by
College-Hill Press, Little, Brown. (Reprinted by permission.)

duce the sounds" (369) since sounds are not taught in isolation but only as contrastive units
within words.

The selection of management targets requires the determination of specific sound
classes which the child has difficulty producing. Blache divided the sounds of English into
six major sound classes that reflect developmental levels: (1) primitive (nonspeech sounds),
(2) vocalic, (3) stop-nasal, (4) semivowel, (5) continuant, and (6) sibilant. The primitive and
vocalic are expected to be acquired by the third year, with others following thereafter.

A therapeutic model is recommended in which features that comprise the most salient contrasts are focused on first, followed by successive steps to finer distinctions. Blache (1989) identified the following feature comparisons occurring in the stop-nasal sound class, which proceed from larger to finer contrasts and are presented in Table 8.6.

Summary of Distinctive Features Approaches

Background Statement.   Distinctive feature approaches to phonological remediation are based on the theory that speech sounds are comprised of individual bundles of features, each phoneme having a unique set of features from the pool of features that characterize segmental productions. Further, if a client has several sounds in error, an efficient strategy in treatment may be to identify or teach an exemplar that contains the absent feature(s), and monitor generalization from that exemplar to other sounds in the same class that are in error.

Unique Features.   This approach is designed to capitalize on patterns or commonalities among error productions that the clinician needs to be aware of in planning the most efficacious treatment plan. Although features are taught in segments, feature analysis and remediation represent a more integrated approach than a traditional approach to individual segments in error.

Strengths and Limitations.   An attraction of distinctive feature–oriented therapy is that it is designed to identify phonological patterns that may underlie several individual errors. A major limitation, however, relates to our earlier discussion indicating that distinctive features were not designed to be used for purposes of clinical intervention. Rather, they were derived from a set of features developed to classify and identify sound segments among language systems of the world. Feature systems have not been developed to classify speech sound errors, and thus not all errors can be described within this framework. In addition, the

TABLE 8.6   Contrast Ordering for Stop–Nasal Sound Class

No.	Pair	Feature	Sample Words
1.	[t-k]	front–back lingual	*tea–key, tape–cape, ten–Ken*
2.	[n-ŋ]	front–back lingual	*win–wing, fan–fang, ton–tongue*
3.	[p-b]	voiced–voiceless	*pea–bee, pig–big, pat–bat*
4.	[t-d]	voiced–voiceless	*toe–doe, time–dime, tot–dot*
5.	[k-g]	voiced–voiceless	*curl–girl, coat–goat, cap–gap*
6.	[b-m]	nasal–nonnasal	*beet–meat, bat–mat, bike–Mike*
7.	[d-n]	nasal–nonnasal	*D–knee, deck–neck, dot–knot*
8.	[g-ŋ]	nasal–nonnasal	*wig–wing, bag–bang, log–long*
9.	[b-d]	labial–lingual	*big–dig, bark–dark, bow–dough*
10.	[d-g]	front–back lingual	*deer–gear, date–gate, doe–go*

Source: "A Distinctive Feature Approach" by S. E. Blache, in *Assessment and Remediation of Articulatory and Phonological Disorders* (p. 377). N. Creaghead, P. Newman, and W. Secord, eds., Columbus, Ohio: Charles E. Merrill, 1989.

linguistic feature classification systems that have been applied clinically are easy to use with sound substitutions, but sound omissions and distortions are difficult to describe within such feature systems. In spite of the fact that distinctive feature approaches as described here are not typically employed, they are included because they encompass the concepts of pattern analyses and treatment focused on linguistic contrasts. This type of intervention serves as the basis of almost all linguistic approaches to treatment.

Research Support.   Data to support a distinctive feature approach to therapy may be gleaned from studies that report the treatment approaches described here. McReynolds and Bennett (1972) reported that all three of their subjects reflected distinctive feature generalization from the exemplar sounds they were taught to other sounds, although the amount of feature generalization varied across subjects. Similarly, Weiner and Bankson (1978) reported that their subject generalized [+ frication] to nontrained items. Costello and Onstein (1976) also reported that their instructional approach was successful in teaching their subject to generalize the [+ continuant] feature. These data support the finding that feature generalization is seen with distinctive feature approaches to remediation, although the amount of generalization varied considerably across subjects. The number of subjects involved in these studies was small and additional data regarding the efficiency of this approach are needed.

Minimal Pair Contrast Therapy

A remediation approach commonly identified as a linguistic approach is known as **minimal pair contrast therapy**. Contrast therapy employs pairs of words that differ only by a single phoneme (e.g., b*at*–p*at*, mo*v*e–moo*d*, *s*un–*t*on). The underlying concept of this type of therapy is that by focusing on word-pairs that typically differ by a single phonemic contrast, the client will be taught that different sounds signal different meanings in words. Investigators have reported changes in children's phonological systems (Weiner, 1981; Elbert and Gierut, 1986; Gierut, 1989, 1990) following training focused on word-pair contrasts. While contrast therapy usually focuses on reduction in the use of phonological processes, it can also be used for treatment based on distinctive features and/or a traditional approach to substitution errors.

An example of a contrast approach to treatment can be observed through remediation strategies employed with a client who deletes final consonants. In this instance, stops may be produced correctly in word-initial position, but deleted in word-final position (lack of syllable closure). In such a circumstance, the clinician can assume that the final consonant deletions are probably not a production (motor or phonetic) problem. Rather, final consonant deletion in this case likely reflects a process or conceptual problem related to syllable structure (use of the open syllable). Treatment for this problem would focus on getting the client to recognize that the presence of a consonant in word-final position is a necessary contrast to distinguish certain word-pairs in the language (e.g., *two–tooth*; *bee–beet*). In this instance, the motoric production of a target consonant is already within a child's productive repertoire, and thus motor production of the sound is not the primary focus of instruction. Rather, the focus of instruction is the development of cognitive awareness of final consonant contrasts/syllable closure.

The most commonly employed type of contrast training typically contrasts a substituted or deleted sound with a target sound. For example, if a client substitutes /t/ for /k/ in word-initial position, contrast training words might include *tea–key* and *top–cop*. Similarly, if a child deletes the final /t/, contrast pairs might include *bow–boat* and *see–seat*. Minimal contrast instruction is appropriate when two contrasting sounds in the adult language are collapsed into a single sound unit with the result that no contrast is made (e.g., /t/ replaced /k/), or where segments are deleted, such as in final consonant deletions. Training is designed to establish sound contrasts that mark a difference in meaning. Such contrasts are often selected for remediation because of their relationship to phonological processes or error patterns seen in children's phonology (i.e., they become exemplars to facilitate generalization to other segments).

Minimal contrast instruction may focus on either perception of contrasts or production of contrasts. A training task that focuses on perceptual training utilizing contrast pairs was first proposed by La Riviere and colleagues (1974). In the minimal contrast application of this procedure, subjects are taught to identify sound categories where the target sounds and errors are presented in word-pairs. For example, if a child deletes /s/ in /s/ clusters (cluster simplification), the clinician verbally presents minimal pairs like *spool–pool* or *spill–pill* to the client. The client is required to sort each lexical item into one of two categories (/s/ singletons or /s/ clusters).

A production-based task would require the client to verbally produce minimal pairs. For example, a client who deletes final consonants might ask the clinician to give him or her the picture of either a *bee* or a *beet*, then be reinforced by the clinician's response for the appropriate production. In this task, the client must be able to perceive the distinction between *bee* and *beet*, and in addition, be able to produce such a distinction. As stated earlier, the reverse of this procedure (i.e., the clinician asks the client to give him or her certain pictures) can be used to establish perceptual contrasts.

Weiner (1981) reported a study where minimal contrast training was used to reduce the frequency of selected phonological patterns. Weiner used minimal pairs in activities where accurate word productions were required for the child to communicate successfully. For example, Weiner used a game to teach final [t] in a minimal contrast format. He placed into minimal pairs such words as *bow* and *boat*. Sample stimuli consisted of several pictures of *bow* and several pictures of *boat*. The instructions for the game were as follows:

> "We are going to play a game. the object of the game is to get me to pick up all the pictures of the *boat*. Every time you say boat, I will pick one up. When I have all five, you may paste a star on your paper." If the child said *bow*, the clinician picked up the *bow* picture. At times he would provide an instruction, e.g., "You keep saying *bow*. If you want me to pick up the *boat* picture, you must say the [t] sound at the end. Listen, *boat*, *boat*, *boat*. You try it. Okay. Let's begin again" (98).

He reported that such training reduced the use of the phonological simplifications (processes) and that generalization to nontrained words was observed.

A variety of treatment materials (word lists, pictures) have been published which are oriented toward minimal contrast therapy. An example of such material is *Contrasts: The Use of Minimal Pairs in Articulation Training* (Elbert et al., 1980), which contains a com-

TABLE 8.7   Contrasts for /t/–/ʃ/ Initial Position

A. *Traditional Articulatory Classification*
   Category: Manner
   Contrast: /t/–/ʃ/ Initial

/i/	/ɪ/	/e/	/ɛ/	/æ/
T	tip / ship	tape / shape	Ted / shed	tad / shad
tea / she	tin / shin	take / shake	tell / shell	tack / shack
tee	till / shill	tame / shame	tear / share	tax / shacks
teak / sheik	tear / shear	tail / shale		tag / shag
teeth / sheath	sheer			tam / sham
teeth / sheathe				tank / shank
tease / she's				
teen / sheen				

/ɑ/	/ʌ/	/u/	/ʊ/	/o/
top / shop	Tut / shut	to / shoe	took / shook	toe / show
tot / shot	tuck / shuck	too / shoe		tone / shone
Tod / shod	ton / shun	two / shoo		toll / shoal
tock / shock		toot / shoot		
tarp / sharp				
tarred / shard				

/ɔ/	/ɝ/	/ɔɪ/	/au/	/aɪ/
tall / shawl	term / Sherm		tout / shout	tie / shy
tore / shore				tine / shine
torn / shorn				
tort / short				

Source: Adapted from M. Elbert, B. Rockman, and D. Saltzman. *Contrasts: The Use of Minimal Pairs in Articulation Training.* Austin, Tex.: Exceptional Resources, Inc. 1980. Used with permission.

prehensive list of minimal pairs designed to facilitate the establishment of phonological contrasts. These monosyllabic minimal pair lists were generated for training production and/or perceptional contrasts between phonemes. (See Table 8.7 for the /t/–/ʃ/ contrast.) An example of a protocol employing a minimal pair training procedure is as follows:

1. Select a sound contrast to be trained based on the client's phonological errors. For example, if the child substitutes /t/ for /ʃ/ (stopping), one might select *tea–she, toe–show,* and *tape–shape* as target contrast words reflecting the stopping pattern. Select five pictures for each of the target words. (In this example, that would include a total of 30 pictures.)

2. Engage the client in minimal contrast training at a *perceptual* level (e.g., "I want you to pick up the pictures that I name. Pick up _____.").

3. Pretest the client's motor production of each of the target words containing the error sound, and if necessary instruct him or her in production of the target phoneme.

4. Have the client imitatively produce each target word.
5. Engage the client in minimal contrast training at a *production* level (e.g., "I want you to tell me which picture to pick up. Every time you say *toe*, I will pick up this picture.").
6. Engage the client in a task designed to incorporate each of the contrast words in a carrier phrase (e.g., "I want you to point to a picture and say 'I found a *tea*'.").
7. Continue the carrier phrase task, only this time incorporating both words into the phrase (e.g., "I found a *tea* and a *she*.").

Clinicians can use their creativity and clinical knowledge to modify a protocol such as that just presented. As stated earlier, there are several descriptions in the literature of minimal pair treatment approaches as well as several commercially available sets of materials designed to facilitate this treatment approach. Another example of a commercially available set of materials to facilitate contrast training is that of *Picture Pairs* and *More Picture Pairs* by Schrader (1987, 1989).

A variation of contrast therapy is one that employs phonemic contrasts that involve **maximal** as opposed to **minimal** oppositions. In this instance, the word-pairs contrast the target sound with a second sound and this second sound contains as many featural differences from the target sound as possible. For example, if a child replaces /ʃ/ with /t/, the target words might be *shoe* and *moo* rather than *shoe* and *two*. In this case, /ʃ/ and /m/ are more dissimilar than are /ʃ/ and /t/, and thus the phoneme oppositions are greater (maximal opposition) rather than smaller (minimal opposition). A second difference between maximal and minimal oppositions is that in maximal oppositions a target sound is not contrasted with the error sound (an approach characteristic of minimal opposition contrast approaches). An underlying assumption of the maximal contrast approach is that phonological oppositions of greater disparity may be easier to acquire than minimal oppositions and will facilitate the client's acquisition of more feature contrasts. Examples of minimal and maximal oppositions are as follows:

Minimal Oppositions	*Feature Differences*
*s*un–*t*on	manner of production
*th*umb–*s*um	place of production
*ch*ew–*sh*oe	manner of production

Maximal Oppositions	*Feature Differences*
*ch*ain–*m*ain	manner of production, nasality, place of production
*c*an–*m*an	manner of production, place of production, nasality
*g*ear–*f*ear	manner of production, voicing, place of production

The usage of maximal oppositions is supported by clinical data from Gierut (1989, 1990). Others (Van Riper, 1939; Winitz, 1975), operating from somewhat different clinical frameworks, have also suggested that learning to perceive or discriminate sound contrasts can be facilitated by first focusing on sound contrasts that evidence maximal opposition of features. It appears that linguistic functioning, particularly acquisition of phonemic contrasts at a perceptual or productive level, may be facilitated by first teaching maximal (as opposed to minimal) contrasts.

The treatment methodologies outlined earlier for minimal contrast therapy are applicable to maximal contrast training. The difference between the two types of instruction is the nature of the contrasts in the word-pairs. Gierut suggested that maximal contrast training facilitates a greater overall change in the phonological system than does minimal contrast training.

Two final notes on contrast therapy: (1) occasionally clinicians employ contrast training at the syllable level (e.g., /sa/–/ʃa/ before moving on to words, to reduce interference from meaningful words and to provide production practice), and (2) for those instances where meaningful minimal pairs cannot be found to reflect a particular contrast, *near* minimal pairs are sometimes used (e.g., [væn–ʃæn]).

Summary of Minimal Pair Contrast Training

Background Statement.   Contrast training is a linguistic approach to phonological remediation designed to facilitate acquisition of phonological contrasts. Instruction typically involves perceptual and production tasks related to word-pairs reflecting phonemic contrasts. Contrast training procedures represent techniques to facilitate the reorganization of the phonological system to reduce the use of phonological processes, and to establish phonemic contrasts and syllable shapes.

Unique Features.   Contrast training is communication oriented. That is, the listener-speaker must perceive-produce a particular phonemic contrast in order to communicate (act or get someone else to act appropriately).

Strengths and Limitations.   The approach is designed for those clients who have certain sounds in their repertoire but fail to use them contrastively. It is also recommended for use with any client who needs to establish phonemic contrasts, regardless of whether errors have a motor component or not. This is especially important, however, for clients with a linguistic component to their phonological delay. By focusing on communication-oriented teaching activities, the training steps are generally less tedious than more drill-oriented activities. Clinicians need to be creative in using this approach and must have a plan for fitting contrast training in with other treatment activities and steps.

Research Support.   Data to support the efficacy of contrast training are available (Ferrier and Davis, 1973; Weiner, 1981; Elbert and Gierut, 1986; Gierut, 1989, 1990). It is anticipated that research in this area will be ongoing and will assist in developing a stronger theoretical base for understanding and treating phonological disorders.

Cycles Approach

The **cycles approach** (Hodson and Paden, 1991; Hodson, 1997), a combination of linguistic and traditional approaches to remediation, was designed for unintelligible children and has been reported to be especially useful with unintelligible children. The cycles approach targets deficient phonological patterns for instruction in order to increase intelligibility. The procedures for this treatment method include (1) auditory stimulation with slight amplification (the client is made aware of the auditory characteristics and to focus attention on the target sounds); (2) production practice (to help the child develop new kinesthetic images); and (3) participation in play activities involving picture and object naming activities that incorporate the target pattern for the day. A cycle is completed after all targeted phonological patterns have been presented for at least one hour each.

The remediation plan is organized around *treatment cycles* that can range from 5 to 6 weeks in length to 15 to 16 weeks, depending on the client's number of deficient patterns and the number of stimulable phonemes within each pattern. Hodson's (1989) suggestions for treating behaviors during cycles included the following:

> Each phoneme within a pattern should be targeted for approximately 60 minutes per cycle (i.e., one 60-minute, two 30-minute, or three 20-minute sessions) before progressing to the next phoneme in that pattern and then on to other phonological patterns. Each pattern is targeted for 2 to 6 hours, depending on the number of sounds targeted within that pattern. Furthermore, it is desirable to provide stimulation for two or more target *phonemes* (in successive weeks) within a pattern before changing to the next target *pattern* (i.e., each deficient phonological pattern is stimulated for two hours or more within each cycle). Only *one* phonological pattern should be targeted during any one session so that the client has an opportunity to focus, and patterns should not be intermingled (324).

A cycle is complete when all phonological patterns selected for remediation at a given point in time have been treated. Following completion of one cycle, a second cycle begins that will again cover those patterns not yet emerging and in need of further instruction. Phonological patterns are recycled until the targeted patterns emerge in spontaneous utterances. Hodson (1989) indicated that three to six cycles of phonological remediation, involving 30 to 40 hours of instruction (40 to 60 minutes per week) are usually required for a client with a disordered phonology to become intelligible. Within each cycle, a pattern is the focus of instruction for two to four weeks with a different phoneme targeted each week. Processes targeted for remediation should occur in at least 40 percent of the instances in which the opportunity for their occurrence is present, based on a 50-item single-word naming task (Hodson and Paden, 1991).

Phonological patterns are targeted for remediation based on the child's "phonological deficiencies" and those patterns on which he or she is most stimulable. Hodson (1989) identified the following "primary potential target patterns/phonemes": early developing phonological patterns, posterior-anterior contrasts, /s/ clusters, and liquids. These patterns are the focus of therapy until posterior/anterior contrasts and all early developing patterns are established and /s/ clusters are emerging in conversation.

An example of the Hodson-Paden approach follows. If fronting of velars occurs at least 40 percent of the time and if velars are stimulable (can be imitated with assistance of auditory and visual cues), velars would be selected as a target pattern for remediation. Following this, a target velar (e.g., /k/) would be selected as an instructional target and the focus of instruction for approximately one hour. Following work on this instructional goal, a second velar (e.g., /g/) would be targeted.

The instructional sequence for each session is as follows:

1. *Review.* At the beginning of each session, the prior week's production practice word cards are reviewed.
2. *Auditory bombardment/Listening activity.* This step requires listening for about 2 minutes while the clinician reads approximately 12 words containing the target sound. This auditory stimulation is done at the beginning and end of each session and includes the use of amplification (mild gain assistive listening device). The clinician may also demonstrate the error and contrast it with the target.
3. *Target word cards.* The client draws, colors, or pastes pictures of three to five target words on large index cards. The name of the picture is written on each card.
4. *Production practice.* The client participates in production practice activities through experiential-play activities. The client is expected to have a very high success rate in terms of correct productions. Shifting experiential-play activities every 5 to 7 minutes helps to maintain a child's interest in repetition of the target words. The client is also given the opportunity to use target words in conversation during a break. Production practice incorporates auditory, tactual, and visual stimulation as needed for correct production at the word level. Usually five words per target sound are used in a single session and the client is instructed to produce the words. A variety of games is used in each session.
5. *Stimulability probing.* The target phoneme in the next session for a given pattern is selected based on stimulability probing (checking to see what words a child can imitate), which occurs at this point in the treatment session.
6. *Auditory bombardment/Listening activity.* Auditory bombardment with amplification is repeated using the 12-item word list from the beginning of the session.
7. *Home program.* Parents are instructed to read the 12-item word list used in the auditory bombardment task to the child at least once a day. The five cards used during the week for production practice are also sent home for the child to practice daily.

The client is not required to meet a criterion level prior to moving on to treatment of other patterns within a cycle. When patterns persist after a single cycle of training, they are recycled for treatment at a later time.

Hodson (1994) reports that she also incorporates metaphonological aspects such as rhyming, syllable and phoneme segmentation and blending, and syllable and phoneme manipulation, because children who are unintelligible have relatively poor rhyming segmentation skills. In addition, some children with delayed phonologies have more difficulty than their normal peers developing literacy skills (see Stackhouse, 1997).

Ingram (1986) suggested that a theoretical rationale for the cycles approach may be gleaned from preliminary data from studies in cross-linguistic phonological acquisition. Just as children acquire the sounds that occur most frequently in their language (e.g., French children learn [v] early, American children learn [v] later), so children receiving repeated auditory bombardment may come to acquire speech sounds presented through this approach. In addition, the recurring focus on particular sounds that occurs with this cyclical approach may allow for the gradual acquisition of phonological contrasts. Ingram suggested that learning in this treatment approach is not unlike that in the normal acquisition process, in which children learn the contrasts that they hear most frequently.

Summary of Cycles Approach

Background Statement.   The cycles approach is based on the phenomenon of gradualness (moving ahead, recycling, moving ahead) as observed in normal phonological acquisition. The emphasis on acquisition of phonological patterns stems from a linguistic perspective of phonological behavior. Production practice of exemplars (target sounds) along with auditory bombardment (listening tasks) reflects more traditional approaches to intervention.

Unique Features.   The most distinctive feature of this approach is its focus on cycling of remediation targets and the fact that behaviors are worked on without continuing instruction to the point of mastery. Focusing on pattern *acquisition* rather than on the more usual concept of elimination of developmentally inappropriate patterns is an appropriate way to conceptualize intervention. The overall blending of traditional and linguistic assessment/treatment methodologies is a unique feature of this procedure.

Strengths and Limitations.   The attributes identified above are all strengths of this approach. Although it was designed for unintelligible children, aspects of this approach can be used with less severely impaired clients. The cycles approach has been adapted for use with children with cleft palates (Hodson, Chin, Redmond, and Simpson, 1983), developmental dyspraxia (Hodson and Paden, 1983), recurrent otitis media and hearing impairments (Gordon-Brannan, Hodson, and Wynne, 1992), and developmental delay.

Research Support.   While the authors have a wealth of clinical experience to support this approach to intervention, published data, particularly of a comparative nature, are lacking. This approach, like many others, represents a composite or "package" of various instructional components. However, it has seen widespread adoption among clinicians for unintelligible and phonologically delayed children.

Language-Based Approaches

Children with severe phonologic disorders frequently have difficulty with other aspects of language, particularly semantics and syntax (Camarata and Schwartz, 1985; Panagos and Prelock, 1982; Hoffman, Schuckers, and Daniloff, 1989). Severe impairments of phonology that coexist with other language impairments suggest that many children have difficulty with the broader aspects of the language learning process. Although the precise nature of the relationship between phonology and other aspects of language is unknown (Fey, 1986), an idea gaining increasing acceptance is that phonologic delay, especially when it coincides with other language impairments, is best remediated by employing a language-based intervention approach (Gray and Ryan, 1973; Matheny and Panagos, 1978; Hoffman, Norris, and Monjure, 1990). Hoffman and colleagues (1990) state that "descriptive research continues to show the importance of language organization levels that are higher than the word level upon sound production, suggesting that remediation of speech disorders outside of a more generalized context of language development may not be the most efficacious tack" (102).

Storytelling

Norris and Hoffman (1990) have described a language-based approach to phonologic intervention based on client generation of narratives. In this approach, preschool children construct verbal stories in response to pictures from action-oriented children's stories and share these with a listener(s). The clinician's primary role in this type of treatment is to engage the child in constructing and talking about the pictures. The goal for each child is to produce meaningful linguistic units, syllable shapes, phonemes, and gestures that are shared with a listener. The clinician seeks to expand each child's language-processing ability by asking children to produce utterances that exceed their current level of functioning.

Norris and Hoffman (1990) also suggested that language-oriented intervention needs to be naturalistic and interactive as the clinician seeks to simultaneously improve semantic, syntactic, and phonologic knowledge. In terms of treatment priorities, phonology is the last component emphasized since intelligibility is a real concern after children have language to express. Such interactions need to be based on spontaneously occurring events, utterances, and communicative situations that arise in the context of daily play routines and instructional activities. They outline three steps for intervention by the clinician: (1) providing appropriate organization of the environment/stimulus materials for the child to attend to, which enables the clinician to alter language complexity systematically throughout the course of therapy; (2) providing a communicative opportunity, including scaffolding strategies that consist of various types of prompts, questions, information, and restatements that provide support to the child who is actively engaging in the process of communicating a message; and (3) providing consequences or feedback that are directly related to the effectiveness of the child's communication.

Norris and Hoffman (1990) described an "interactive storytelling" technique in which the clinician points to a picture and models language for the client, then gives the child an opportunity to talk about the event. If the child miscommunicates the idea, the adult provides feedback to the child designed to assist the child in reformulating the message. The clinician can use three primary responses with the child:

1. *Clarification.* When the child's explanation is unclear, inaccurate, or poorly stated, the clinician asks for a clarification. The clinician then supplies relevant information to be incorporated in the child's response, restates the event using a variety of language forms, and asks the child to recommunicate the event. Hoffman, Norris, and Monjure (1990) presented the following example of this type of response: If a child described a picture of a man cooking at a grill by saying, "Him eating," the clinician might say:

> No, that's not what I see happening. The man isn't eating yet, he's cooking the food. See his fork, he is using it to turn the food. I see him—he is cooking the food. He will eat when he's done cooking, but right now the food is cooking on the grill. He is cooking the food so that they can eat (105).

Then the clinician provides an opportunity for the child to restate the information (e.g., ". . . so tell that part of the story again"). Thus, feedback is based on meaning rather than structure.

2. *Adding events.* If the child adequately reports an event, the clinician points out another event to incorporate in the story using a variety of language models. The child is then given the opportunity to retell the story. In an example from Hoffman, Norris, and Monjure (1990), the clinician points to specific features in the picture and says something like:

> That's right, the man is cooking. He is the dad and he is cooking the hamburgers for lunch. Mom is putting plates on the table. Dad will put the hamburgers on the plates. So you explain the story to the puppet (105).

3. *Increasing complexity.* If the child adequately describes a series of events, the clinician seeks to increase the complexity of the child's story by pointing out relationships among events such as motives of the characters, cause-effect relationships among the individual events, time and space relationships, and predictions. The child is given the opportunity again to reformulate his or her own version of the story. Another example from these authors is: If the child said, "The daddy is cooking hamburgers and the mommy is setting the table," the clinician might prompt the child to link these two events in time and space by saying:

> That's right, mommy and daddy are making lunch for the family. When daddy finishes cooking the hamburgers he will put them on the plates, so tell that part of the story to the puppet (105).

While the concepts expressed by Hoffman, Schuckers, and Daniloff (1989) and Norris and Hoffman (1990) have appeared relatively recently, they are not totally unlike some of the notions espoused by Backus and Beasley (1951) several decades ago. Backus and Beasley expressed the need to work from whole to part to whole in a social context (i.e., language discourse to specific components of language and back to overall communication). More recently, Low, Newman, and Ravsten (1989) have extended the communication focus of Backus and Beasley by developing what they call a communication-centered instruction (CCI) approach to articulation remediation. CCI emphasizes the social use of language with the focus on a speech sound in a word that is part of a socially useful communicative utterance. CCI is applicable to other disorders besides phonologic ones.

Guidelines that Low and colleagues (1989) developed for planning treatment activities based on this approach are as follows:

1. Teaching activities should simulate the client's daily communication experiences.
2. Activities should encourage clients to use correct phonology to clarify communication in preference to teaching them directly (though requiring responses such as imitation may be included in instruction).
3. Positive group interaction is essential to the approach.
4. To facilitate generalization, practice of target behaviors is repeated in several communication-centered activities, all of which are slightly different.

5. Individual therapy should be viewed as a supplement to group therapy that allows for isolating target sounds and engaging in more traditional phoneme-related instruction. Such traditional instruction should be followed by rehearsing the phonemic behaviors in communicative utterances to be used in subsequent group lessons.

Recent studies have questioned the indirect effect that language-based intervention has on correction of phonologic errors. In a study conducted by Fey, Cleave, Ravida, Long, Dejmal, and Easton (1994), 30 preschool children displaying mild to severe speech and language impairments received either clinician or parental language intervention. Treatment in both settings focused on language-based stimulation in highly naturalistic tasks that were designed to facilitate grammar (i.e., making sandwiches, planting beans, play, etc.).

Baseline and treatment measures of phonology and expressive grammar were obtained at regular intervals. The results indicated that although gains in the children's grammatical output were observed, phonologic gains remained insignificant. Fey and colleagues (1994) stated: "We found no support for our prediction that effective facilitation of grammar would lead to spontaneous improvements in phonological output in children with speech and language impairments" (605).

Fey and colleagues (1994) indicated that the lack of an indirect effect of language-based intervention on phonology could have resulted from the intervention style employed and the severity level of the speech and language impairments. Their subjects appeared to be more severely involved than those of Hoffman, Norris, and Monjure (1990). Fey and colleagues (1994) concurred with the findings of Tyler and Sandoval (1994), who also reported that language-based instruction had little effect on children with moderate to severe problems in both domains. Both of these studies concluded that clinical attention needed to be focused on both speech and language when impairments in these areas coexisted. This could be accomplished by simultaneously treating phonology and grammar or by shifting intervention focus from one objective to another.

Summary of the Language-Based Approaches

Background Statement.   Language-based approaches are generally founded on two basic premises: (1) Phonology is a part of the overall language system and should be treated in a language context; and (2) improvement in phonologic behaviors occurs more rapidly when instruction is focused on the overall use of language as a tool of communication, rather than on specific aspects of language (syntax, semantics, phonology).

Unique Features.   Unique features of this approach relate to the heavy emphasis on facilitating overall language improvement as opposed to correction of specific phonemes. The instructional style is different than the traditional practice of working directly on phonology.

Strengths and Limitations.   From a theoretical perspective, the rationale behind this approach is attractive. It remains to be seen, however, just how and with which clients this approach can be beneficial. The role of traditional phonologic intervention in conjunction with this approach has not been adequately explored.

Research Support.   Preliminary data from Hoffman, Norris, and Monjure (1990) suggested that a whole language approach was a more efficacious approach to language-phonology intervention than was phonologic intervention by itself but the subjects appeared to have mild/moderate phonologic delay and included a small number of subjects.

Remediation Guidelines for Linguistic Approaches

1. A linguistic approach is recommended when there are multiple sound errors that reflect phonologic error patterns and these patterns are not motor based. These approaches are very useful with young children who are unintelligible but are generally less useful with residual errors.

2. A linguistic approach is also recommended when there are few errors but the errors reflect a single phonologic rule.

3. Once error patterns have been identified, a review of the child's phonetic inventory will assist in the identification of target sounds (exemplars) and key words. This review should include such factors as facilitative contexts, word-position, stimulability, frequency of occurrence, and developmental occurrence.

4. Selection of training words should reflect the syllabic word shapes the child uses. For example, if the child uses only CV and CVCV syllable shapes, multisyllabic target words are inappropriate. Obviously this guideline is not appropriate, however, if the focus of remediation is the unstressed syllable deletion process or other processes focusing on syllable structure simplifications.

5. Treatment efficiency may be increased by selecting target words that facilitate the reduction of two or more processes simultaneously. For example, if a child uses stopping and deletes final fricatives, the selection of a final fricative for training may aid in the simultaneous reduction of the processes of stopping and final consonant deletions.

6. When phonologic errors reflect errors in several sound classes (e.g., final consonant deletion may affect stops, fricatives, and nasals), at least one exemplar should be selected for training from each sound class.

7. Instruction related to process reduction should focus on deletion of the process rather than the phonetic accuracy of sounds used in reorganizing the phonologic system. For example, if a child deletes final consonants but learns to say [dɔd] for [dɔg], the /d/ for /g/ replacement should be overlooked at the *initial* stage of instruction because the child has begun to change his or her phonologic system to incorporate final consonant productions.

8. In using a linguistic approach to remediation, the clinician probably will need to devise specific treatment protocols and procedures since few complete remediation programs based on this approach have been published.

9. Minimal contrast therapy, focusing on both perception and production, is recommended as part of a remediation program when phonemic contrasts are collapsed.

10. Treatment focused on other aspects of language may result in positive changes in phonology. For example, working on plural and morphological endings may reduce the deletion of final consonants.

11. Teaching behaviors from a linguistic perspective may be quite similar to certain methods used in more traditional approaches.

12. Correction of phonologic errors based on treatment of overall language behavior does not seem to be an effective strategy for moderate and severe phonologic-impaired children, but more encouraging results have been reported in children with mild phonologic delay.

Making Progress in Therapy: Response Generalization

Generalization

Once target behaviors are in a client's repertoire and can be produced with some ease, the next task is to facilitate generalization to other linguistic contexts and, eventually, to non-clinical settings. Generalization is a process that is *facilitated* rather than taught, and it is relevant to correction of phonologic errors that may be viewed as motor and/or linguistic in nature. Generalization is a critical and all-important step in the learning process for all children who receive treatment for phonologic delay. Our discussion of generalization will include an introduction to the concept, followed by a review of (1) across-position generalization, (2) across-context generalization, (3) across-linguistic unit generalization, (4) across-sound and feature generalization, and (5) across-situation generalization.

Generalization has been defined by Stokes and Baer (1977) as

> the occurrence of relevant behavior under different non-training conditions (i.e., across subjects, settings, people, behavior, and/or time) without the scheduling of the same events in those conditions as had been scheduled in the training conditions. Thus, generalization may be claimed when no extra training manipulations are needed for extra training changes (350).

In other words, generalization (sometimes called *transfer*) is the principle that learning one behavior in a particular environment often carries over to other similar behaviors, environments, or untrained contexts. For example, if one learns to drive in a Ford automobile, there is a high probability that one can also drive a Plymouth. Generalization of training occurs from one stimulus—driving apparatuses in the Ford—to another—driving apparatuses in the Plymouth. In terms of articulation remediation, if a client learns to produce /f/ in the word *f*ish, that [f] production will probably generalize to other words that contain /f/, such as *f*un. If generalization did not occur, it would be necessary to teach a sound in every word and context—an impossible task.

The clinician must rely on a client's ability to generalize in order to effect a change in phonologic usage. Generalization, however, does not occur automatically, nor do all persons have the same aptitude for it. People vary in their ability to achieve generalization, but certain activities can increase the likelihood of generalization.

One type of generalization is **stimulus generalization**, which occurs when a learned response to a particular stimulus is evoked by similar stimuli. The importance of reinforcement in such generalization cannot be overemphasized. Behaviors that have been reinforced in the presence of a particular stimulus may be said to have generalized when they occur in the presence of novel but similar stimuli, even though the response was not reinforced. Consider this example: A client who utilizes the process of "fronting" has been taught, through the use of an auditory model and appropriate reinforcement, to produce /k/ correctly at the word level in response to the auditory stimulus, "Say kangaroo." The client is later shown a picture of a kangaroo and asked to name it, but no model is provided. If the client says "kangaroo" with [kʰ] produced correctly in response to the picture, stimulus generalization has occurred.

Response generalization is another type of generalization that is especially relevant to speech remediation. This is the process in which taught responses carry over to other behaviors that are not taught. An example of response generalization is as follows: A client with /s/ and /z/ errors is taught to say [s] in response to an auditory model of [s]. He or she is then presented with an auditory model [z] and asked to imitate it. If the client emits a correct [z], response generalization has occurred. Such generalization is well documented in the literature, including an early study by Elbert, Shelton, and Arndt (1967) in which children with /s/, /z/, and /r/ errors were taught to say [s] correctly. Generalization was evident by correction of the untrained /z/, which has many features in common with /s/. However, no generalization to the untrained [r] was noted. Obviously, sounds in the same sound class and having similar features with the target sound are those where response generalization is most likely to occur.

Several different types of generalization may occur during phonologic remediation, including generalization from one position to another, from one context to another, to increasingly complex linguistic levels, to nontrained words, to other sounds and features, and to various speaking environments and situations. Clinicians often attempt to facilitate generalization by sequencing instructional steps from simple to more complex behaviors. By proceeding in small progressive steps, the clinician seeks to gradually extend the behavior developed during the establishment period to other contexts and situations.

The amount of training required for generalization has not been established and seems to vary considerably across subjects. Elbert and McReynolds (1978) have reported data from five children indicating that from 5 to 26 sessions were required before generalization occurred. They speculated that the error patterns exhibited by children affected both the time required and the extent of transfer which occurs.

For those clients who begin remediation with an established target behavior in their repertoire, generalization may be the primary task of instruction. Following is a discussion of the various types of generalization that are expected in the articulation remediation process.

Across–Word Position Generalization

Generalization of correct sound productions across word-positions is well documented (Elbert and McReynolds, 1975, 1978; Powell and McReynolds, 1969). This term refers to generalization from a word-position that is taught (initial, medial, or final) to a word-position that is not taught. By teaching a sound in a particular position (e.g., initial position), generalization may occur to a second position (e.g., final position). Speech-language pathologists have traditionally taught target sounds first in the initial position of words, followed by either the final or medial position. One rationale for beginning with the initial position is that, for most children, many sounds are first acquired in the prevocalic position (the most notable exception is certain fricatives that appear first in word-final position).

In the process of investigating the paired-stimuli approach to articulation remediation,

Weston and Irwin (1971) examined position generalization. They observed that when a sound was taught in the prevocalic position, generalization usually occurred to the postvocalic position. Similarly, they observed that sounds taught in the postvocalic position usually generalized to the prevocalic position. In contrast, McLean (1970) found, in a study involving retarded children, that although instruction and practice in the initial (prevocalic) position resulted in generalization to initial position in other words, little transfer occurred to other word-positions. Likewise, Compton (1975) reported little generalization from initial to final word-position in a case study involving a child with normal intelligence.

Ruscello (1975) studied the influence of training on generalization across word-positions. Two groups, each containing three subjects, were presented training programs that differed with respect to the number of word-positions practiced in each session. Ruscello reported significantly more generalization across training sessions for those subjects who practiced a target sound in the initial, medial, and final word-positions than the group who practiced a target sound only in the word-initial position. Weaver-Spurlock and Brasseur (1988) also reported that simultaneous training of /s/ in the initial, medial, and final positions of familiar words was an effective training strategy for across-position generalization in probe words.

Olswang and Bain (1985) reported different amounts of position generalization for /s/ and /l/ in two subjects. For both subjects, improvement in initial /l/ had little influence on final /l/. In other words, improvement on initial /l/ did not seem to facilitate improvement of final /l/. By contrast, when /s/ was trained in one word-position in one subject, it seemed to facilitate production of the sound to other positions. They attributed the differences in position generalization between /l/ and /s/ to the greater allophonic variation between initial and final /l/ compared to that of initial and final /s/.

Wolfe, Blocker, and Prater (1988) reported that generalization of sounds in the medial word position may be related to whether the word reflects a sound in the traditional medial position (e.g., /k/ in bacon), or is related to inflection (e.g., /k/ in picking). In their study greater generalization occurred with medial inflection, which they attributed to factors of coarticulation, perceptual salience, and representational integrity of the word.

It can be inferred from the available data that for children with normal intelligence, generalization from initial to final position is just as likely to occur as generalization from final to initial. A preferred word-position that would maximally facilitate position generalization has not been established. Thus, the word-position in which a target sound is trained does not seem to be a factor in position generalization. In terms of clinical management, unless the pattern of errors suggests a particular word-position for initial training (such as final consonant deletion), it is recommended that the clinician train the word-position that the client finds easiest to produce, check for generalization to other positions, and then proceed to train the other word-positions if generalization has not already occurred. Except for selected fricative sounds, the easiest position to teach often is the initial position. However, contextual testing may result in the identification of contexts that are more facilitating for an individual child than those which can be predicted from developmental phonological data.

Across-Context Generalization
Technically, position generalization may be viewed as a type of contextual generalization. The term *contextual generalization*, however, more commonly refers to phonetic context

transfer—for example, generalization from /s/ in *ask* to /s/ in *biscuit* or to /s/ in *fist*. This type of generalization where a production transfers to other words without direct treatment is an example of response generalization as described above.

When preliminary testing has indicated specific contexts in which an error sound may be produced correctly, clinicians will frequently attempt to stabilize such productions—that is, see that a target sound can be consistently produced correctly in that context—and then provide instruction designed to facilitate generalization of the correct sound to other contexts. As with all types of generalization, the client must exhibit transfer to untrained contexts at some point for the remediation process to be complete.

In a study of phoneme generalization, Elbert and McReynolds (1978) reported that although facilitative phonetic contexts have been posited as a factor in generalization, their data did not support the idea that certain contexts facilitate generalization across subjects. Instead, they found a great deal of variability in facilitative contexts across subjects. The authors also reported that once a child imitated the sound, generalization occurred to other contexts. They concluded that the client's possession of the sound in his or her productive repertoire had more to do with generalization than did contextual factors.

Elbert, Powell, and Swartzlander (1991) examined the number of minimal word-pair exemplars necessary for phonologically impaired children to meet a generalization criterion. They reported that for most children, generalization occurred using a small number of word-pair exemplars (five or less for 80 percent of the children) but there was substantial variability across subjects. The occurrence of response generalization subsequent to teaching a small number of exemplars is consistent with findings from previous treatment reports (Elbert and McReynolds, 1978; Weiner, 1981).

Across–Linguistic Unit Generalization

A third type of generalization involves shifting correct sound productions from one level of linguistic complexity to another (e.g., from syllables to words). For some clients, the first goal in this process is to transfer isolated sounds to syllables and words; others begin at the syllable or word level and generalize target sound productions to phrases and sentences.

Van Riper and Erickson (1996) recommended that the transfer sequence be initiated with sounds in isolation, followed by syllables, words, and finally sentences. This hierarchy of production complexity has been widely adhered to as a treatment sequence.

Instruction at the transfer phase of the instructional continuum begins at the highest level of linguistic complexity at which a client can produce a target behavior on demand. Instruction progresses from that point to the next level of complexity. Winitz (1975) speculated that when sounds are taught in isolation, the effects of coarticulation are absent, and therefore the potential for generalization to syllables and words is relatively poor. This notion received some support from a study reported by McReynolds (1972), in which the transfer of /s/ productions to words was probed after each of four sequential teaching steps: (1) /s/ in isolation, (2) /sa/, (3) /as/, and (4) /asa/. Although no transfer to words was observed following training on /s/ in isolation, over 50 percent transfer to words was observed following training on /sa/. It should be recognized, however, that the training of /s/ in isolation prior to syllables may have had a learning effect and influenced the generalization observed following syllable instruction.

Some clinicians prefer initially to teach sounds in isolation or in syllables rather than in words in order to decrease interference from previous learning. To avoid interference from previously learned behaviors, the use of nonsense syllables or nonsense (nonce) words to facilitate generalization has been recommended.

Van Riper and Erickson (1996) and Winitz (1975) recommended that sounds be taught in nonsense syllables before they are practiced in meaningful words, thereby reducing the interference of previous error productions on the target sound. This view contrasts with another notion that phonologic contrasts are more readily established at the word or lexical level since *meaningful* contrasts are a key to normal phonologic acquisition.

Powell and McReynolds (1969) studied generalization in four subjects who misarticulated /s/. They reported that when two of the subjects were taught consonant productions in nonsense syllables, transfer of the target sound to words occurred without additional training. The other two subjects had to be provided instruction at each level of linguistic behavior because generalization from nonsense syllables to words did not occur.

Elbert, Dinnsen, Swartzlander, and Chin (1990) reported that when preschool children were taught target sounds within a minimal pair contrast training paradigm, generalization occurred to other single-word productions as well as to conversational speech. These findings would suggest that these children learned more than motor production skills during treatment because correct forms were stored and retrieved on demand. Based on a three-month posttreatment probe, they reported that subjects continued to improve and increase the number of correct productions.

To facilitate generalization, Gerber (1973) outlined an instructional sequence that relied heavily on the use of nonsense syllables. Gerber arranged nonsense materials according to a hierarchy of complexity in the following sequence:

1. Simple CV, VCV, and VC syllables
2. More complex syllables, including consonant clusters in the pre-, post-, and intervocalic positions: CCV, VCC, and VCCV
3. Simple nonsense words: CVC
4. More complex nonsense words specifically tailored to contexts difficult for the client
   a. Multisyllabic configurations such as *sikesoo*, *lanasos*
   b. Variations in abutting consonants in releasing and arresting positions such as *kapset*, *kikso*
5. "Phrases" composed of nonsense words
6. "Conversations" in nonsense words
7. Nonsense material embedded in meaningful units

In summary, it appears that some clients will generalize from one linguistic unit to another without specific training; others will require specific instructional activities for transfer from one linguistic unit to another. The process of generalization seems to vary across individuals for most types of generalization and is true also for linguistic unit generalization.

Across-Sound and Across-Feature Generalization

A fourth type of generalization is observed when correct production of a target sound generalizes from one sound to another. Generalization most often occurs within sound classes and/or between sounds that are phonetically similar (e.g., /k/ to /g/; /s/ to /z/ and /ʃ/). Clinicians have long observed that training on one sound in a cognate pair frequently results in generalization to the second sound (e.g., Elbert et al., 1967). McNutt (1994), in a study of bilingual children, reported that correction of /s/ in English generalized to correction of a defective /s/ in French.

Powell and Elbert (1984) investigated the generalization patterns of two groups of three children each, with misarticulations. Specifically, they wanted to see if the group receiving instruction on earlier developing consonant clusters (stop + liquid) would exhibit generalization patterns different from those of the group receiving instruction on later-developing consonant clusters (fricative + liquid). The authors reported that no clear overall pattern was observed; instead, the six subjects exhibited individual generalization patterns. All subjects evidenced some generalization to both the trained and untrained consonant clusters. The most interesting finding was that generalization to both cluster categories occurred on the final probe measure in five of six subjects regardless of the treatment received. Powell and Elbert (1984) attributed the generalization across sound and class seen in three subjects in part to their good pretreatment stimulability skills.

Weiner (1981) also reported across-sound generalization in teaching final consonants to children who deleted them. He trained subjects to produce word-final stops and found generalization to word-final fricatives. He also showed that when stopping of fricatives was reduced, the process of fronting of stops was also reduced.

Generalization of correct production from one sound to another is expected when remediation targets are selected on the basis of place, manner, and voicing analysis, distinctive feature analysis, or phonologic process analysis. Often in these approaches, target behaviors, or exemplars, reflecting processes common to several error productions are selected for training. This is done on the assumption that generalization will occur from exemplars to other error sounds within the same sound class or, in some instances, across sound classes.

Sound generalization, as stated earlier, is sometimes explained on the basis of feature similarity among sounds. An underlying assumption of distinctive feature analysis and remediation is that features will generalize from one sound production to another production containing the same features. An example of such generalization can be seen in the client who initially did not correctly produce any sounds containing [+ stridency], yet after learning to produce /s/, was able to correctly articulate /ʃ/ and /z/, which also contain the feature [+ stridency].

A client can learn a feature and transfer the feature without necessarily correcting a sound. For example, a client who substitutes stops for fricatives may learn to produce /f/ and begin using it in his or her speech for several fricative sounds. Although the client no longer substitutes stops for fricatives, he or she now substitutes /f/ for other fricatives (e.g., [sʌn] → [fʌn]; [ʃou] → [fou]; in other words, the client has incorporated a feature into his or her productions but still misarticulates several of the same sounds.

McReynolds and Bennett (1972) studied three subjects who received training to facilitate feature generalization. Instruction for each subject focused on a specified sound that was selected to reflect a particular feature. Specifically, one subject was taught an exemplar containing the [+ stridency] feature, another the [+ voicing] feature, and the third the [+ continuancy] feature. Feature generalization to other error sounds was assessed through deep testing of those phonemes not taught. Results for the three subjects indicated that the feature generalized to several sounds even though training was limited to a single sound exemplar.

Feature generalization is a critical element in most treatment based on a phonologic process approach since elimination of a process may be dependent upon acquisition of a feature in a client's repertoire. The examples presented previously, in which stops were substituted for fricatives (stopping), reflect this phenomenon: By teaching the [+ frication] feature, the client acquired a feature that resulted in the reduction of the stopping in untrained fricatives.

Frequently, the establishment of feature contrasts is part of the effort to reduce and eliminate process usage; thus, feature teaching and process reduction approaches are inextricably intertwined. The notion of feature and sound generalization, like other types of generalization, is critical to the remediation process.

Across-Situations Generalization

The fifth and final type of generalization to be discussed in this chapter, called *situational generalization*, involves transfer of behaviors taught in the clinical setting to other situations and locations, such as school, work, or home. This type of generalization is critical to the remediation process because it represents the terminal objective of instruction (i.e., correct phonologic productions in conversational speech in nonclinical settings). Such generalization has also been called *carryover* in the speech-language pathology literature.

Most clinicians focus on activities to facilitate situational transfer during the final stages of remediation. Some, including the authors, have argued that clinicians should incorporate these activities into early stages of instruction. For example, once a client can produce single words correctly, efforts should be made to incorporate these words into nonclinical settings. Although much emphasis is placed on facilitating situational generalization, little experimental data are available to provide specific guidance to the clinician.

Studies by Costello and Bosler (1976) and Bankson and Byrne (1972) have shown that situational generalization can be facilitated through training, but the extent of such transfer varies greatly from one individual to another. Costello and Bosler (1976) investigated whether certain clinical situations were more likely to facilitate generalization than others. Using a program designed by Carrier (1970), they observed the extent of transfer that occurred from training in the home environment to probes obtained in the following four settings:

1. A mother administered the probe while sitting across from her child at a table in a treatment room of the speech clinic.
2. An experimenter (who was only vaguely familiar to the child) administered the probe while sitting across from the child at the same table in the same room as setting 1.
3. The same experimenter administered the probe while she and the child were seated at separate desks facing each other in a large classroom outside the speech clinic.
4. A second experimenter (unknown to the child prior to the study) administered a probe while she and the child were alone and seated in comfortable chairs in the informal atmosphere of the clinic waiting room.

Although all three subjects generalized from the teaching setting to one or more experimental settings, there was no evidence that one setting was more facilitative than another. These findings point out the complexity of the transfer process. It may be that the variables differ so much from person to person that it is impossible to predict which environments are most likely to facilitate situational transfer.

Costello and Bosler (1976) also reported more situational generalization of training words than untrained words. One might infer from this finding that more situational generalization might be facilitated through the use of a large number of training words than fewer words.

Olswang and Bain (1985) monitored situational generalization for three 4-year-old children in two different settings during speech sound remediation. They examined connected speech samples recorded in conversational activities in a clinic treatment room and connected speech samples audio recorded by parents during conversational activities at home. They reported similar rates and amounts of generalization of target sounds for both settings.

Bankson and Byrne (1972) reported that four out of five subjects generalized correct sound production in words from a motor-based remediation procedure to conversational samples gathered both in the training setting (school) and the home environment. While the amount of generalization seen in the home and school training probes varied from day to day for each subject, the daily fluctuations were consistent between settings for each subject. The overall extent to which generalization occurred varied greatly across individuals and fluctuated within subjects from day to day.

One strategy that has been suggested to facilitate situational generalization is the use of self-monitoring (self-evaluation). Self-monitoring techniques have included hand raising (Engel and Groth, 1976), charting (Diedrich, 1971; Koegel, Koegel, and Ingham, 1986), and counting of correct productions, both within and outside the clinic (Koegel, Koegel, Van Voy, and Ingham, 1988). Bennett, Bennett, and James (1996) suggested the following steps to facilitate self-monitoring:

1. External monitoring and verbal feedback
2. External monitoring with cues provided for revision (e.g., raise hand)
3. Self-revision by client when errors occur
4. Anticipating when errors may occur
5. Automatic usage of correct production

Koegel and colleagues (1988) examined generalization of /s/ and /z/ in seven children. They reported that when children self-monitored their conversational productions in the clinic, no generalization of the correct target production outside the clinic occurred. However, when children were required to monitor their conversational speech outside the clinic, "rapid and widespread generalization" occurred across subjects, although at slightly different rates. They reported high levels of generalization for all subjects. In contrast, when Gray and Shelton (1992) field tested the self-monitoring strategy of Koegel and colleagues (1988), the results did not replicate the positive generalization treatment effect reported by Koegel and colleagues (1988). As a result, additional research is needed to determine which clients are most likely to benefit from a self-monitoring strategy to facilitate generalization.

Shriberg and Kwiatkowski (1987), in a retrospective study of efficacy of intervention strategies, identified self-monitoring procedures as a potentially effective component to facilitate generalization to continuous speech. A subsequent experimental study (Shriberg and Kwiatkowski, 1990), included self-monitoring instruction. They reported that seven of the eight preschool subjects generalized from such self-monitoring instruction to spontaneous speech. They concluded, however, that while self-monitoring facilitated generalization, it varied in terms of type, extent, and point of onset. Thus, while self-monitoring would appear to be a critical skill in generalization, these data did indicate that speech sound generalization could not be predicted from the onset of self-monitoring behaviors.

Despite a paucity of data on situational generalization, available evidence indicates that, as with other forms of generalization, the extent to which it occurs in different settings varies greatly among individuals. There is also the suggestion that situational generalization may be influenced by age and how intact the child's phonologic system is (Elbert et al., 1990).

Several investigators have suggested that productive phonologic knowledge influences children's generalization learning (Dinnsen and Elbert, 1984; Elbert and Gierut, 1986; Gierut, Elbert, and Dinnsen, 1987; Gierut, 1989). They have inferred that phonologic knowledge accounts for some of the individual differences that occur in generalization. Gierut and colleagues (1987) reported that greater generalization occurred on sounds where children exhibited more knowledge (correct productions in a wide array of contexts) as opposed to less knowledge (correct productions in fewer contexts; more positional constraints), but generalization was restricted to those sounds for which training was provided. They also reported that when intervention was directed toward sounds where the child evidenced the least phonologic knowledge, generalization learning occurred across the child's phonologic system. These investigators recommended that clinicians choose sounds for treatment that reflect the least phonologic knowledge (inventory constraints). Even though training on sounds in which children showed most knowledge facilitated greater generalization within a sound class, training on sounds for which children exhibited least knowledge resulted in more broad-based generalization. Gierut and colleagues (1987) inferred from these findings that training on sounds in which children displayed least knowledge resulted in more systemwide changes and reorganization of the child's phonologic system than did training on sounds in which children showed most knowledge.

Williams (1991) examined generalization of nine children who exhibited least phonologic knowledge as reflected by inventory constraints (i.e., the children did not produce /s/ and /r/ on a conversational sample or on a 306-item probe test). The misarticulated [s] and [r] were trained in consonant clusters. Williams reported three different generalization and learning patterns across the subjects and hypothesized that differences in generalization reflected different levels of phonological knowledge, even though all error targets were classified in the least phonologic knowledge category. Williams questioned if Gierut and colleagues' (1987) category of least knowledge was too broad to capture subtle differences in children's knowledge and recommended acoustical measurements to supplement transcription to further differentiate the amount of phonologic knowledge demonstrated for sounds in the least knowledge category of this system. This observation is consistent with recommendations from Weismer, Dinnsen, and Elbert (1981); Smit and Bernthal (1983); and Tyler, Edwards, and Saxman (1990).

Parental Assistance with Generalization

Clinicians have long recognized that the generalization process in articulation remediation might be facilitated if individuals from the client's environment could be drawn into the generalization phase of the treatment process. The assumption has been that persons significant to the client—parents, spouse, teachers, or peers—could engage in selected activities designed to extend what the clinician was doing in the clinical setting. Several programs include instructional activities designed for parents to use with their children at home (Mowrer, Baker, and Schutz, 1968; Gray, 1974). Sommers (1962) and Sommers and colleagues (1964) studied several variables related to articulation instruction. Greater improvement between pre- and posttest scores was reported for children whose mothers were trained to assist with instruction than for a control group of children whose mothers had not received training. Carrier (1970) reported a study comparing a group of ten children 4 to 7 years old who participated in an articulation training program administered by their mothers and a similar control group who received minimal assistance from their mothers. The experimental group obtained significantly higher scores on four phonologic measures than the control group.

Other investigations in which parents provided directed articulation instruction for their children were reported by Shelton, Johnson, and Arndt (1972) and Shelton, Johnson, Willis, and Arndt (1975). In the first investigation, eight school-age children received instruction and monitoring by their parents in the home. Repeated measures involving baseline and treatment probes on sound production tasks, reading samples, and conversational samples reflected varying results. Significant changes on the sound production tasks were not found although scores were higher on the posttest. On the other hand, significant differences were found between mean baseline scores and scores on final reading samples and conversational samples. Four-month posttreatment scores indicated that gains made during the program were maintained.

The second investigation was similar to the first, but younger children (4- to 6-year-olds) were studied. In contrast to the earlier study, these children improved significantly on the sound production tasks. It should be pointed out that the pretest scores for these younger children were lower than for the older group; in other words, the younger group had more room for improvement and hence a higher probability of significant differences. The younger children, however, showed less improvement on the conversational samples. Shelton and his colleagues (1975) speculated that the monitoring-reinforcement procedure had greater influence on the conversational scores of subjects who had higher scores on the sound production task at the time the procedure was initiated.

Generalization Guidelines

1. To facilitate position and context generalization, the clinician usually begins instruction with target behaviors in positions or contexts in the client's repertoire.
2. Since word productions form the basis of position generalization, productions at this level should be incorporated into the instructional sequence as quickly as possible.
3. The more alike that two or more sounds are in their phonetic characteristics, the more likely that generalization will occur from one to another. For example, teaching [ɝ] usually results in generalization to the unstressed [ɚ] and the consonantal [r]; teaching one member of a cognate sound-pair, such as [s], will usually result in the client's use of the cognate [z].
4. Teaching a distinctive feature in the context of one sound, such as continuancy in [f], should result in some generalization of that feature in other untreated sounds, such as [ʒ], especially within the same sound class.

5. Data are lacking to support a particular order for teaching sounds in various word-positions. The traditional procedure—teaching sounds first in the initial position and then in the final and medial positions—is not supported by available research (even though the initial position develops earliest in most sounds, except for fricatives). Teaching a sound in all positions simultaneously may be an approach to more rapid sound position generalization.

6. To facilitate generalization, target behaviors selected for remediation should represent exemplars of error patterns in clients with multiple errors. In selecting sounds to target for reduction of phonologic processes, select at least one sound for each sound class in which the process occurs because generalization is most likely to occur among sounds in the same sound class.

7. Nonsense syllables may facilitate production of sounds in syllable contexts during establishment of sound production because nonsense syllables pose less interference with previously learned behaviors than words. Meaningful words may generalize more rapidly than nonsense syllables because they reflect actual phonemic contrasts and are reinforced in the environment.

8. Activities to facilitate situational generalization are advised as soon as the client can say a sound in words, rather than waiting until sounds are produced at the sentence level. However, in the case of preschool children, generalization frequently takes place without including a plan to facilitate generalization in treatment.

9. When sounds are taught in which clients demonstrate least knowledge, they are more likely to generalize to correct production of other sounds than when clients are taught sounds in which they demonstrate most knowledge. More rapid generalization to other words and contexts occurs when sounds that reflect most knowledge are treated.

10. Parents and others in the child's environment can be used effectively to facilitate phonologic change in children. The clinician must be sensitive to the role parents or other nonprofessionals can assume in the treatment process. First, if parents are to judge the accuracy of sound productions, they must be able to discriminate the sounds correctly. Second, the clinician must demonstrate to the parents the procedures to be used in the program; then the parents must demonstrate to the clinician the procedures to be used to insure that parents can carry out the procedures. Third, recognize that parents have only a limited amount of time; consequently, programs should be designed for short periods. Fourth, written instructions of the specific tasks should be provided to the caregivers—parents. Finally, clinicians should keep in mind that parents probably function better as monitors of productions than as teachers. Often, parents lack the patience and objectivity necessary to teach their own child. However, if parents or other individuals in the child's environment have the desire, skill, time, and patience to work with their children, the clinician may have a helpful facilitator of the generalization process.

Dismissal from Instruction

The final phase of phonologic instruction occurs when the client habituates new target behaviors and otherwise assumes responsibility for self-monitoring of target phonologic productions. This phase of therapy is an extension of the generalization phase.

During the final phase of therapy, sometimes referred to as the *maintenance phase* (a motor learning perspective), clients decrease their contact with the clinician, and sometimes this phase is viewed as the final stage of instruction. Shelton (1978) labeled the terminal objective of articulation remediation as **automatization** and described it as automatic usage of standard articulation patterns in spontaneous speech. The term *automatization* implies that phonologic productions can be viewed as motor behavior that develops into an automatic response. When phonologic errors are linguistic in nature, maintenance may be viewed as the mastery of phonologic rules and phonemic contrasts. In reality, both the motor production and phonologic rules become part of a person's everyday productive behavioral responses by this point in treatment. The maintenance phase may be considered complete once the client can consistently use target behaviors in spontaneous speech.

During maintenance, the client usually receives intermittent reinforcement for the new speech patterns because this type of schedule results in behavior that is most resistant to extinction. Clients are also required to monitor their own articulation procedures during maintenance. Self-monitoring tasks can be checked by having the client keep track of target productions during specified periods of the day.

To determine the extent to which a client has maintained target behaviors, the clinician must assess a client's behavior during conversational speech. Diedrich (1971) described procedures for counting and charting speech behaviors but recognized that there are many times when speech patterns cannot be externally monitored. He suggested that three-minute "Talk" samples are a good way to begin monitoring speech during conversation and that counting correct and incorrect target sound productions during a 3-minute time period is an effective way to monitor productions. Prior to dismissal from treatment, Diedrich also advised, the monitoring period should be increased to include a majority of the speaking time.

In a study cited earlier, Bankson and Byrne (1972) reported a treatment procedure designed to facilitate generalization and maintenance of correct target sound productions. This procedure involved repetitive readings of a list of target words at increasingly rapid rates. Although generalization to conversational speech occurred from this motor task, none of the subjects developed correct target sound productions to the point of producing their error sounds correctly 95 percent of the time or more in conversation.

Manning and his colleagues (1976, 1977) have suggested that the extent to which a client automatizes a response is related to his or her ability to articulate correctly under conditions of noise. These authors measured the articulatory skills of children who misarticulated either /s/ or /r/. Subjects were divided into a low acquisition group (score below 80 percent correct on the *Deep Test of Articulation*) and a high acquisition group (score above 80 percent correct on the *Deep Test of Articulation*). The children were administered the *Deep Test of Articulation* while competing speech noise was presented binaurally through earphones; subjects were also administered the same task in a quiet condition (absence of noise). A difference score, based on the articulation test scores under the two conditions, was obtained. Children in the high acquisition group demonstrated a significantly smaller difference score between the noise and quiet conditions than the children in the low acquisition group. The authors concluded that as children acquired correct production of /s/ and /r/, they simultaneously automatized the correct articulatory gestures for sounds, as evidenced by higher test scores and less influence of the noise. These data must be interpreted cautiously, however, because noise was not presented at a constant hearing level and the stimulus conditions were not counterbalanced.

Information from the learning literature offers insights into the maintenance or retention of newly acquired phonologic patterns. **Retention**, in the context of phonologic remediation, refers to the continued and persistent use of responses learned during instruction. Once an individual learns a new phonologic pattern or response, he or she must continue to use (retain) the response. In clinical literature, retention is sometimes discussed in terms of intersession retention and sometimes in terms of habitual retention. *Intersession retention* refers to the ability to produce recently taught responses correctly. Speech clinicians frequently observe "between-session forgetting" in many clients. Mowrer (1977) pointed out that lack of intersession retention is a particular problem with mentally retarded children. *Habitual retention* is the persistent and continued use of the response after instruction has been terminated. The term *maintenance* is frequently used to refer to this phenomenon. Speech clinicians occasionally dismiss clients from instruction only to have them return for additional therapy some months later. Such individuals obviously did not habituate or retain their newly learned responses.

Sommers (1969) reported that articulation errors are particularly susceptible to regression. In a follow-up study of 177 elementary school children who had been dismissed from articulation instruction during a six-month period, he found that approximately one-third had regressed. Based on conversational samples of target sound productions, 59 percent of those who had worked on /s/ and /z/ had regressed, but only 6 percent of those who had worked on /r/ had regressed. He does not report dismissal criteria or the level of performance prior to dismissal.

In contrast, Elbert and colleagues (1990) reported that learning continued in preschool children beyond treatment as subjects' speech continued to improve on both single-word and conversational speech samples obtained three months post-treatment. These data support the idea that young children are actively involved in the learning process and seem to make changes more easily in their phonologic system. Such changes seemed to occur even after treatment was terminated.

Little is known about the reasons for regression in habitual retention or maintenance, but it is quite likely that variables affecting habitual retention affect intersession retention as well. On the basis of memory studies, Winitz (1969) proposed that interference, which results in competition between the error sound and the newly acquired sound, may explain why individuals forget articulatory responses. Winitz pointed out that the years of motor production practice using an incorrect articulatory gesture, such as /t/ for /tʃ/, will interfere with the individual's ability to produce a newly learned /tʃ/. Similarly, speech clinicians frequently observe individuals who, during the early stages of instruction, insert a /θ/ following a newly learned /s/ in a word context (e.g., [sθup]).

Mowrer (1982) pointed out several factors that have been shown to influence the degree to which information will be retained, whether in the child who is dismissed from therapy but returns for lack of long-term maintenance or in the child who seems to have forgotten previous learning in the three days between sessions. First, the meaningfulness of the material used to teach the new responses may affect retention, although there is little empirical evidence in the articulation learning literature on this point. In general, as the meaningfulness of the material increases, the rate of forgetting tends to decrease, and thus the use of meaningful material is recommended during remediation. Thus, names of friends, family members, pets, familiar objects, and animals are appropriate choices. Although meaningfulness of material may be an important aid to long-term retention, the clinician may find, as stated earlier, that nonmeaningful material (e.g., nonsense syllables) may be useful during earlier phases of instruction (i.e., establishment). Leonard (1973) reported that when /s/ had been established in meaningful words, fewer training trials were required to transfer to other words than when nonsense items were utilized. But this finding on generalization must be distinguished from the finding presented earlier in our discussion of interference—that acquisition or establishment of new responses can be accomplished in fewer trials with nonsense items than with meaningful items.

A second factor believed to affect retention is the degree or extent to which something has been learned. In general, the greater the number of trials during the learning process, the greater the retention. Retention improves when some overlearning of verbal material takes place. To avoid unnecessary practice, it is important to determine the minimum amount of learning needed to provide a satisfactory level of retention. The optimum point for stopping instruction occurs when additional training does not produce sufficient change in performance to merit additional practice; however, there is little data to guide the clinician about where this point may be.

A third factor affecting retention is the frequency of instruction or the distribution of practice. Retention is superior when tasks are practiced during several short sessions (distributed practice) than during fewer, longer sessions (massed practice). On the basis of this fact, frequent, short practice sessions are recommended. In his review of this topic, Mowrer (1982) concluded: "On the basis of controlled learning experiments in psychology alone, it could be recommended that clinicians could increase retention by providing frequent instruction; but bear in mind that no data are available from speech research that confirms this recommendation . . . the important factor in terms of frequency of instruction is not how much instruction . . . but the total number of instruction periods" (259).

A fourth factor shown to affect retention is the individual's motivational state. The more motivated a person, the greater the retention of the material that has been learned. Little, if any, experimental work reported in the phonologic literature has attempted to examine motivational state during speech instruction.

Dismissal Criteria

The maintenance phase provides a period for monitoring retention, and it is during this period that dismissal decisions are made. Limited data on dismissal criteria have been reported, and thus evidence is lacking to support a single dismissal criterion. Elbert (1967) suggested dismissal might be based on two questions: (1) Has the maximum change in this individual's speech behavior been attained? (2) Can this individual maintain this level of speech behavior and continue to improve without additional speech instruction? Whatever criteria are used for dismissal, they should be based upon periodic samples of phonologic behavior over time. The maintenance phase provides the final opportunity for the clinician to monitor, reinforce, and encourage the client to assume responsibility for habituation of the new speech patterns.

Diedrich and Bangert (1976) reported data on articulatory retention and dismissal from treatment. Some of the children studied were dismissed after reaching a 75 percent criterion level for correct /s/ and /r/ productions, as measured on a 30-item probe word test plus a 3-minute sample of conversational speech. Four months later, 19 percent of the subjects had regressed below the 75 percent criterion level. No greater retention was found, however, among those children who remained in treatment until achieving higher than 75 percent criterion level on the probe measure. Diedrich and Bangert concluded that most speech clinicians tend to retain children with /s/ and /r/ errors in articulation instruction longer than necessary. It is unclear whether similar conclusions would have been reached if a higher criterion level (e.g., 95 to 100 percent) had been used.

Maintenance and Dismissal Guidelines

1. Because the client is seen less frequently for clinical instruction during the maintenance phase, the client should assume responsibility for self-monitoring.
2. The reinforcement schedule for correct responses should be intermittent during maintenance, just as during the latter stages of generalization. Either a variable ratio or variable interval schedule of reinforcement is recommended.
3. Little information is available on dismissal criteria; therefore, the matter is left up to clinicians and clients. It has been suggested that clinicians may tend to keep clients enrolled for phonologic remediation longer than is necessary. In other words, the cost-benefit ratio for intervention may significantly decline after a certain point is reached in treatment.

Intervention for Children with Developmental Verbal Dyspraxia (DVD)

The topic of developmental verbal dyspraxia (DVD) was introduced in Chapter 5 in our discussion of factors related to the presence of phonologic disorders. In this section, we will add to the historical and descriptive background presented in that chapter by addressing issues relevant to clinical intervention with this subpopulation of the phonologically impaired.

DVD appears to involve both motor and linguistic components, with wide variation in symptoms across children. Aram (1984) suggested that the problem be viewed as a syndrome that includes a severe and persistent phonologic disorder coupled with an expressive syntactic disorder, with variable neurological and articulatory findings. Velleman and Strand (1994) proposed a hierarchical hypothesis of DVD, suggesting that children may be capable of producing the individual aspects of speech production (i.e., articulatory postures, phonemes, words), but have great difficulty "bridging among the various elements that constitute language performance" (120). Thus the problem has been viewed as a combined motor and linguistic problem.

Assessment

Assessment of this population is not unlike that used with any child with a phonologic disability and typically includes a case history, hearing screening, and review for deficits in other areas of communication (language, voice, fluency). There are, however, specific aspects of evaluations of the DVD population that warrant elaboration.

The oral mechanism examination should review strength, tone, and stability of the oral structure (e.g., can the child move the tongue independently of the mandible? Does the child do anything special to stabilize the mandible, such as thrust it forward?). Review of a child's feeding history may be of interest in this regard. Overall motor skills, both automatic and volitional, including the ability to perform imitative and rapidly alternating tongue movements, plus diadokokinetic rates should be included. Velleman and Strand (1994), in a review of the literature, suggested that DVD children have difficulty with transitions between sounds. While static articulatory positions (sounds in isolation) may not be difficult to produce, rapid combinations of movements may be difficult. The rapid successive movements of connected speech entail constant approximations of specific articulatory targets because there are no absolute or static positions associated with speech sounds. For children with DVD, the inherent dynamic overlapping movement involved in producing sequential motor speech elements is a problem. Velleman and Strand (1994) indicated that sequencing difficulties may not manifest themselves in phonemic sequencing errors per se, but rather are more evident at the articulatory level, affecting the relative timing of glottal and articulatory gestures. These latter factors result in perceived errors of voicing and vowels, especially diphthongs.

In analyzing speech performance, the clinician must keep in mind the nature of DVD as a disorder involving the hierarchical levels of speech and language. Movements, transitions, and timing should be observed as speech is assessed at a variety of linguistic levels (i.e., semantics, syntax, phonetic/phonemic levels). For children with a very limited verbal repertoire, an independent analysis of a phonological sample is recommended. For those with higher verbal skills, a traditional phonologic assessment battery (relational analysis) is recommended, with particular attention to the analysis of speech sounds within syllabic units. In this instance, the connected speech sample will allow the examiner to review syllable and word shapes produced by the child. Phonologic assessment should also include imitation of words that increase in number of syllables (e.g., *please*, *pleasing*, *pleasingly*).

Because children with DVD evidence problems with the dynamic organization of communication efforts, it is not unusual for problems to be present with the suprasegmental aspects of speech. Coordinating the laryngeal and respiratory systems with the oral mechanism is often very difficult. This problem may result in difficulty with properly varying intonation contours, modulation of loudness, and maintaining proper resonance. Vowels may be prolonged because the child needs time to organize coordination for the next series of speech sound movements.

A final comment on assessment of children with suspected DVD should be made. Because of the concern about apraxia, and sometimes concomitant dysarthria, it may be prudent to refer the more seriously impaired child to a pediatric neurologist to determine the status of current neurological functioning. Seizure history and/or potential, associated limb apraxias, and general knowledge of neurological functioning may influence the overall management program for a given child and thus warrant such a referral.

Recommended Phonologic Assessment Battery for DVD

1. Case history (including review of feeding history)
2. Hearing screening/testing
3. Screening of voice and fluency characteristics

4. Speech mechanism examination

- Structure and function
- Strength, tone, stability
- Diadokokinetic rate

5. Connected speech sample

- Segmental productions
- Syllable and word shapes production
- Phonologic patterns present and/or lacking
- Intonation, vocal loudness, resonance

6. Segmental productions (citation form testing)

- Consonants, vowels, and diphthongs
- Syllable shapes used in response to stimulus items

7. Phonologic process review

- Patterns used
- Patterns missing

8. Stimulability testing

- Segments
- Syllables
- Words with increasing number of syllables

9. Language evaluation

- Comprehension and production
- Sound productions at various semantic and syntactic levels

A test specifically designed for use with the DVD population is the *Screening Test for Developmental Apraxia of Speech* (Blakely, 1980).

Treatment

The recommended treatment of children with DVD is different from the more traditional motor and/or linguistic approaches to phonologic intervention. Two significant differences between what has been discussed elsewhere in this chapter and what will be presented here are short-term goals of therapy and the production units focused on in therapy.

A major short-term therapy goal is to build a functional vocabulary for a client. Often DVD children have significant intelligibility problems, and efforts need to be directed toward building a core of intelligible words to facilitate the communication process. To the extent possible, the phonologic production activities suggested here should include attention to syllabic structures and combinations of these syllables so that the child will gain some initial verbal building blocks.

A major focus of instructional activities is on the motor-planning component of the disorder. Rather than using drill motor activities that focus on sound or syllable repetitions, a variety of speech and language contexts should be provided for purposes of practicing the organization, transitions, and timing of movements required in the dynamic process of on-going speech. Emphasis is placed on shifting the stimulus materials to incorporate larger patterns of sound sequences. Rosenbeck, Kent, and LaPointe (1984) recommended contin-ually shifting the segmental targets in a succession of syllables beginning with CV or VC, repeating the patterns, and then systematically varying the CV pattern and moving into word combinations. Another technique for facilitating the use of sounds in sequence is known as "touch-cueing" (Bashir, Grahamjones, and Bostwick, 1984). In this procedure, the clinician touches a particular area of the face or neck as each sound in a sequence is pro-duced. Children learn the sound associated with each touching cue. Thus, children can be presented with simultaneous touch, auditory, and sometimes visual cues as they produce sounds in various movement patterns.

Occupational therapy (OT) is a profession that has also had an interest in and been in-volved with children evidencing DVD. The interest of these professionals in apraxias, no-tably limb apraxia, has been extended to oral and verbal apraxias. Some of their techniques, particularly those involving "sensory integration," have been reported to be helpful to clients with various types of apraxia. As a result, some professionals in the field of speech-language pathology have borrowed this methodology for treatment of DVD.

Emphasis is placed on sequential movements involving the articulators, including al-ternating movements such as biting the upper lip, biting the lower lip, and attending to mus-cle tone. Special instruction is necessary to employ some of the OT's techniques since such procedures are not part of the usual portfolio of skills held by speech-language pathologists. A set of guidelines for working with DVD clients is presented in Table 8.8 (Velleman and

TABLE 8.8 Basic Principles of a Speech Production Treatment Program for Children with DVD (Velleman and Strand, 1994) Used by permission.

1. Main focus of treatment should be syllable structure control and organization within a variety of dynamic linguistic contexts.
2. A successful program is one that will facilitate correct production of varying syllable shapes and the organization of these shapes into longer and increasingly complex phonotatic patterns.
3. A sound-by-sound treatment plan that emphasizes phoneme production in isolation prior to moving to words and phrases does *not* address the hierarchical dynamic movement problem in DVD.
4. Auditory discrimination training does *not* address the problem.
5. Frequent, short sessions with breaks are most successful. Because DVD is a dynamic disorder, system fatigue is a problem.
6. Sessions should be divided into short parts:
   a. Warm-ups: Imitation of body and/or oral motor sequences.
   b. Practicing the scales: Syllable sequence drill activities. Establish consistent connected syllable productions from within the child's repertoire. Include sequences that vary articulatory positions, for example, from front to back ([bʌdʌgʌ] or "buttercup") or vice versa ([gʌ dʌ bʌ] or "go to bed").
   c. Learning the song: Meaningful single-word activities to include a core group of words that would increase overall intelligibility of speech.
   d. Changing the song: Short sentence activities starting with a key carrier phrase and changing one word, gradually increasing in length and complexity.

Strand, 1994). For children who are very young or severely impaired, gestures and pantomime should be encouraged, and an augmentative communication system may be recommended. Facilitating communication through these techniques is often viewed as a means to facilitate verbal communication as well as the development of other aspects of language.

Phonologic Awareness and the Speech-Language Pathologist

Investigators have suggested that children's failure to acquire basic reading skills is frequently related to phonologic processing skills (Moats and Lyon, 1996). More specifically, there is increasing evidence to suggest that young children's phonologic awareness skills are predictors of later reading and spelling performance. In other words, children who demonstrate poor phonologic awareness skills experience greater difficulty learning to read. It has been reported that children with moderate to severe phonologic problems frequently exhibit limited phonologic awareness skills. Hodson (1994) pointed out that children who are unintelligible at the time they enter kindergarten are particularly at risk for reading problems. Webster and Plante (1992) reported that in a comparison of performance on four phonologic awareness tasks between a group of moderate to severely unintelligible children and a group of phonologically normal children, the normal children scored significantly higher than did the phonologically impaired group. Because of a possible relationship between speech sound production problems and literacy (reading problems), phonologic awareness is of interest to speech-language pathologists. In addition, speech-language pathologists are frequently asked to provide consultation to classroom teachers or provide direct intervention to children who are experiencing reading problems in combination with poor phonologic awareness skills.

Phonologic awareness (also termed phoneme segmentation, phoneme analysis, and metaphonology) is the ability to identify and manipulate the sounds of the language. Phonologic awareness includes the ability to segment ongoing speech into words, syllables, intrasyllabic units (onset and rime), and individual phonemes (van Kleeck, 1995). One of the keys to learning to read is the ability to *identify* the different sounds (phonemes) that constitute words and then to associate these sounds with the written word. Besides being able to identify the sounds in words, a reader must be able to *manipulate* these sounds. The manipulation of sounds includes tasks such as being able to segment words into their constituent sounds, being able to rhyme words, and being able to blend sounds; skills that are all essential to the reading process. Ball (1993) stated that "phonological awareness is the metalinguistic ability that involves the more or less explicit understanding that words are made of discrete units" (130).

One of the primary goals of reading instruction in early elementary grades is to teach students the relationship among speech sounds, the phonology of their language, printed symbols, and the written alphabet. Swank (1994) and van Kleeck (1995) in summarizing the literature made the following summary statements about the relationship between phonologic awareness and literacy skill development:

- A significant relationship exists between phonologic analysis and reading development.
- Performance on phonologic awareness tasks may have predictive value for later reading development.

- Training in phonologic awareness skills may facilitate reading and spelling achievement.
- Training in phonologic awareness skills has been shown to be effective before formal reading instruction begins.
- Children need instruction in both phonologic awareness and letter-sound correspondence to make maximal gains in literacy skills.

Assessment of Phonologic Awareness

Ball (1993) recommended five phonologic tasks to be included in an assessment of phonologic awareness:

1. *Rhyming*—a skill that may facilitate reading but in itself is not sufficient for reading acquisition. Tasks to assess rhyming might include: (a) instructing the child to provide a rhyming word for a word presented by the teacher or clinician; (b) categorizing words according to rhyme (child must pick out the word that does not belong); and (c) judging whether or not a pair of words rhyme.
2. *Alliteration*—identification of words that begin with a certain sound, such as determining whether words begin with the same sound; selecting, from a group of words, the word that has a different beginning sound.
3. *Phoneme blending*—blending two or more sounds into a word when the sounds are presented separately.
4. *Invented spellings*—analyzing children's spelling when they have been asked to spell some easy and/or common words.
5. *Phoneme segmentation*—breaking a word into its constituent phonemes. These tasks are those most highly correlated with reading success, but performance may be related to reading instruction. There are commercially available assessment instruments for this task, such as the *Auditory Conceptualization Test* (Lindamood and Lindamood, 1979).

Several overall phonologic awareness instruments are available commercially, including the *Test of Phonological Awareness* (Torgeson and Bryant, 1993), and the *Phonological Awareness Profile* (Robertson and Salter, 1995).

Intervention

Certain phonologic awareness skills need to be developed prior to formal reading instruction (van Kleeck, 1995). Such skills include segmenting sentences into words, segmenting words into syllables, and being aware of subsyllabic units (units intermediate between syllables and phonemes called *onsets* and *rimes*). The *onset subsyllabic unit* is the initial consonant or consonant cluster of a syllable. The *rime* includes the remainder of the syllable, including a vowel and possibly a final consonant or consonant cluster (e.g., in the word "front," "fr" is the onset and "ont" is the rime). Swank (1994) posits two stages of phonologic awareness: One is the awareness that occurs before formal reading instruction begins, and the other is the phonologic awareness that develops as a result of learning to read.

Skills developed during the final stage of phonologic awareness are typically facilitated through activities that are engaged in at home, in preschool, or during the kindergarten year.

Sound play activities involving nursery rhymes, finger plays, poems, rhyming stories, stories with alliterations, and stories with nonsense words are all examples of activities which focus a child's attention on the sound structure of the language. These are the kinds of activities that the speech-language pathologist may employ and expand upon before formal reading instruction begins.

During the second stage of awareness, which may overlap with formal reading instruction, awareness tasks to be developed include segmentation and blending of phonemes. Clinicians might begin by teaching children to divide words into syllables. Instruction might begin with compound words such as *hotdog*. In this task, the word is segmented into two words, *hot* and *dog*, and then the child is instructed to blend the two words into a single word. Once children understand how to divide words into syllables, they should be taught to divide syllables into phonemes. It is often helpful to use tokens or blocks to represent individual phonemes in words. Blackman (1989) describes a technique called "say it and move it" in which children are taught to segment and blend words using blocks (also see Catts and Vartiainen, 1993). In these activities, instruction should begin with CV or CVC words containing continuent sounds. More complex words containing stop consonants can be introduced later.

Role of the Speech-Language Pathologist

Many activities designed to facilitate phonologic awareness can be incorporated into phonologic and/or language treatment. These activities can be conducted both in a pull-out model of intervention or in an inclusive classroom in which the classroom teacher and/or the speech-language pathologist provides instruction about the sound structure of words. Catts (1991) suggested that the speech-language pathologist should incorporate speech sound awareness training in the management of all children who are language impaired because of their risk for academic failure.

References

Aram, D., "Assessment and treatment of developmental apraxia." *Seminars in Speech and Language, 5* (1984): 2.

Aungst, L., and J. Frick, "Auditory discrimination ability and consistency of articulation of /r/." *Journal of Speech and Hearing Disorders, 29* (1964): 76–85.

Backus, O., and J. Beasley, *Speech Therapy with Children*. Boston, Mass.: Houghton Mifflin, 1951.

Baker, R. D., and B. P. Ryan, *Programmed Conditioning for Articulation*. Monterey, Calif.: Monterey Learning Systems, 1971.

Ball, E., "Assessing phoneme awareness." *Language, Speech, and Hearing Services in Schools, 24* (1993): 130–139.

Bankson, N. W., and M. C. Byrne, "The effect of a timed correct sound production task on carryover." *Journal of Speech and Hearing Research, 15* (1972): 160–168.

Bashir, A., F. Grahamjones, and R. Bostwick, "A touch-cue method of therapy for developmental apraxia." *Seminars in Speech and Language, 5* (1984): 127–137.

Bennett, B., C. Bennett, and C. James, "Phonological development from concept to classroom." Paper presented at the Speech-Language-Hearing Association of Virginia Annual Conference, Roanoke, Virginia, 1996.

Bernthal, J. E., M. Greenlee, R. Eblen, and K.

Marking, "Detection of mispronunciations: A comparison of adults, normal-speaking children with articulation errors." *Journal of Applied Psycholinguistics, 8* (1987): 209–222.

Blache, S. E., "A distinctive feature approach." In N. Creaghead, P. Newman, and W. Secord (Eds.), *Assessment and Remediation of Articulatory and Phonological Disorders.* Columbus, Ohio: Charles E. Merrill, 1989.

Blache, S. E., "Minimal word-pairs and distinctive feature training." In M. Crary (Ed.), *Phonological Intervention: Concepts and Procedures.* San Diego, Calif.: College-Hill Press, 1982.

Black, L., "So you want to dismiss 80 percent of your caseload." Paper presented at the 1972 North Carolina Special Education Conference, Raleigh, N.C., 1972.

Blackman B., "Phonological awareness and word recognition: Assessment and intervention." In A. Kamhi and H. Catts (Eds.), *Reading Disabilities: A Developmental Language Perspective.* Boston, Mass.: Allyn and Bacon, 1989.

Blakely, R., *Screening Test for Developmental Apraxia of Speech.* Tigand, Ore.: C.C. Publications, 1980.

Bradley, D., "A systematic multiple-phoneme approach." In N. Creaghead, P. Newman, and W. Secord (Eds.), *Assessment and Remediation of Articulatory and Phonological Disorders.* Columbus, Ohio: Charles E. Merrill, 1989.

Camarata, S., and R. Schwartz, "Production of object words and action words: Evidence for a relationship between phonology and semantics." *Journal of Speech and Hearing Research, 26* (1985): 50–53.

Carrier, J. K., "A program of articulation therapy administered by mothers." *Journal of Speech and Hearing Disorders, 33* (1970): 344–353.

Catts, H., "Facilitating phonological awareness: Role of speech-language pathologists." *Language, Speech, and Hearing Services in Schools, 22* (1991): 196–203.

Catts, H., and T. Vartiainen, *Sounds Abound*, East Moline, Ill.: Linguasystems, 1993.

Compton, A. J., "Generative studies of children's phonological disorders: A strategy of therapy." In S. Singh (Ed.), *Measurements in Hearing, Speech, and Language.* Baltimore, Md.: University Park Press, 1975.

Costello, J., and C. Bosler, "Generalization and articulation instruction." *Journal of Speech and Hearing Disorders, 41* (1976): 359–373.

Costello, J., and J. Onstein, "The modification of multiple articulation errors based on distinctive feature theory." *Journal of Speech and Hearing Disorders, 41* (1976): 199–215.

Curtis, J. R., and J. C. Hardy, "A phonetic study of misarticulation of /r/." *Journal of Speech and Hearing Research, 2* (1959): 244–257.

Diedrich, W. M., "Procedures for counting and charting a target phoneme." *Language, Speech, and Hearing Services in Schools, 2* (1971): 18–32.

Diedrich, W. M., and J. Bangert, "Training and speech clinicians in recording and analysis of articulatory behavior." Washington, D.C.: U.S. Office of Education Grant No. OEG-0-70-1689 and OEG-0-71-1689, 1976.

Dinnsen, D., and M. Elbert, "On the relationship between phonology and learning." In M. Elbert, D. Dinnsen, and G. Weismer (Eds.), *Phonological Theory and the Misarticulating Child*, ASHA Monographs. Rockville, Md.: ASHA, 1984.

Elbert, M., "Dismissal Criteria from Therapy." Unpublished manuscript, 1967.

Elbert, M., D. A. Dinnsen, P. Swartzlander, and S. B. Chin, "Generalization to conversational speech." *Journal of Speech and Hearing Disorders, 55* (1990): 694–699.

Elbert, M., and J. Gierut, *Handbook of Clinical Phonology Approaches to Assessment and Treatment.* San Diego, Calif.: College-Hill Press, 1986.

Elbert, M., and L. V. McReynolds, "Transfer of /r/ across contexts." *Journal of Speech and Hearing Disorders, 40* (1975): 380–387.

Elbert, M., and L. V. McReynolds, "An experimental analysis of misarticulating children's generalization." *Journal of Speech and Hearing Research, 21* (1978): 136–149.

Elbert, M., T. W. Powell, and P. Swartzlander, "Toward a technology of generalization: How many exemplars are sufficient?" *Journal of Speech and Hearing Research, 34* (1991): 81–87.

Elbert, M., B. Rockman, and D. Saltzman, *Contrasts: The Use of Minimal Pairs in Articulation Training.* Austin, Tex.: Exceptional Resources, Inc., 1980.

Elbert, M., R. L. Shelton, and W. B. Arndt, "A task for education of articulation change." *Journal of Speech and Hearing Research*, *10* (1967): 281–288.

Engel, D. C., and L. R. Groth, "Case studies of the effect on carry-over of reinforcing postarticulation responses based on feedback." *Language, Speech, and Hearing Services in Schools*, *7* (1976): 93–101.

Ferrier, L., and M. Davis, "A lexical approach to the remediation of final sound omission." *Journal of Speech and Hearing Disorders*, *38* (1973): 126–130.

Fey, M. E., *Language Intervention with Young Children.* San Diego, Calif.: College-Hill Press/Little Brown, 1986.

Fey, M. E., "Articulation and phonology: Inextricable constructs in speech pathology." *Language, Speech, and Hearing Services in Schools*, *23* (1992): 225–232.

Fey, M. E., P. L. Cleave, A. I. Ravida, S. H. Long, A. E. Dejmal, and D. L. Easton, "Effects of grammar facilitation on the phonological performance of children with speech and language impairments." *Journal of Speech and Hearing Research*, *37* (1994): 594–607.

Gerber, A., *Goal: Carryover.* Philadelphia, Penn.: Temple University Press, 1973.

Gierut, J., "Maximal opposition approach to phonological treatment." *Journal of Speech and Hearing Disorders*, *54* (1989): 9–19.

Gierut, J. A., "Differential learning of phonological oppositions." *Journal of Speech and Hearing Research*, *33* (1990): 540–549.

Gierut, J., M. Elbert, and D. Dinnsen, "A functional analysis of phonological knowledge and generalization learning in misarticulating children." *Journal of Speech and Hearing Research*, *30* (1987): 462–479.

Gordon-Brannan, M., B. Hodson, and M. Wynne, "Remediating unintelligible utterances of a child with a mild hearing loss." *American Journal of Clinical Practice*, *1* (1992): 28–38.

Gray, B., "A field study on programmed articulation therapy." *Language, Speech, and Hearing Services in Schools*, *5* (1974): 119–131.

Gray, B., and B. Ryan, *A Language Program for the Nonlanguage Child.* Champaign, Ill.: Research Press, 1973.

Gray, S. I., and R. L. Shelton, "Self-monitoring effects on articulation carryover in school-age children." *Language, Speech, and Hearing Services in Schools*, *23* (1992): 334–342.

Hodson, B., "Phonological remediation: A cycles approach." In N. Creaghead, P. Newman, and W. Secord (Eds.), *Assessment and Remediation of Articulatory and Phonological Disorders.* Columbus, Ohio: Charles E. Merrill, 1989.

Hodson, B., "Helping individuals become intelligible, literate, and articulate: The role of phonology." In B. Hodson (Ed.), From Phonology to Metaphonology: Issues, Assessment and Intervention. *Topics in Language Disorders*, *14* (1994): 1–16.

Hodson, B., L. Chin, B. Redmond, and R. Simpson, "Phonological evaluation and remediation of speech deviations of a child with a repaired cleft palate: A case study." *Journal of Speech and Hearing Disorders*, *48* (1983): 93–98.

Hodson, B. W., "Disordered phonologies: What have we learned about assessment and treatment?" (pp. 197–224). In B. Hodson and M. Edwards (Eds.), *Perspectives in Applied Phonology.* Gaithersburg, Md.: Aspen Publishers, Inc., 1997.

Hodson, B., and E. Paden, *Targeting Intelligible Speech: A Phonological Approach to Remediation.* San Diego, Calif.: College-Hill Press, 1983.

Hodson, B., and E. Paden, *Targeting Intelligible Speech: A Phonological Approach to Remediation*, 2nd ed. Austin, Tex.: PRO-ED, 1991.

Hoffman, P., J. Norris, and J. Monjure, "Comparison of process targeting and whole language treatments for phonologically delayed preschool children." *Language, Speech, and Hearing Services in Schools*, *21* (1990): 102–109.

Hoffman, P., G. Schuckers, and R. Daniloff, *Children's Phonetic Disorders: Theory and Treatment.* Boston, Mass.: Little, Brown, 1989.

Ingram, D., "Explanation and phonological remediation."

Child Language Teaching and Therapy, 2 (1986): 1–19.

Koegel, L. K., R. L. Koegel, and J. C. Ingham, "Programming rapid generalization of correct articulation through self-monitoring procedures." *Journal of Speech and Hearing Disorders*, 51 (1986): 24–32.

Koegel, R., L. Koegel, K. Van Voy, and J. Ingham, "Within-clinic versus outside-of-clinic self-monitoring of articulation to promote generalization." *Journal of Speech and Hearing Disorders*, 53 (1988): 392–399.

La Riviere, C., H. Winitz, J. Reeds, and E. Herriman, "The conceptual reality of selected distinctive features." *Journal of Speech and Hearing Research*, 17 (1974): 122–133.

Leonard, L. B., "The nature of deviant articulation." *Journal of Speech and Hearing Disorders*, 38 (1973): 156–161.

Lindamood, C. H., and P. C. Lindamood, *Lindamood Auditory Conceptualization Test*. New York: Teaching Resources Corporation, 1979.

Locke, J. L., "The inference of speech perception in the phonologically disordered child. Part I. A rationale, some criteria, the conventional tests." *Journal of Speech and Hearing Disorders*, 40 (1980): 431–444.

Low, G., P. Newman, and M. Ravsten, "Pragmatic considerations in treatment: Communication centered instruction." In N. Creaghead, P. Newman, and W. Secord (Eds.), *Assessment and Remediation of Articulatory and Phonological Disorders*. Columbus, Ohio: Charles E. Merrill, 1989.

McCabe, R., and D. Bradley, "Systematic multiple phonemic approach to articulation therapy." *Acta Symbolica*, 6 (1975): 1–18.

McDonald, E. T., *Articulation Testing and Treatment: A Sensory Motor Approach*. Pittsburgh, Penn.: Stanwix House, 1964.

McLean, J. E., "Extending stimulus control of phoneme articulation by operant techniques." In *ASHA Monographs*, 14, Washington, D.C.: American Speech-Language-Hearing Association, 1970.

McNutt, J., "Generalization of /s/ from English to French as a result of phonological remediation." *Journal of Speech-Language Pathology and Audiology/Revue d'orthophonie et d'audiologie*, 18 (1994): 109–114.

McReynolds, L. V., "Articulation generalization during articulation training." *Language and Speech*, 15 (1972): 149–155.

McReynolds, L. V., and S. Bennett, "Distinctive feature generalization in articulation training." *Journal of Speech and Hearing Disorders*, 37 (1972): 462–470.

McReynolds, L. V., and D. Engmann, *Distinctive Feature Analysis of Misarticulations*. Baltimore, M.D.: University Park Press, 1975.

Manning, W. H., N. Keappock, and S. Stick, "The use of auditory masking to estimate automatization of correct articulatory production." *Journal of Speech and Hearing Disorders*, 41 (1976): 143–150.

Manning, W. H., M. L. Wittstruch, R. R. Loyd, and T. F. Campbell, "Automatization of correct production at two levels of articulatory acquisition." *Journal of Speech and Hearing Disorders*, 42 (1977): 77–84.

Masterson, J., "Classroom-based phonological intervention." *American Journal of Speech-Language Pathology: A Journal of Clinical Practice*, 2 (1993): 5–9.

Matheny, N., and J. Panagos, "Comparing the effects of articulation and syntax programs on syntax and articulation improvement." *Language, Speech, and Hearing Services in Schools*, 9 (1978): 57–61.

Moats, L. C., and G. Lyon, "Wanted: Teachers with knowledge of language." *Topics in Language Disorders*, 16 (1996): 73–86.

Monnin, L., and D. A. Huntington, "Relationship of articulatory defects to speech-sound identification." *Journal of Speech and Hearing Research*, 17 (1974): 352–366.

Mowrer, D. E., *Methods of Modifying Speech Behaviors*. Columbus, Ohio: Charles E. Merrill, 1977.

Mowrer, D. E., *Methods of Modifying Speech Behaviors*, 2nd ed. Columbus, Ohio: Charles E. Merrill, 1982.

Mowrer, D. E., R. Baker, and R. Schutz, *S-Programmed Articulation Control Kit*. Tempe, Ariz.: Educational Psychological Research Associates, 1968.

Norris, J., and P. Hoffman, "Language intervention within naturalistic environments." *Language, Speech, and Hearing Services in Schools*, 2 (1990): 72–84.

Olswang, L. B., and B. A. Bain, "The natural occurrence

of generalization articulation treatment." *Journal of Communication Disorders, 18* (1985): 109–129.

Panagos, J., and P. Prelock, "Phonological constraints on the sentence productions of language-disordered children." *Journal of Speech and Hearing Research, 24* (1982): 171–177.

Powell, J., and M. Elbert, "Generalization following the remediation of early- and later-developing consonant clusters." *Journal of Speech and Hearing Disorders, 49* (1984): 211–218.

Powell, J., and L. McReynolds, "A procedure for testing position generalization from articulation training." *Journal of Speech and Hearing Research, 12* (1969): 625–645.

Powers, M. J., "Clinical and educational procedures in functional disorders of articulation." In L. Travis (Ed.), *Handbook of Speech Pathology and Audiology.* Englewood Cliffs, N.J.: Prentice-Hall, 1971.

Robertson, D., and W. Salter, *The Phonological Awareness Profile.* East Moline, Ill.: LinguiSystem, 1995.

Rosenbeck, J. C., R. D. Kent, and L. L. LaPointe, "Apraxia of speech: An overview and some perspectives. In J. C. Rosenbeck, M. R. McNeil, and A. E. Aronson (Eds.), *Apraxia of Speech: Physiology, Acoustics, Linguistics Management* (pp. 1–72). San Diego, Calif.: College-Hill Press, 1984.

Ruscello, D. M., "The importance of word position in articulation therapy." *Language, Speech, and Hearing Services in Schools, 6* (1975): 190–196.

Ruscello, D., "Motor learning as a model for articulation instruction." In J. Costello (Ed.), *Speech Disorders in Children.* San Diego, Calif.: College-Hill Press, 1984.

Ruscello, D., and R. Shelton, "Planning and self-assessment in articulatory training." *Journal of Speech and Hearing Disorders, 44* (1979): 504–512.

Rvachew, S., "Speech perception training can facilitate sound production learning." *Journal of Speech and Hearing Research, 37* (1994): 347–357.

Savin, H. B., "What the child knows about speech when he starts to learn to read." In J. F. Kavanaugh, and I. G. Mattingly (Eds.), *The Relationships Between Speech and Reading.* Cambridge, Mass.: M.I.T. Press, 1972.

Schrader, M., *Picture Pairs.* San Antonio, Tex.: Communication Skill Builders, 1987.

Schrader, M., *More Picture Pairs.* San Antonio, Tex.: Communication Skill Builders, 1989.

Schwartz, R. G., "Clinical applications of recent advances in phonological theory." *Language, Speech, and Hearing Services in Schools, 23* (1992): 269–276.

Scripture, M. K., and E. Jackson, *A Manual of Exercises for the Correction of Speech Disorders.* Philadelphia, Penn.: F. A. Davis, 1927.

Secord, W., "The traditional approach to treatment." In N. Creaghead, P. Newman, and W. Secord (Eds.), *Assessment and Remediation of Articulatory and Phonological Disorders.* Columbus, Ohio: Charles E. Merrill, 1989.

Shelton, R., "Disorders of articulation." In P. Skinner, and R. Shelton (Eds.), *Speech, Language, and Hearing.* Reading, Mass.: Addison-Wesley, 1978.

Shelton, R. L., A. F. Johnson, and W. B. Arndt, "Monitoring and reinforcement by parents as a means of automating articulatory responses." *Perceptual and Motor Skills, 35* (1972): 759–767.

Shelton, R. L., A. F. Johnson, V. Willis, and W. B. Arndt, "Monitoring and reinforcement by parents as a means of automating articulatory responses: II. Study of pre-school children." *Perceptual and Motor Skills, 40* (1975): 599–610.

Shelton, R., A. Johnson, and W. Arndt, "Delayed judgment speech-sound discrimination and /r/ or /s/ articulation status and improvement." *Journal of Speech and Hearing Research, 20* (1977): 704–717.

Shriberg, L., "A response evocation program for /ɝ/." *Journal of Speech and Hearing Disorders, 40* (1975): 92–105.

Shriberg, L. D., and J. Kwiatkowski, "A retrospective study of spontaneous generalization in speech-delayed children." *Language, Speech and Hearing Services in Schools, 18* (1987): 144–157.

Shriberg, L. D., and J. Kwiatkowski, "Self-monitoring and generalization in preschool speech-delayed children." *Language, Speech and Hearing Services in Schools, 21* (1990): 157–170.

Shriberg, L. D., and J. Kwiatkowski, "Phonological disorders III: A procedure for assessing severity of involvement." *Journal of Speech and Hearing Disorders, 47* (1982): 256–270.

Smit, A. B., and J. Bernthal, "Voicing contrasts and their phonological implications in the speech of articulation-disordered children." *Journal of Speech and Hearing Research, 26* (1983): 19–28.

Sommers, R. K., "Factors in the effectiveness of mothers trained to aid in speech correction." *Journal of Speech and Hearing Disorders, 27* (1962): 178–186.

Sommers, R. K., "The therapy program." In R. Van Hattum (Ed.), *Clinical Speech in the Schools.* Springfield, Ill.: Charles C Thomas, 1969.

Sommers, R. K., A. K. Furlong, F. H. Rhodes, G. R. Fichter, D. C. Bowser, F. H. Copetas, and Z. G. Saunders, "Effects of maternal attitudes upon improvement in articulation when mothers are trained to assist in speech correction." *Journal of Speech and Hearing Disorders, 29* (1964): 126–132.

Sommers, R. K., M. H. Schaeffer, R. H. Leiss, A. J. Gerber, M. A. Bray, D. Fundrella, J. K. Olson, and E. R. Tomkins, "The effectiveness of group and individual therapy." *Journal of Speech and Hearing Research, 9* (1966): 219–225.

Stackhouse, J., "Phonological awareness: Connecting speech and literacy problems." In B. Hodson and M. Edwards (Eds.), *Perspectives in Applied Phonology* (pp. 157–196). Gaithersburg, Md.: Aspen Publishers, Inc., 1997.

Stoel-Gammon, C., and C. Dunn, *Normal and Disordered Phonology in Children.* Baltimore, Md.: University Park Press, 1985.

Stokes, T. F., and D. M. Baer, "An implicit technology of generalization." *Journal of Applied Behavior Analysis, 10* (1977): 349–367.

Swank, L., "Phonological coding abilities: Identification of impairments related to phonologically based reading problems." *Topics in Language Disorders, 14* (1994): 56–71.

Torgeson, J., and B. Bryant, *Phonological Awareness Training for Reading.* Austin, Tex.: PRO-ED, 1993.

Tyler, A., M. Edwards, and J. Saxman, "Acoustic validation of phonological knowledge and its relationship to treatment." *Journal of Speech and Hearing Disorders, 55* (1990): 251–261.

Tyler, A. A., and K. T. Sandoval, "Preschoolers with phonological and language disorders: Treating different linguistic domains." *Language, Speech, and Hearing Services in Schools, 25* (1994): 215–234.

Van Hattum, R. J., "Program scheduling." In R. Van Hattum (Ed.), *Clinical Speech in the Schools.* Springfield, Ill.: Charles C Thomas, 1969.

van Kleeck, A., "Emphasizing form and meaning repeatedly in prereading and early reading instruction." *Topics in Language Disorders, 16* (1995): 27–49.

Van Riper, C., *Speech Correction: Principles and Methods.* Englewood Cliffs, N.J.: Prentice-Hall, 1939.

Van Riper, C., *Speech Correction: Principles and Methods,* 6th ed. Englewood Cliffs, N.J.: Prentice-Hall, 1978.

Van Riper, C., and L. Emerick, *Speech Correction: An Introduction to Speech Pathology and Audiology.* Englewood Cliffs, N.J.: Prentice-Hall, 1984.

Van Riper, C., and R. Erickson, *Speech Correction: An Introduction to Speech Pathology and Audiology,* 9th ed. Englewood Cliffs, N.J.: Prentice-Hall, 1996.

Velleman, S., and K. Strand, "Developmental verbal dyspraxia." In J. Bernthal, and N. Bankson (Eds.), *Child Phonology: Characteristics, Assessment, and Intervention with Special Populations* (pp. 110–139). New York: Thieme Publishers, 1994.

Weaver-Spurlock, S., and J. Brasseur, "Position training on the generalization training of [s]." *Language, Speech, and Hearing Services in Schools, 19* (1988): 259–271.

Weber, J., "Patterning of deviant articulation behavior." *Journal of Speech and Hearing Disorders, 35* (1970): 135–141.

Webster, P. E., and A. S. Plante, "Effects of phonological impairment on word, syllable, and phoneme segmentation and reading." *Language, Speech, and Hearing Services in Schools, 23* (1992): 176–182.

Weiner, F., "Treatment of phonological disability using the method of meaningful minimal contrast: Two case studies." *Journal of Speech and Hearing Disorders, 46* (1981): 97–103.

Weiner, F., and N. Bankson, "Teaching features." *Language, Speech, and Hearing Services in Schools, 9* (1978): 29–34.

Weismer, G., D. Dinnsen, and M. Elbert, "A study of the voicing distinction associated with omitted, word-final stops." *Journal of Speech and Hearing Disorders, 46* (1981): 91–103.

Weston, A. J., and J. V. Irwin, "Use of paired-stimuli in modification of articulation." *Perceptual and Motor Skills, 32* (1971): 947–957.

Williams, A. L., "Generalization patterns associated with training least phonological knowledge." *Journal of Speech and Hearing Research, 34* (1991): 722–733.

Williams, G., and L. V. McReynolds, "The relationship between discrimination and articulation training in children with misarticulation." *Journal of Speech and Hearing Research, 18* (1975): 401–412.

Winitz, H., *Articulatory Acquisition and Behavior.* Englewood Cliffs, N.J.: Prentice-Hall, 1969.

Winitz, H., *From Syllable to Conversation.* Baltimore, Md.: University Park Press, 1975.

Winitz, H., "Auditory considerations in articulation training." In H. Winitz (Ed.), *Treating Articulation Disorders for Clinicians by Clinicians.* Baltimore, Md.: University Park Press, 1984.

Wolfe, V. I., S. D. Blocker, and N. J. Prater, "Articulatory generalization in two word-medial and ambisyllabic contexts." *Language, Speech, and Hearing Services in Schools, 19* (1988): 251–258.

$$Chapter \quad 9$$

Instrumentation in Clinical Phonology

JULIE J. MASTERSON,
Southwest Missouri State University

STEVEN H. LONG,
Case Western Reserve University

EUGENE H. BUDER,
University of Memphis

The widespread availability and use of computers has had an impact on the manner in which both clinicians and researchers are able to analyze phonological samples. In this chapter we discuss two basic types of computer-based instrumentation. The first is computerized phonological analysis (CPA), in which the clinician or researcher enters keyboard characters that represent the target and phonetic forms for the words included in a sample and then performs various analyses on these data. The second is computerized acoustic phonetic analyses (CAPA), in which the speech signal itself is input into the computer for analysis. Both of these technologies can be of great benefit to both clinicians and researchers who are interested in phonological analysis.

Computerized Phonological Analysis

Talking with speech-language pathologists over the years, we have heard various descriptions of a dream for clinical technology. In this dream a clinician records a speech sample from a child, drops the tape into a sleek hi-tech box, presses a few buttons, and then collects a printed phonetic transcript and analysis of phonological patterns. Regrettably, this IS only a dream and we have little idea when, if ever, it will be realized. In the meantime, clinicians should become aware of **computerized phonological analysis** (CPA) methods that do exist and the different ways in which they work. This knowledge will help practitioners to make wise consumer decisions in acquiring computer hardware and software and to make appropriate clinical use of the available technology.

A number of advantages have been claimed for CPA, but two stand out above the others: (1) it saves time, and (2) it provides greater detail of analysis. Clinicians usually have large caseloads, and it is impossible to spend several hours analyzing samples from each client. Some CPA packages can derive a phonetic inventory and perform a substitution and phonological rules analysis on a 400-word sample in less than a minute. Although some time is required for data entry, this leaves most of the clinician's time available for interpreting results and planning appropriate therapy, two things that a computer alone cannot do.

To organize our discussion of CPA, we have identified five parameters by which various programs can be evaluated and judged. These are: (1) method of data entry, (2) method of data processing, (3) options for output of analyses, (4) hardware requirements, and (5) documentation and support. From the consumer's perspective, these five features largely determine whether a program is affordable, practical to use, and yields analyses that are clinically valuable.

In our discussion of these five issues, we will refer to seven currently available CPA packages. These are Automatic Articulation Analysis Plus (AAAP) (Weiner, 1993, 1995); Computer Analysis of Phonological Processes Version 1.0 (CAPP) (Hodson, 1985); Computerized Profiling (CP) (Long and Fey, 1993); Interactive System for Phonological Analysis (ISPA) (Masterson and Pagan, 1993); Logical International Phonetic Programs Version 1.03 (LIPP) (Oller and Delgado, 1990); Pye Analysis of Language Version 2.0 (PAL) (Pye, 1987); and Programs to Examine Phonetic and Phonologic Evaluation Records Version 4.0 (PEPPER) (Shriberg, 1986).

Data Entry

From the user's perspective, a critical feature of any CPA program is its scheme of data entry. This scheme determines, in large part, how easy the software is to learn and to use. Below we discuss some of the variables in organizing data entry among the different CPA programs.

Phonetic Characters

CPA software must provide a means for inputting phonetic transcriptions from a computer keyboard, displaying this data on the screen, and printing the transcriptions on paper. Microcomputers can be programmed to work with either text characters (letters and numbers) or graphics. In the past, text programs were simpler to create and required less hardware to operate than graphics programs; however, this difference has lessened in recent years. All Macintosh computers run graphics programs and virtually all PC computers produced since 1990 will run them.

Text characters are entered by pressing keys on the keyboard and are represented on the screen and on paper by a set of codes stored in the machine. The limitations of text programming for CPA software are that (1) not all IPA characters and diacritics are available as text characters, and (2) characters must be displayed in a left-to-right sequence. This left-to-right display does not permit diacritics to be positioned above, below, or to the upper right of sound segments. Text programs for CPA (PAL, CP for PC computers) get around these limitations by substituting available characters for those IPA symbols that are not available (e.g., the schwa vowel may be represented with the symbol @). Diacritics are always placed to the right of the consonant or vowel segments they modify. To operate a program written in this way, the user must learn an alternate system of phonetic representation and be able to switch back and forth between this system and the IPA. At first, there is likely to be some confusion and mental effort, which decreases as the user becomes more familiar with the other transcriptional system.

Graphics programs for CPA (ISPA, LIPP, PEPPER, AAAP, CP for Macintosh) use special fonts to represent all IPA symbols. The standard method for inputting phonetic symbols is to retain all the key-to-symbol correspondences that exist on the computer keyboard (e.g., typing a lower-case *p* inputs the symbol for a voiceless bilabial stop) and to use unique key combinations for entering all other symbols (e.g., holding down the Control key while typing *s* may produce the symbol for a voiceless palatal fricative /ʃ/). The user must learn the keyboard mapping scheme of the software, and touch typing may be somewhat difficult because of the need to press more than one key simultaneously.

Correspondence Between Target and Production Forms

Substitution and omission analyses are accomplished by comparing target sounds with transcriptions of a client's productions. CPA software must be able to determine "what corresponds to what." For example, if [ti] was produced for the target /klin/, the program must recognize that the target cluster /kl/ was realized as [t], the target was vowel /i/ as [i], and the /n/ was omitted.

Software must either establish correspondences between target sounds and production forms or rely on the user to specify the correspondences. If the user is to specify the correspondences, the data must be entered in a format that somehow indicates the boundaries of phonological units in both the target and production forms. One way to accomplish this is to require that the two forms be vertically aligned. For example, in the case of /smok/ → [mot] the forms are entered as:

TARGET: smok
PRODUCTION: mot

In this format, used by programs such as ISPA and LIPP, target and production units can be compared column by column in order to determine which sounds have changed and which have been produced correctly (e.g., /sm/ → [m], /o/ produced correctly, /k/ → [t]).

CP determines correspondences automatically by identifying the vowels in a string of sounds and then considering everything else to be a consonant. For example, in the case of /wægən/ → [wædə], the program can scan both the target and production forms for vowels:

TARGET: wægən
                  V V
PRODUCTION: wædə
                  V V

All other segments are then identified as consonants and the two forms are aligned in accordance with their vowels:

TARGET: wægən
               CVCVC
PRODUCTION: wædə
               CVCV

If the program finds that the number of vowels in the target and production forms differ, it will know that a change in syllable structure has occurred (e.g., "weak syllable deletion") or that a mistake was made in data entry.

This need for one-to-one correspondence between target forms and production forms poses several difficulties for computer-aided phonological analysis. One difficulty occurs when consonants are deleted or added. For example, when clusters are reduced, it must be decided which segment(s) are deleted. If /ski/ was produced as [ti], both user-determined and automatic methods of correspondence establishment would identify cluster reduction. However, the classification of the error as stopping or fronting would depend upon whether correspondence was established between [t] and /s/ or [t] and /k/. This, in turn, might lead to slightly different judgments about the nature of a client's phonological difficulties.

Another problem inherent in segmental comparisons is the occurrence of errors that are not based upon segment-to-segment relationships. For example, in coalescence, features of each consonant in the cluster are included in a third consonant that is substituted for the entire cluster, such as /slip/ → [fip]. Segmental comparison would count one segment as deleted and might not even recognize the relationship between the remaining cluster member and the substituted sound.

Every CPA program contains a set of definitions (which may or may not be modifiable) for determining phonological rules. These definitions are often stated in terms of specific segmental substitution patterns. For example, a program may count any occurrence of a /k/ → [t] substitution as fronting of velars. Occasionally, this approach can be misleading. A child might produce /kot/ as [tot] because of alveolar assimilation rather than velar fronting. Velars produced in words that did not contain alveolar targets would be produced correctly if the pattern was alveolar assimilation. Many programs will count such an error as assimilation but will also count it as an occurrence of velar fronting. If results are offered only in terms of percentages, the user may misinterpret the child's phonological pattern. Programs such as PEPPER and ISPA count this substitution as an example of both fronting and assimilation. These programs output all words that have been classified as being affected by a particular process. The user can then determine whether the classifications are appropriate.

Single-Word or Connected Speech
CPA software can allow data to be entered either as single words or connected speech. Both methods can analyze data elicited as single words or connected speech; however, each method approaches the task in a different manner. For instance, in single-word programs such as ISPA, data from a standardized single-word articulation test are entered word by word:

ENTRY 1	horse
PHONETIC TARGET:	hors
TRANSCRIPTION:	hot

ENTRY 2	pig
PHONETIC TARGET:	pɪg
TRANSCRIPTION:	pɪd

Data from a connected speech sample are entered as a series of single words. The sentence *Goats eat hay* would be entered in the following manner:

ENTRY 1	goats
PHONETIC TARGET:	gots
TRANSCRIPTION:	dots

ENTRY 2	eat
PHONETIC TARGET:	it
TRANSCRIPTION:	it

ENTRY 3	hay
PHONETIC TARGET:	he
TRANSCRIPTION:	he

In connected speech programs, such as PEPPER and CP, words from an articulation test can be entered as a single item and placed on one line:

ENTRY 1	horse	pig	clock	host	yellow	block
PHONETIC TARGET:	hors	pɪg	klak	gost	jɛlo	blak
TRANSCRIPTION:	ho t	pɪd	k ak	gos	jɛwo	b at

Similarly, data from a spontaneous speech sample are entered as follows for a connected speech program:

ENTRY 1	He	raises	horses
PHONETIC TARGET:	hi	rezɪz	horsɪz
TRANSCRIPTION:	hi	redɪ	hortɪ

The sentence must be broken up and treated as a series of individual items when using a program designed to analyze single words.

ENTRY 1	He
PHONETIC TARGET:	hi
TRANSCRIPTION:	hi

ENTRY 2	raises
PHONETIC TARGET:	rezɪz
TRANSCRIPTION:	redɪ

ENTRY 3   horses
TARGET: horsɪz
TRANSCRIPTION: hortɪ

To our knowledge, none of the programs on the market analyze rules that operate across word boundaries (though LIPP has the potential to do so). Thus, even a program designed to allow connected speech input ultimately segments each sentence into individual words and performs the analysis based on word-to-word comparisons. A connected speech program is advantageous only in that it maintains the integrity of the utterances as they were transcribed.

Closed versus Open Set of Targets

CPA software is designed either to handle a specific set of targets (*closed set*) or to allow users to enter their own targets (*open set*). If the software employs a closed set, it may not allow missing data (null responses); that is, the clinician must obtain a response for every item in the data set or else the program will not yield accurate analyses.

CAPP and AAAP are examples of CPA programs that work only with a closed set of targets. Because the targets do not change from one analysis to the next, the programs operate with a smaller set of variables, which leads to faster data output. For example, the segmentation of each target into individual sounds can be stored in the program so that the information is already available for data analysis. In addition, analyses based on phonetic or feature classes are greatly simplified because the program will "know" which word items are relevant to a particular analysis. If the program contains a closed set of 75 words and only items 9, 16, 33, 37, 48, and 64 contain velar consonants, then only these items need to be examined for velar substitution and velar fronting.

In summary, closed-set programs have the advantage of being easy to learn and operate. Closed-set programs may also output data faster than open-set programs; however, the availability of rapid processors, such as the PowerPC and Pentium chips, have minimized the differences in speed between the two types of programs. The disadvantages of using closed-set programs are that (1) the stimulus set available in the program may not be appropriate for a given client; (2) the limited number of stimuli may not allow for an adequate sample; (3) they usually require a complete set of production forms, which may be difficult to obtain; and (4) they cannot be used to analyze connected speech. A sample collected from spontaneous conversation can be analyzed only with an open-set program.

Time-Saving Features

As the previous examples show, CPA data entry involves at least two and sometimes three types of entries: the *gloss* (orthographic) form, the *target* (phonetic) form, and the *production* (phonetic) form. Program features that automatically supply one or more of these items can result in considerable time savings.

If a program works with a closed set of targets, the target forms are embedded in the program and are not modifiable. If, however, the program allows an open set of target forms, it stores these forms on disk. This feature allows the user to create files consisting of gloss and/or target forms for use with different clients.

Some CPA programs, such as LIPP and CP, include a phonetic dictionary that contains pairs of gloss and target forms. The user enters the orthographic forms of the words produced in a sample and the program looks up the corresponding target forms in the dictionary. If a word is not in the dictionary, the user must enter the phonetic target. The requirement to enter the phonetic target is likely to slow down the data entry process significantly.

Data Processing

All CPA programs perform a **relational** (substitution and omission) **analysis** and many perform an **independent** (catalogue of phonetic productions) **analysis** as well. The manner in which these analyses are done varies because of differences in program assumptions or models. In the paragraphs that follow, four such assumptions are discussed.

The Structural Unit

The structural unit of phonological analysis is either the syllable or the word. CPA software will analyze sound positions in words and consonant clusters differently depending upon which structural unit is employed. For example, as shown here, the words *grandma*, *spoonful*, and *airplane* all contain adjacent consonants that would be analyzed as medial consonant clusters by PEPPER and CAPP, which use the word as the basic structural unit.

grændma	spunfʊl	ɛrplen
-CCC-	-CC-	-CC-

If the syllable is assumed to be the structural unit, as in CP, the consonants are classified as initial, medial, and final singletons, or clusters, based on their position in the syllable:

grænd ma	spun fʊl	ɛr plen
-CC C-	-C C-	-CC-

A word-based structure allows a programmer to use straightforward logic: Consonants at the beginning of a word are identified as initial, those at the end of a word as final, and all others as medial. In contrast, a syllable-based structure requires *phonotactic* information (sound sequences that are permitted in English). ISPA, for instance, consults a list of "allowable" consonant clusters whenever a word-medial sequence of consonants is encountered. If a sequence is not on the list but consists of more than two consonants, then a search commences to find any juxtaposed sounds that are on the list. For example:

græ ndma	sequence of consonants [ndm] found;
[ndm] not on list;	[nd] on list
græ nd ma	word sequenced as shown

Another syllable-based program, CP, leaves the decision up to the user. A juncture symbol is entered that causes the program to separate units appropriately. For instance, if the word *grasshopper* is entered as

TARGET: græs+hapɚ
PRODUCTION: gwæs+hapɚ

the program would analyze the sound changes in /græ s/ → [gwæ s] and /hapɚ/ → [hapɚ].

It is crucial to learn, by reading the documentation and experimenting with data files, whether the CPA software is syllable or word based. If the program makes segmentation decisions automatically, the user should take special note of multisyllabic word targets. If the program treats all word-medial consonants as medial position, the user can work around this limitation by entering portions of the target as separate items. For example: *butterfly* could be entered as two entries: (1) *butter*, (2) *fly*. This tactic will work as long as the user segments the production form correctly and remembers that any statistics based upon word counts will be inflated.

Operation of Multiple Rules

Some sound changes reflect the operation of more than one phonological rule. For example, a clinician might find a child who produces /slip/ as [tip]. The initial sound change, from a cluster to a stop, can be interpreted as resulting from two underlying processes: one that reduces clusters to singletons (cluster reduction) and one that substitutes stops for fricatives. Ideally, CPA software should be able to identify such instances of multiple-step sound changes.

Phonological rule identification can be accomplished in more than one way. In the simplest method, which applies only to sound substitutions, a program will search for all the substitution patterns that serve as manifestations of a particular phonological pattern. For example, a program can identify instances of velar fronting by locating the following substitutions: /ŋ/ → [n], /k/ → [t], /g/ → [d] (other substitutions also might be included /ŋ/ → [d], /k/ → [d], etc., depending on how the process is defined). This method, used in CP, is effective in detecting single-step patterns of substitution or omission. However, it may not identify sound changes that occur as a result of more than one rule. It is possible to assign definitions for two-step patterns. For instance, a program could search for /ʃ/ → [t] and always categorize it as an instance of palatal fronting and stopping. One might be dissatisfied with this interpretation, however, unless there was evidence that these two processes were operating independently in other substitution patterns. The program would need to cross-check other patterns in the data, which becomes a formidable programming task. In another method, used in ISPA and LIPP, the program works from a featural description of each phone and a featural description of the phonological rule (e.g., velar → alveolar). Rule identification then occurs in two steps: First, the program scans the target forms for phones that match the featural description (e.g., all velar sounds); then the program scans the corresponding production forms for a match with the other term in the featural description (e.g., all alveolar sounds). In this manner a segment can serve as an opportunity for multiple rules and a substitution can be counted as representing more than one rule. For example, final /g/ in the word *log* is classified as a velar and thus an opportunity for fronting; a final consonant and therefore, an opportunity for final consonant deletion; and a voiced segment and thus an opportunity for devoicing of final consonants. This method does allow the determination of multiple-step rules but has the disadvantage of potentially inflating percentages of occurrence for individual rules.

Clearly, both methods have associated pros and cons. Clinicians should remember that the purpose of CPA software is to organize the data in a way that aids interpretation. It is not surprising that a given program may not perform the organization and interpretation in a manner that suits all users. The key to using CPA software effectively is to recognize the prescribed organization. Multiply determined sound simplifications are a good example. If these are not analyzed, then the user should find out what the program does with them. If such sound simplifications are listed in a general category such as "Idiosyncratic" or "Other" substitutions, it is possible for the user to complete the analytical work.

User-Determined Processing

Clinicians have their own needs and preferences in phonological assessment and analysis. If these preferences are not met by a specific CPA program, then the user must either adapt to the program or modify the software.

Modifications of a program may range from customizing the output to altering the basic decisions made in the program. Users may wish to change terminology in the output so that it conforms to their preferences. For example, one might prefer "plosive" to "stop," "cluster" to "blend," or "liquid simplification" to "gliding." Clinicians also may wish to re-define certain categories. For example, a user may want to exclude the omission of postvo-calic liquids in the analysis of final consonant deletion.

The simplest way to create an open design for CPA software is to organize the program so that selected variables are stored on disk and loaded each time the program is run. It is then possible for the user either to modify variables directly (e.g., by editing them with a word processor) or by means of a utility module. Programs that allow for this kind of user input, such as LIPP and CP, are more difficult to create because they must ensure that the user cannot inadvertently crash the program as modifications are made. Modifications of any program should always be done on a working copy of the master program disk(s). Hence, no user-modifiable program should be copy protected.

Speed

One of the principal reasons for using CPA software is the potential for saving time. Compared to analysis by hand, all CPA software will provide greater efficiency. The speed of a program is the product of factors related to both hardware and software. The language in which a program is written will have some effect on how quickly it will run. All recent programs are compiled, however, which tends to minimize such speed differences.

The speed of a computer's microprocessor will determine the rate at which a program's instructions are executed. As improved microprocessors have been developed, they have been incorporated into newer model microcomputers. In some instances it is possible to enhance performance of an older microcomputer by adding accelerator boards that contain the newer microprocessor.

The speed of input/output operations may be of little or great consequence, depending on the design of a particular CPA program. If the program performs a large number of disk operations, such as reading in data and variables, storing data in temporary files, and writing the program output to a disk file, then more efficient input/output will have a significant effect. The greatest variable in input/output is the speed with which the disk drives operate. A hard disk drive will perform much faster than a floppy drive. RAM disks or RAM caches—bits of electronic memory that simulate a mechanical disk drive—will also improve speed, though they also carry the risk of information loss in the event of a power outage or machine malfunction.

The user can be given some control over the speed of an analysis by organizing a program so that its various analyses (phonetic inventory, correspondence, rule structure, etc.) are performed in a series of independent operations. The user can then select which of the analyses are to be done and eliminate time spent on unwanted analyses. PEPPER, LIPP, CP, and ISPA all offer the user this kind of control.

Users should consider the issue of speed in relation to their own time requirements and work habits. CPA software might be used with the intention of rapidly analyzing test data so that results can be interpreted and presented to clients. In this case, speed is a very important requirement and may even outweigh other considerations in the selection of a program. On the other hand, when the primary purpose of CPA software is to gain greater detail of analysis, speed of execution is less significant.

If speed is important, the user might consider enhancement through hardware upgrades. The cost of a hard disk drive or accelerator board may be small compared to the improved efficiency it can bring to a frequently used program.

Output

The types of output available and the format in which they may be viewed are important considerations for CPA software. Optimally, output should be under the control of the user and permit querying of results. It should be possible to have the results shown only on the screen, printed, or stored in a disk file.

User Control

The kinds of analyses available are important features for CPA packages that offer several different types. For example, some programs offer phonetic, substitution, and rules analyses. The user may not need all of these analyses, and the option to select only the ones desired is, therefore, valuable.

Querying of Results

Many times clinicians will examine preliminary results from the phonetic or rules analysis and desire additional information. For example, they may want to query the data for selected subsets of the findings, such as substitutions or phonological rules that occurred in specific phonetic contexts or under phonotactic constraints. Users may want to look at all words in which a certain substitution was used or in which a certain target phoneme or feature occurred. They may also be interested in examining groups of words in which a particular rule was potentially operative. Upon selection of one of the subsets, the availability of further analysis options (e.g., effects of phonetic environment) may assist the user in determining the contexts in which the rules or substitutions occur. ISPA and CP are examples of programs that allow such queries to be made.

Storage of Results

CPA software should allow users to output results to a monitor, printer, or disk files. If data output are in graphic mode, screen and printer compatibility are important. Analysis results stored on a disk are particularly beneficial because they can be imported by most word processing programs and included in reports, IEPs, manuscripts, and the like. LIPP, ISPA, and CP all provide the option of disk file output.

Hardware Requirements and Cost

Most current CPA packages are designed to run on IBM-compatible or Macintosh microcomputers. A few versions remain that run on the Apple II series (II, IIe, IIc, IIGS). There is a range of prices for phonological analysis programs and, as with many other products, a high cost does not ensure a quality program or one that is well suited to an individual clinician's needs. Cost and features, therefore, must be evaluated by each potential user. The expense involved with a software package includes more than just the cost of the package. Some programs may involve special hardware components, and the cost of these should be considered.

Documentation and Support

Documentation and support are often referred to as hidden considerations in software evaluation because they are so easily overlooked. The clarity and thoroughness of the manual, the provision of a tutorial program, and the availability of technical support are all important program features.

The Manual

Adequate documentation for a computer program is essential. The level of knowledge expected from the user should be clearly stated, and the manual should be written accordingly. Most manuals assume at least a basic familiarity with phonological analysis and include few suggestions about collection and preliminary transcription of the sample. These manuals typically provide basic information on how to use the software to facilitate analyses with which users are already familiar. Thus, these manuals will not contain information about the theoretical background or applicability of phonological analysis. However, because the definitions of specific rules may vary from one researcher to another, all manuals should state the program's criteria for assigning phonological rules.

The manual also should contain straightforward instructions for operating the software. This should include definitions and functions associated with each menu choice. Examples of option sequences used to perform various analyses should be provided. The user should not have to wade through a lot of information before understanding the basic operation of the program.

Tutorial Program

A tutorial program is another desirable component of a software package. The tutorial is designed to walk the user through the operation of the program, and this hands-on experience often makes subsequent use more easily understood. PEPPER, LIPP, CP, and ISPA offer tutorials. Each describes a series of steps that produce various analyses of interest.

Technical Support
The price of software makes it a substantial investment. All packages should include an address and telephone number in case additional support is needed. The provision of adequate technical support to registered purchasers is one way that software developers have hoped to discourage illegal software copying.

Summary

Table 9.1 provides short descriptions of several CPA programs that are currently available. Each program is considered in terms of the symbols used, level of phonetic transcription allowed, data set, method for handling multiple rules, analysis unit, incorporation of a phonetic dictionary, user-modifiable features, output devices, copy protection schemes, and hardware requirements.

CPA software offers numerous benefits to the clinician. The savings in time are accompanied by a depth of analysis that may otherwise be difficult to achieve. Although there are problems inherent to CPA, most can be overcome by awareness and good judgment on the part of the user. We have tried to illustrate the power and desirability of CPA software while at the same time emphasizing the clinician's responsibility for accurate data entry and interpretation of results. The microcomputer can be a very rapid counter and efficient organizer, but it offers little flexibility. Thus, CPA software can function only as an aide to the professional who must make the decisions about the status of a client's phonological system.

Computerized Acoustic Phonetic Analysis

Though still not in widespread regular use by clinicians, **computerized acoustic phonetic analysis** (CAPA) can provide useful information in the assessment and treatment of phonological and articulatory disorders. Visual displays and quantitative measures of digitized speech samples can facilitate transcription of samples, help distinguish phonological from articulatory disorders on a subperceptual level, support the assessment and diagnosis of disorders, aid treatment (via visual feedback, as with such systems as SpeechViewer II by IBM Corp. and Video Voice by Micro Video), and provide records for tracking efficacy and documenting functional outcomes.

Historically available only in well-funded and sophisticated laboratories and employed by research scientists, CAPA can now be performed on standard-issue desktop or even laptop microcomputers using a variety of commercially available software programs. With the advent of multimedia capability as a standard feature of microcomputers, digital sound acquisition and playback capability are the norms for most systems, and many current speech analysis programs make use of these features. By supplementing the cost of basic computer equipment by approximately $500, a clinician can perform acoustic phonetic analysis as a basic technique for understanding and managing articulation and phonological disorders.

TABLE 9.1 Features Available for Currently Available Computerized Phonological Analysis Programs

	AAAP	CAPP	PEPPER	ISPA	CP-Mac	CP-IBM	LIPP	PAL
Symbols	IPA[a]	transliterated	IPA	IPA	IPA	transliterated	IPA/user determined	transliterated
Level of representation	broad	broad	broad/ narrow	broad/ narrow	broad/ narrow	broad/ narrow	broad/ narrow superbroad	broad/ narrow
Data set	fixed	fixed	open	open	open	open	open	open
Multiple rules	no	no	no	yes	no	no	yes	no
Analysis unit	word	word	word	word/ syllable	word/ syllable	word/ syllable	user determined	word
Phonetic dictionary	no	no	no	no	yes	yes	yes	yes
User modifiable features	no	no	num./type of analyses	num./type of analyses; keyboard[b]	num. of analyses; keyboard[b]	num./type of analyses; rule defs.	num./type of analyses[d]; keyboard	no
Output devices	monitor printer[a]	monitor printer	monitor[c] printer disk file	monitor printer disk file	monitor printer disk file	monitor printer disk file	monitor printer disk file	monitor printer disk file
Hardware requirements	Apple II 1 floppy	IBM/com; hard drive	IBM/com; 640K RAM; 2 floppy drives or hard drive; Math proc. specific monitors, printers	Mac Plus or higher; floppy or hard drive	Mac Plus or higher; hard drive	IBM/com 256K RAM; 2 floppy drives or hard drives	IBM/com 640K RAM; EGA/VGA; mouse	IBM/com 256K RAM; floppy or hard drive

[a]Printed output uses transliteration, not IPA symbols.
[b]Keyboard remapped with MacroMaker files.
[c]Reports appear sideways on the monitor.
[d]Available only with Upper LIPP.

Because technical and budgetary constraints are no longer major stumbling blocks to the use of computerized acoustic phonetic analysis (CAPA), the infusion of this technique into clinical practice is now more easily accomplished. What are some of the best goals for applications of CAPA? How can these goals be achieved with some sense of security that the methods are sound? These questions have become acute with the increased availability of the software programs. Unfortunately, though some answers to these questions are becoming clearer, both questions remain unresolved. In fact, vigorous debate over the relevance and accurate application of acoustic analysis to speech and language disorders in general can be found in the pages of journals like the *Journal of Speech and Hearing Research* and the *Journal of the Acoustical Society of America*. For example, various and sometimes contrasting perspectives on coarticulation and its development are provided by researchers using different acoustic analysis frameworks (compare, e.g., Hodge, 1989; Nittrouer, Studdert-Kennedy, and McGowan, 1989; Sussman, Minifie, Buder, Stoel-Gammon, and Smith, 1996). Furthermore, some long-standing acoustic measures that seemed easy to apply to correlates of pathology, such as the perturbation measurements for voice disorders, have become increasingly suspect, both on technical grounds regarding issues of calibration (Green, Buder, Rodda, and Moore, 1997; Titze, 1995), and on interpretive grounds such as the problem of finding perceptual correlates (Rabinov, Kreiman, Gerratt, and Bielamowicz, 1995). Nonetheless, excellent data on speech parameters (e.g., formant frequencies, durations, f_0, intensity, etc.) and their variability have been gathered for normal phonologies in children and adults (Eguchi and Hirsh, 1969; Kent and Forner, 1979; Smith, 1978), and the scope of such studies is now rapidly increasing.

The main goal of this section will be to identify some of the chief benefits and difficulties of using modern microcomputer-based acoustic analysis programs. By touching on some desirable basic capabilities and analyses afforded by such programs, this section should also assist the reader in selecting a program. It is not within the scope of this chapter to provide a thorough introduction to modern acoustic phonetic analysis techniques; hence, it will be assumed that the reader has some familiarity with speech sound acoustics and the types of displays (such as spectrograms) of such speech sounds. Competence in acoustic analysis requires familiarity with such matters as the nature of sound as a pressure wave, the spectral components of periodic sounds (e.g., fundamental frequency and harmonics), and the features used to identify various resonances in the vocal tract that shape sound sources into acoustic features (e.g., formants and frequency centers of fricative and burst turbulence noises). Other texts are available for further study in acoustic or other instrumental analysis of speech; see, for example, Baken (1987) for clinical instrumentation in general and Kent and Read (1992) for acoustic phonetics in particular. Chapter 1 of this volume also provides useful background information (see especially the section on acoustic considerations).

Though often performed to validate perceptual observations, acoustic analysis can be especially valuable when used to distinguish articulatory patterns that may otherwise appear to be equivalent. This kind of analysis can show that what appears to be complete phoneme substitution may be only partially so. For example, the clinician may originally think that a child is employing initial consonant voicing. However, this may not be the case if the intruding consonant used for the voiceless target has a different voice onset time (VOT) than the target voiced consonant (Weismer, 1984). The monograph chapter by

Weismer (1984) is highly recommended for ideas on acoustic measures suitable for verifying the presence of acoustic features that are not easily perceived by the listener. As we will see, such investigations can provide a helpful perspective for distinguishing whether speech errors are predominantly phonological or articulatory in nature.

This section is designed to help guide clinicians and researchers toward making good recordings, digitizing samples, and analyzing and quantifying some of the basic acoustic parameters of speech samples. Specific examples will be illustrated for selected segmental and suprasegmental measures with applications in child phonology, and the illustrations will be developed using two of PC-based CAPA systems: CSL and CSpeechSP (see Table 9.2 for further information on these and other comparable systems).

Recordings

The number of ways in which recordings can be analyzed depends on the quality of the recording. Chapter 6 of this volume cites excellent recommendations by Allen (1984). Many measures can be performed on speech from basically adequate recordings, such as those made with a table or floor-standing microphone and a reasonably good quality audiocassette recorder. While even basic transcription is greatly facilitated with high-quality stereo recordings using microphones that are attached to the client or subject, the range of valid acoustic analysis measures is especially enhanced. We would, therefore, add to Allen's recommendations by suggesting the use of attachable microphones and high-quality recording equipment when available.

High quality can be obtained with audiocassettes but is usually superior with other media like DAT tapes or Hi Definition sound on videocassette. Though not so frequently considered for acoustic recordings, simultaneous video recording can assist with later glossing or transcribing or even for validation of orofacial posture during speech. Even the practice of recording directly to the hard drive of a microcomputer (a *digital* form of recording) is becoming reasonable because of inexpensive high-capacity storage devices and the widespread availability of sound input and output on computers.

Stereo sound can be achieved simply by also attaching a microphone to any therapist, family member (e.g., child's mother), or researcher who is also participating in a recording situation. This signal can then be sent to the unoccupied channel of the child's recording. Alternatively, the second channel can be taken from a room microphone. As Allen (1984) indicates, stereo is desirable for the improvement of intelligibility and comprehension because of many factors: binaural presentation assists the localization of sound, and it is also helpful to hear what other people in a conversation are saying in order to provide context for the transcription of disordered speech.

Attaching a microphone to the client helps for both transcription and analysis, chiefly by reducing the variations in intensity that come with varying microphone-source distances and also by reducing room noise and reverberation effects. Options include lavaliere microphones worn on clothing (which can be effective with children if hidden or sewn into the clothing) or headset microphones worn with a boom extending the microphone a certain distance from the lips (more reasonable with adults). The practice of attaching a microphone is especially valuable for small children, who may speak more in mobile free-play than when seated. Wireless microphones make this option feasible.

TABLE 9.2   A List of Speech Analysis Systems (adapted from Buder & Kent, 1995)

Systems for the PC	Systems for the Macintosh
CSL Kay Elemetrics Corp. 2 Bridgewater Lane Lincoln Park, NJ 07035-1488 USA Tel: 800 289-5297 (USA or Canada) or 201 628-6200 Fax: 201 628-6363	Signalyze InfoSignal Inc. C.P. 73, CH-1015 Lausanne, SWITZERLAND Fax: 41-21-691-1372 Email: 76357.1213@compuserve.com U.S. Distributor: Network Technology Corporation 91 Baldwin St. Charlestown, MA 02129 Tel: 617 241-9205 Fax: 617 241-5064
CSpeechSP Paul H. Milenkovic 118 Shiloh Dr. Madison, WI 53706 USA Tel: 608 833-7956	
CSRE AVAAZ Innovations, Inc. P.O. Box 8040 1225 Wonderland Rd. North London, Ontario N6G 2B0, CANADA Tel: 519 472-7944 Fax: 519 472-7814 Email: info@avaaz.com	SoundScope GW Instruments, Inc. 35 Medford St. Somerville, MA USA Tel: 617 625-4096 Fax: 617 625-1322 Email: d0268@appleLink.apple.com
SpeechStation Sensimetrics Corporation 26 Lansdowne St. Cambridge, MA 02139 USA Tel: 617 225-2442 Fax: 617 225-0470 Email: sensimetrics@sens.com	
Dr. Speech Tiger Electronics, Inc. P.O. Box 85126 Seattle, WA 98145 USA Tel: 206 499-5757 Fax: 206 367-2672	

Digitizing

Digitizing occurs when speech is transferred into the computer as an electrical signal, whether from a microphone or from the playback of a recording. (In fact, DAT tapes already record sounds as digitized data, and these recordings can sometimes then be passed directly into the computer as digital sound "files.") Basically, all speech sounds are originally pressure variations over time. There are, therefore, two continuous dimensions: time and pressure. Digitizing, whether by DAT or the computer, takes continuous (*analog*) quantities and "discretizes" them by reducing them to discrete (*digital*) quantities.

One way of understanding the difference between analog and digital is to consider that an analog number can have an infinite number of significant decimal places, while a digital number will always have a set, finite number of place columns. *Discretizing*, or selecting a digital number to represent an analog quantity, is done on both dimensions of the sound wave: (1) *time*, called sampling, and (2) *intensity*, called quantization. The main specification for time sampling is its rate, measured in Hz (frequency). The main specification for intensity is quantization, defined by the number of places in the digital number, measured in bits. The two specifications of sampling rate and quantization indicate how rapidly in time the digital samples are taken and how precisely the level of sound pressure is measured in that sample.

The bits specification (i.e., bits quantization) is usually optimal at about 15 or 16. Sixteen (16) bits allow 96 decibels (or 65,536 levels) of intensity to be coded. With this fine level of resolution, virtually all the relevant details of speech can be included. It is especially valuable to have this many levels of resolution in looking at fine variations in signals that are very low in intensity. For example, nonsibilant fricatives are usually extremely low in intensity, and 16-bit quantization is particularly valuable when digitizing this class of sounds.

It is the sampling rate specification—in kilohertz—that can be most critical for optimal analysis of child speech. A sampling rate of 44.1 kHz is considered "CD-quality" sound. Sampling rates store energy at frequencies up to about 20,000 Hz which is more than adequate for accurately representing speech.

Speech may be intelligible in very small frequency bands, as in telephone transmissions (e.g., 300–3,000 Hz), but complete acoustic analysis can only be performed in more full-frequency bands. In young children's speech, third formant frequencies can exceed 5 kHz and fricative energy is often 10 kHz or higher. A sampling rate of 22 kHz is likely to be adequate for most situations.

The range of frequencies in a signal becomes visible in a *spectrum analysis*, which breaks down the total intensity of a sound into its respective sinusoidal frequency component and creates a frequency-domain representation. The discrete Fourier transform is the most common means of obtaining a spectrum from digitized speech and is the usual basis for the power spectrum display as well as for the three-dimensional, time-varying spectrogram. Spectrograms can be used to compare frequency ranges of the same word spoken by persons of different gender and age, as in Figure 9.1, which displays four spectrograms with three different speakers saying the word "shoe" /ʃ/. This display is from the CSL system and contains panels (or "views") from a single screen display. (There is also a set of dropdown command menus across the top of the screen not included in this cropping). The range in each panel is 10 kHz. Panels A and B contain different views of the same word spoken by an adult man, and Panels C and D contain the word spoken by a woman and by a 30-month-old child, respectively.

To interpret a spectrographic display, the viewer must take into account the effective bandwidth of the analysis filter. To remind the reader of the basic effect of bandwidth of analysis on the spectrogram, Panel A was calculated with a *narrowband* setting of 28 Hz (with many samples going into the Fourier transform), and Panel B was calculated with a

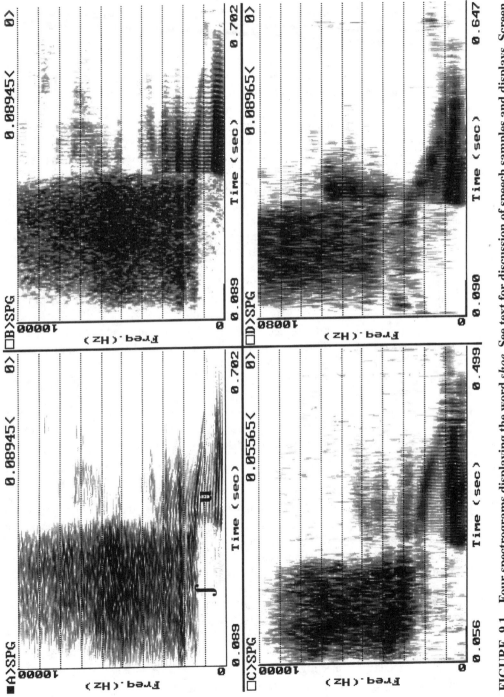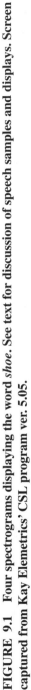

FIGURE 9.1 Four spectrograms displaying the word *shoe*. See text for discussion of speech samples and displays. Screen captured from Kay Elemetrics' CSL program ver. 5.05.

wideband setting of 146 Hz (fewer samples going into the Fourier transform). Panel A (the wideband) shows good frequency resolution of the harmonics in the periodic voiced speech, and Panel B (the narrowband) shows good temporal resolution of the glottal pulses in the voiced portion. It is important to understand bandwidth of analysis because it is dependent on f_0 and, therefore, age and gender. The distinction between what is "narrow" and what is "wide" is really best defined according to whether the harmonics or the glottal pulses are resolved rather than by a strict absolute number. The bandwidth of analysis in Hz that exceeds f_0 will be that bandwidth of analysis that becomes "wide" (e.g., 146 Hz for a low-pitched male voice as in Panel B), because this bandwidth will be broader than the difference between harmonics. It is also exactly at this point that the size (in samples) of the transform is no longer as long as a glottal pulse, allowing the details of the glottal cycle itself to be resolved.

In summary, to analyze men, women, and children at "equivalent" bandwidths, an analyst should generally increase the actual bandwidth of analysis according to the increase of average f_0 in these subjects (though some exception to this may be taken for certain formant analysis situations, as discussed later). Panels C and D of Figure 9.1 show wideband analyses of the woman- and child-spoken samples of *shoe*. In these examples, to retain a display of glottal pulses and not harmonics, the bandwidths of analysis have been increased to exceed peak f_0 in these samples. Note that this results in broader formant analyses, especially in the child sample.

As a whole, Figure 9.1 also helps to illustrate the increasing range of frequencies required for a full display of the basic sample features in moving from the adult male to the small child. Note that the first five formants of the adult male sample fall within the first 4 kilohertz of the spectrogram. In the woman's speech (Panel C), 5 or 6 kilohertz are required to span these formants, and the child's fifth formant approaches 7 kilohertz. Perhaps more importantly for full analysis of consonant structure, the center frequencies of the frication are above 8 kHz. These observations emphasize the need for high sampling rates when digitizing child speech. Higher sampling rates are usually advantageous for all speech analysis when increased computer storage demand is not a problem.

Parameter Analysis

The wealth of detail visible in a spectrogram helps to emphasize the need to extract specific quantities, or *parameters*, representing aspects of speech that are most relevant to the speaker's articulatory or phonological patterns. Parameters that are descriptive of speech sounds include segment durations, vowel formants, fundamental frequency, intensities, spectral shapes, and the like. For purposes of illustrating CAPA, we will focus on segment duration, fundamental frequency, and spectral shape. Two kinds of analyses are performed, one in which two of a child's utterances are compared with one another and one in which the child's utterance is compared with an adult model.

Within-Speaker Comparisons

Figure 9.2 depicts two spectrograms, each of a different utterance by the same 30-month-old child. The selection of samples here is inspired by the types of analyses described in Weismer (1984). The child was transcribed (for broad purposes) as having substituted /s/ for

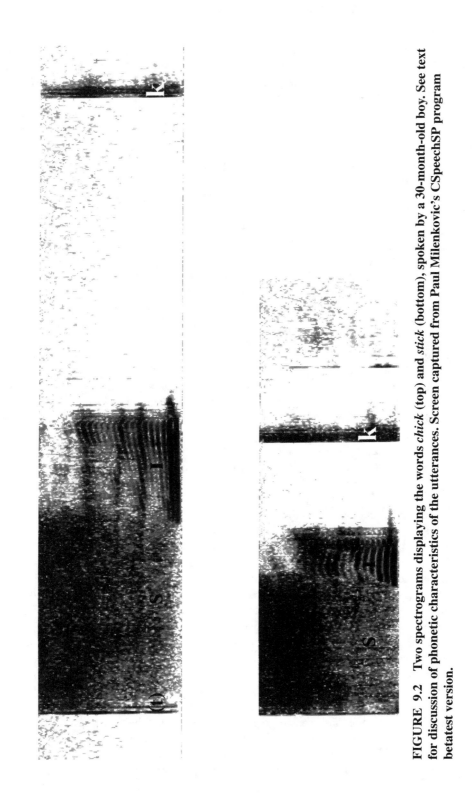

FIGURE 9.2 Two spectrograms displaying the words *chick* (top) and *stick* (bottom), spoken by a 30-month-old boy. See text for discussion of phonetic characteristics of the utterances. Screen captured from Paul Milenkovic's CSpeechSP program betatest version.

the complex word-initial consonants in each case (/tʃ/ → [s], /st/ → [s]). Indeed, the spectral energy of the fricative in both cases is concentrated above the midline—that is, at least above 5 kHz—and is, therefore, likely heard as a good /s/. However, in the *chick* production, a small, though clear, stop release initiates the frication. By focused listening, with cursors demarcating the attack and gating out most of the following frication to avoid a backward masking effect on the audibility of the attack, a low-intensity stop burst is clearly heard, indicating that the child seems to have recognized the phonological requirement for an affricate but perhaps did not fully realize the pressure required for a well-formed stop plus fricative sequence. In addition, the frication is quite high in resonant frequencies, consistent with an alveolar rather than a palatal place of articulation. This also would not be unusual if the child's focus had indeed been an alveolar placement for the stop component of the affricate. In sum, though the affricate is not articulatorily well formed, it would not appear phonologically to be a simple /s/.

The same child's utterance for *stick* is depicted in the lower panel of Figure 9.2. The two panels are time aligned, with just under 1 second for the whole screen. We can, therefore, see a difference in rate of production with a marked slowing in the top utterance. However, the fricative segment of the affricate in the top word occupies only about 44 percent of the whole word length, while the fricative segment of the lower word occupies over 66 percent of the whole word. The extension and prolongation of this segment relative to its following vowel is especially marked, and this prolongation is consistent with the notion that the child is aware of a contrast between the affricative /tʃ/ and the cluster /st/, even though both are heard as /s/. To validate this interpretation, we might require comparison with the child's articulation of true /s/, and many more samples, to judge the consistency of the effect. Three points are established by this illustration: (1) as Weismer (1984) pointed out, segment duration analysis can be of diagnostic value in judging the completeness of a substitution; (2) spectrogram viewing can alert us to difficult-to-hear features that may also address the issue of complete substitution (as in the low-intensity burst in the child's attempted affricative); and (3) an independent acoustic analysis comparing a child's utterances with one another can be informative.

Segment duration measurement is not always clear-cut. The chief reason is that sequential, discrete, and phonologically identified phonemes can be difficult to find in acoustic and physiological records of speech. The famous analogy by Hockett (1955) comparing articulated phonemes to smashed and mingled eggs well describes the situation the clinician faces when trying to sort out segmental durations by placing boundaries between phonemes.

A few analysis practices can enhance the user's ability to use acoustic displays to delineate segments and measure their durations. In fact, these practices should enhance any measurements that rely on effective display and interpretation of speech displays. First, the user should combine as many relevant displays as possible. Many temporal measurements can be made from the waveform; and because the waveform is simply the time-domain representation of untransformed data samples, it is maximally precise for decisions regarding discrete temporal events. However, the user can never be sure what a particular waveform pattern or feature represents without examining its frequency structure spectrally. For example, until the user has a spectrographic representation of the background noise surrounding a speech signal, it may not be possible to discern low-intensity fricatives such as /θ/.

A related second point is always to ensure that a display is optimal, both in the parameters that control the analysis algorithm generating the display as well as in the settings for the display itself. Basically, the user should always be aware of whether the gain is adequate; if the display is too dim, features may be missed and duration measures may be based on the wrong events. It is also possible that a too-dark display may obscure subtle variations within and across variations or even make background noises appear to be speech events. Obtaining optimal display gain begins with the digitizing; the louder portions of the input signal should fill the range of bits. However, all programs include display gain adjustments of one type or another; and these are especially important for the spectrogram.

A third practice for effective analysis is to use the ear as a source of information and often as the final basis for judgment. Though signal processing techniques and visual displays are powerful for teasing out and objectifying detailed aspects of the acoustic record, even inaudible ones, most speech measurements are made to affirm perceptible features. Using a CAPA program, the analyst can greatly refine such perceptions simply by using cursors to delimit portions of the waveform for playback of selected segments of the signal (thus avoiding the masking effects that normally obscure many rapid or low-intensity components of the signal). In duration measurement or segmentation tasks, for example, we may be interested in identifying perceived segment length, not necessarily all the audible behavior associated with an utterance. Specifically, there may be vocal fold vibration for a considerable period of time at the end of an open syllable, even while vocal tract behavior is lapsing from speech back to simple exhalation; the ear can be one guide to determining when the audible behavior is no longer associated with the production of a speech segment.

This latter point suggests that the analyst needs to consider the linguistic intentions of the speaker, which raises the final, and perhaps most important, point about speech measurement. A good analyst is never enslaved to a particular "reading" generated by the computer but is always using all senses in combination with his or her knowledge of the speaker and the context to correctly interpret the displayed sample. Moreover, the object of the analysis will itself dictate the criteria for "correctness." If a neurogenic, physiological speech motor disturbance or other articulatory error pattern is under investigation, then all acoustic data relative to the speaker's production pattern should be examined, subliminal or otherwise. If, on the other hand, phonological units based on a listener's perspective are the goal of analysis, the analyst's focus should be on the general features of the signal, disregarding clearly unintended random variations introduced by a momentarily uncontrolled part of the vocal apparatus.

In the preceding example we examined a child's strident fricatives for evidence that an affricate or a cluster was intended instead of the simple fricative. The following example illustrates vocal behavior that seems uncontrolled, raising issues for syllable duration measurement and concerns for the stability of the child's voicing ability. An analysis that compares the token to an adult model is required to help interpret the signal. In both cases, the analyst needs to become something of a mind reader to discern those physiological behaviors that are intentional and linguistically controlled from the background of uncontrolled audible behaviors. Acoustic phonetic analysis is only a tool in this process and does not alleviate an investigator from decision-making, even for the simplest measures.

Between-Speakers Comparisons

Figure 9.3 contains a waveform, f_0 contour, and spectrogram of the word "monkeys" /mʌŋkiz/ spoken by a 30-month-old girl. The spectrogram provides fairly clear criteria for the main articulatory events of interest. The first main sonorance begins with the nasal (of

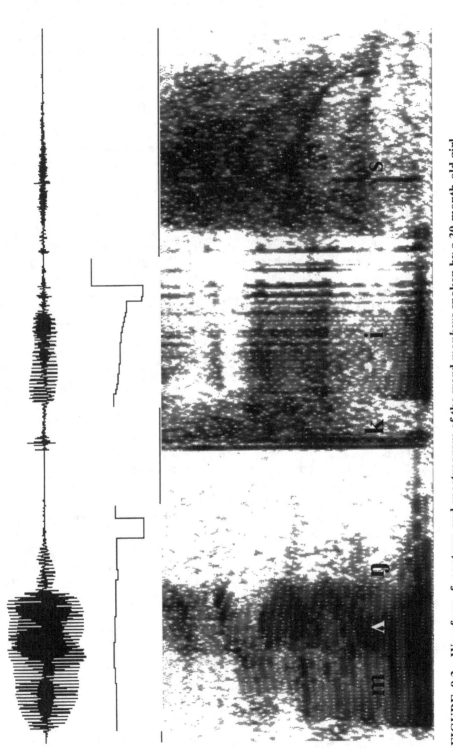

FIGURE 9.3 Waveform, f₀ contour, and spectrogram of the word *monkeys* spoken by a 30-month-old girl.

slightly lower intensity in higher frequencies), opens into the low middle vowel, and then attenuates again into the lower intensity syllable final nasal. A stopgap is followed by an aspirated velar release, followed by voicing in a high-front vowel. However, prior to the final frication, voicing seems to break up; and the final consonant appears (and is heard to be) devoiced. Is this a case of final consonant devoicing or voice pathology, or does it reflect normal articulatory and phonological patterning?

Considering now that this word was uttered phrase final, we might expect some declination of tone, prolongation of the final syllable, and devoicing of the final consonant (especially in English). The phrase-final prosodic marker has the phonological effect of devoicing the final fricative (/z/ → [s]), an example of tier interaction (Bernhardt and Stoel-Gammon, 1994). For such suprasegmental factors we examine the prosodic parameters of f_0 and intensity: f_0 is displayed in Figure 9.3 below the waveform.

Perhaps the most salient features of the f_0 plot are what appear to be errors. This display was selected purposefully to violate the expectation that computer analysis programs should automatically give a sensible result that does not require inspection. However, the program used to generate this analysis, CSpeechSP, has 11 control parameters that can be used to modify the algorithm, and this plot was obtained with analysis parameter settings in default positions. The situation demonstrates once again the need for an active analyst.

Though not all the parameter adjustments bear discussion here, some discussion of the results displayed in Figure 9.3 is merited. The cataclysmic-appearing drop in f_0 at the end of the first syllable actually occurs during the transition from a nasal to a full stop; note the drastically reduced intensity in the waveform. Although parameter settings are available to "sensitize" the algorithm to a low-intensity fundamental in the vicinity of the values preceding and following the "gap," a simpler strategy would be to acknowledge that the sound energy here is not perceptually salient and disregard the f_0 readings altogether. This could be implemented by the adjustment of a dB threshold parameter that excludes low intensity waveforms as "unvoiced." Of greater concern is the clearly aperiodic phonatory pattern in the latter part of the second syllable.

Before examining the f_0 extraction any further, an adult model might be examined in order to calibrate the clinician's expectations. Figure 9.4 provides this relational perspective, depicting a phrase-final production of the word *monkeys* spoken by an adult female from the same geographic region as the child. This spectrogram provides a useful perspective, containing three parallels to the child utterance: (1) the final consonant is devoiced, (2) there is a lack of continuity in the voicing of the final syllable just prior to the final consonant, and (3) the f_0 trace shows the same characteristic drop in this final syllable. Apparently what was potentially aberrant about the child's production is just a different form of a pattern also seen in an adult production. Along with the devoicing and declination of a phrase-final, word-final syllable, it is common to see a glottalized voice and even the double-pulse phonation clearly evident in the adult spectrogram (note the strong vertical lines occurring at the end of the /ɪ/ vowel, with approximately half the frequency of the ordinary glottal pulses earlier in the vowel). Regarding the use of CAPA in these situations, note that the f_0 analysis, as displayed in Figure 9.4, even with the big jump downward in the second syllable, is not, therefore, incorrect. There is indeed a sudden halving of the fundamental frequency. Again, it is a matter of whether the analyst is more interested in identifying acoustically defined cycles or in recovering the speaker's intended intonation contour. From the latter perspective, the sudden step in the f_0 trace may be ignored and

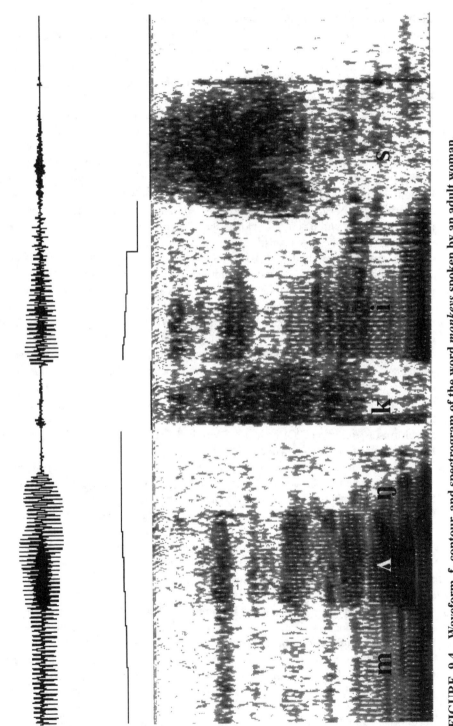

FIGURE 9.4 Waveform, f_0 contour, and spectrogram of the word *monkeys* spoken by an adult woman.

considered to be a symptom of nonmodal phonation occurring in a context where it is not inappropriate (there is really no percept here of a drastic shift in f_0). Does a similar analysis apply to the child?

Figure 9.5 contains a zoomed-in display of the difficult section from the above child data. From this perspective it becomes clear that the fundamental frequency algorithm that produced the contour was thrown off by several irregularities in the phonatory cycling. Can we be sure that the analyses are correct? There is one highly reliable method for checking fundamental frequency analysis: As long as one can identify glottal pulses in the waveform, the fundamental frequency is simply the inverse of one of these glottal periods. This principle is exploited by the CSpeechSP interface, as illustrated in Figure 9.4, by a utility that allows the analyst to place cursors delimiting the glottal pulse and then enter the value of that f_0 in the contour display below (see the bar between the vertical cursors). Because there is evidence here of glottal pulsing at a rate that is close to the general preceding contour in frequency, this episode might still be regarded to have been voiced just up to the onset of frication. The linguistic context, adult model, and presence of glottal pulses in the gap can all be used to justify a coding of this syllable as normal and continuously voiced. It is interesting to note that the glottalized voice in the adult has become very "clean," with only a few double pulses, while the child's syllable-terminal voicing is more irregular. This irregularity notwithstanding, we are less inclined to be concerned either with the "failure" of the f_0 detecting algorithm (it has not actually failed, as there really is no fundamental frequency!) or with the "failure" of the child to maintain even voicing throughout this syllable (adults don't either!). The main point of this final example is to show that some signal processing routines, even when correctly used, can give results that may or may not be desirable, depending on the analyst's purposes.

Other Parameters

Many other speech parameters require the same careful program use and attention to the nature of the signal that we have encountered for consonant articulation, segment duration, and fundamental frequency measures. Good formant frequency analysis in particular can require a solid background in the acoustic theory of speech production as well as a good understanding of the control parameters used in spectral analysis. These matters involve details that exceed the bounds and topic of this chapter; some further details regarding the use of CSL to analyze child speech data for experimental research applications are provided in Buder (1996), and the system described therein has been used for research on vowels and consonants in babbling and early speech (Stoel-Gammon, Buder, and Kehoe, 1995; Sussman at al., 1996).

From a general perspective, essentially the same principles apply as in the discussion of other measurements. We summarize those principles here as a way of reviewing the main points of this section on CAPA. First, multiple displays are best for cross-checking and corroboration of measures. For formant analysis it is advisable to use broad and narrow spectrograms, FFT-based power spectra, and also Linear Predictive Coefficients (LPC)–based power spectra (see Kent and Read, 1992 for further details). Although many systems provide "automatic" LPC-based formant tracking routines, these generally are to be viewed with caution and often require extensive control-parameter adjustments to track disordered or developing speech. Not all systems provide extensive user access to these control parameters.

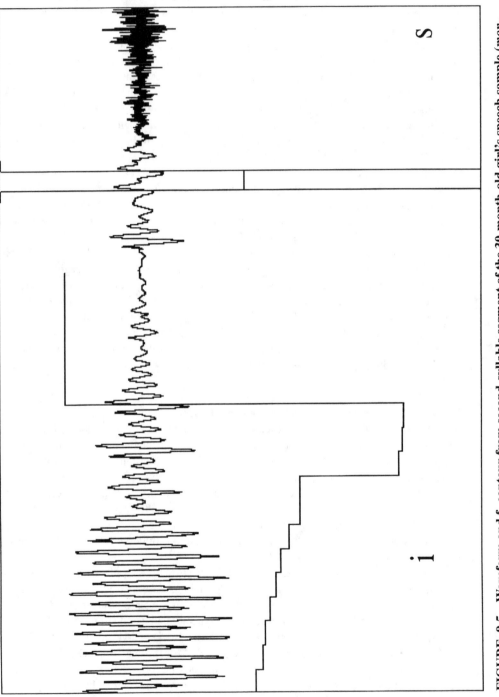
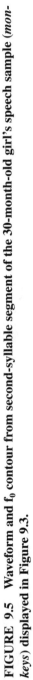

FIGURE 9.5 Waveform and f_0 contour from second-syllable segment of the 30-month-old girl's speech sample (*monkeys*) displayed in Figure 9.3.

Second, the analyst must be sure to maximize the analysis settings, display range, and clarity. The effects of sampling rate and bandwidth of analysis were discussed earlier. Though it is generally advisable to increase bandwidth of analysis for samples with higher fundamental frequency, it may also be necessary to adopt narrowband analysis to obtain the best precision of frequency domain measurement. For frequency measures from a spectro-gram displayed on a computer screen, precision can be further limited simply by the num-ber of pixels devoted to a given frequency range (and hence the finest possible cursor increments). In some cases, this precision can be maximized if it is possible to "zoom" in on a frequency range and thereby pick out finer spectral features.

Third, a good analyst always relies on the ear's ability to evaluate the validity of a mea-sure. It is all too easy to visually regard two harmonics as two different formants when they are in fact excited by one formant, or conversely to see one formant where in fact two have come into close proximity to one another. Both of these situations may arise in the corner vowels /i/ and /u/, where formants have moved into extreme positions; however, one quick listen should be all that is required to steer an attentive analyst back on track.

Finally, a good instrument-user always understands the limitations and failings of his/ her instruments and is not to be fooled or distracted by an erroneous or irrelevant reading. We must always respect the dramatic differences in the capabilities of computer-based in-struments versus fully multimodal conscious human beings and exploit the strengths of each. Computerized acoustic phonetic analysis systems are growing in their capacity to de-liver rapid and perspicuous displays or even to perform sophisticated analysis algorithms. This translates into an enhanced opportunity, and also an obligation, to use all of our knowl-edge of speech and many of our senses to discern patterns of phonological and articulatory behavior.

Summary

In this chapter, we have discussed computer-based tools for facilitating optimal phonolog-ical analysis. These tools provide major benefits, particularly in the areas of speed and amount of detail. On the other hand, we have attempted to make clear that instrumentation should serve a supplementary role in any type of analysis. The fact that results of analysis come from a computer does not make them inherently correct. In both phonological analy-sis and acoustic phonetic analysis, results taken from the computer are not valuable unless appropriately interpreted by the clinician or researcher.

References

Allen, G., "Some tips on tape recording speech-language samples." *Journal of the National Student Speech-Language-Hearing Association, 12* (1984): 10–17.

Baken, R. J. *Clinical Measurement of Speech and Voice.* Boston: Allyn and Bacon, 1987.

Bernhardt, G., and C. Stoel-Gammon, "Nonlinear phonology: Introduction and clinical application: Tutorial." *Journal of Speech and Hearing Re-search, 37* (1994): 123–143.

Buder, E. H., "Experimental phonology using acoustic phonetic methods: Formant measures from child speech" (pp. 254–265). In B. Bernhardt, D. Ingram, and J. Gilbert (Eds.), *Proceedings of the UBC*

International Conference on Phonological Acquisition. Somerville, Mass.: Cascadilla, 1996.

Buder, E. H., and R. D. Kent, "Survey of microcomputer-based speech acoustic analysis systems." Poster session presented at the annual convention of the American Speech-Language-Hearing Association. Orlando, Fla., 1995.

Eguchi, S., and I. J. Hirsh, "Development of speech sounds in children." *Acta Otolaryngologic*, Suppl. 257 (1969): 5–48.

Green, J., E. H. Buder, P. Rodda, and C. Moore, "Reliability of measurement across several acoustic voice analysis systems." In M. Cannito, K. Yorkston, and D. Beukelman (Eds.), *Motor Speech Disorders: Neuromotor Speech Disorders: Nature, Assessment and Management.* Baltimore, Md.: Paul H. Brookes, 1997.

Hockett, C. F., "A manual of phonology." In *International Journal of American Linguistics* (Memoir II). Baltimore, Md.: Waverly, 1955.

Hodge, M. M., "A comparison of spectral temporal measures across speaker age: Implications for an acoustical characterization of speech acquisition." Ph.D. thesis. University of Wisconsin–Madison, Madison, Wis., 1989.

Hodson, B., *Computerized Assessment of Phonological Processes: Version 1.0* (Apple II Series Computer Program). Danville, Ill.: Interstate, 1985.

Kent, R. D., and L. Forner, "Developmental study of vowel formant frequencies in an imitation task." *Journal of the Acoustical Society of America, 65* (1979): 208–217.

Kent, R. D., and C. Read, *The Acoustic Analysis of Speech.* San Diego: Singular, 1992.

Long, S., and M. Fey, *Computerized Profiling: Version 1.0* (Macintosh Computer Program). San Antonio, Tex.: The Psychological Corporation, 1993.

Long, S., and M. Fey, *Computerized Profiling: Version 7.0* (MS-DOS Computer Program). San Antonio, Tex.: The Psychological Corporation, 1993.

Masterson, J., and F. Pagan, *Interactive System for Phonological Analysis: Version 1.0* (Macintosh Computer Program). San Antonio, Tex.: The Psychological Corporation, 1993.

Nittrouer, S., M. Studdert-Kennedy., and R. S. Mc-

Gowan, "The emergence of phonetic segments: Evidence from the spectral structure of fricative-vowel sequences spoken by children and adults." *Journal of Speech and Hearing Research, 32* (1989): 120–132.

Oller, K., and R. Delgado, *Logical International Phonetic Programs: Version 1.03* (MS-DOS Computer Program). Miami, Fla.: Intelligent Hearing Systems, 1990.

Pye, C., *Pye Analysis of Language: Version 2.0* (MS-DOS Computer Program). Lawrence, Kan.: 200 Arrowhead Drive, 1987.

Rabinov, C. R., J. Kreiman, B. R. Gerratt, and S. Bielamowicz, "Comparing reliability of perceptual ratings of roughness and acoustic measures of jitter." *Journal of Speech and Hearing Research, 35* (1995): 26–32.

Shriberg, L., *Program to Examine Phonetic and Phonological Evaluation Records, Version 4.0* (MS-DOS Computer Program). Hillsdale, N.J.: Erlbaum, 1986.

Smith, B. L., "Temporal aspects of English speech production: A developmental perspective." *Journal of Phonetics 6* (1978): 37–67.

Stoel-Gammon, C., E. H. Buder, and M. Kehoe, "Acquisition of phonemic and phonetic aspects of vowel duration: A comparison of English and Swedish." *The Proceedings of the XIIIth International Congress of Phonetic Sciences, 4* (1995): 30–37.

Sussman, H., F. Minifie, E. Buder, C. Stoel-Gammon, and J. Smith, "Consonant-vowel dependencies in babbling and early words: A locus equation approach." *Journal of Speech and Hearing Research, 39* (1996): 424–433.

Titze, I., *Summary Statement for the Workshop on Acoustic Voice Analysis.* Iowa City, Iowa: National Center for Voice and Speech, 1995.

Weiner, F. *Automatic Articulation Analysis Plus* (Windows Computer Program). State College, Penn.: Parrot Software, 1993, 1995.

Weismer, G., "Acoustic analysis strategies for the refinement of phonological analysis." In M. Elbert, D. A. Dinnsen, and G. Weismer (Eds.), *Phonological Theory and the Misarticulating Child, ASHA Monographs, 22* (pp. 69–85). Rockville, Md.: ASHA, 1984.

Procedures for Teaching Sounds

Specific Instructional Techniques

As a supplement to the establishment procedures presented in Chapter 8, the following methods for teaching sounds are presented. Clinicians must be familiar not only with general approaches to the establishment of phonemes but also with specific suggestions for teaching sounds. Sources such as Nemoy and Davis (1954) may be consulted for a more extensive list of ideas regarding phonetic placement and successive approximation approaches to sound teaching; however, the material presented on the following pages represents a potpourri of ideas that may be helpful to those who are beginning to develop a repertoire of techniques for evoking and establishing consonant sounds frequently in error. Clinicians who need word lists or drill material are referred to *Articulation Therapy and Consonant Drill Book* by Goda (1970), *Voice and Articulation Drill Book* by Fairbanks (1960), *Better Speech and Better Reading* by Schoolfield (1951), *Phonetic Context Drillbook* by Griffith and Miner (1979), and *Contrasts: The Use of Minimal Pairs in Articulation Training* by Elbert, Rockman, and Saltzman (1980).

Instructions for Correction of an Interdental Lisp

It is important to remember that /s/ may be taught by having the client place his or her tongue behind either the upper teeth or the lower teeth (usually preferred).

1. Instruct the client to protrude the tongue between the teeth and produce a /θ/, and then push the tip of his or her tongue inward with a thin instrument, such as a tongue blade. As a variation, instruct the client to slowly and gradually withdraw the tongue while saying /θ/ and, while still attempting to make /θ/, scrape the tongue tip along the back of the front teeth and upward.

2. Instruct the client to produce /t/ in a word like *tea*. Have him or her pronounce it with a strong aspiration after release of the /t/ prior to the vowel. Instruct the client to slowly slide the tip of the tongue backward from the alveolar ridge following a prolonged release. The result should be [ts]. Then prolong the [s] portion of [ts].

3. Instruct the client to say the following word-pairs, pointing out that the tongue is in a similar position for /t/ and /s/.

tea–sea	*teal–seal*	*tell–sell*	*told–sold*	*tame–same*	*tip–sip*
top–sop	*tight–sight*	*too–Sue*	*tub–sub*	*turf–surf*	*till–sill*

4. Instruct the client to open his or her mouth, put the tongue in position for /t/, drop the tip of the tongue slightly, and send the airstream through the passage. The client can sometimes feel the emission of air by placing a finger in front of his or her mouth.

5. Instruct the client to produce /ʃ/ and then retract his or her lips (smile) and push the tongue slightly forward.

6. Instruct the client to say /i/ and blow through the teeth to produce /s/.

7. Insert a straw in the groove of the tongue and have the client blow to produce /s/.

8. If the client can make a correct /z/, take a word such as *zero* and ask him or her to listen carefully and to feel where the tongue is when whispering the word, prolonging the first sound. This sound can then become the client's model.

9. Instruct the client to use the following phonetic placement cues:
   a. Raise the tongue so that the sides are firmly in contact with the inner surface of the upper back teeth.
   b. Groove the tongue slightly along the midline.
   c. Place the tip of the tongue about a quarter of an inch behind the upper teeth.
   d. Bring the teeth together.
   e. Direct the air stream along the groove of the tongue toward the cutting edges of the lower teeth.

Instructions for Correction of a Lateral Lisp

1. Position a straw so that it protrudes from the side of the mouth. When a lateral [s] is made, the straw should resonate on the side of the mouth where the airstream is directed. When the straw is inserted into the front of the mouth and a correct /s/ is made, the straw will resonate in the front of the mouth.

2. Direct attention to a central emission of the airstream by holding a feather, a strip of paper, or a finger in front of the center of the mouth, or have the client tap the incisor gently with his or her forefinger while [s] is being produced. If the sound is being emitted through a central aperture, a break in continuity of the outflow of the breath will be noted. If the sound is being emitted laterally, no break in the continuity of the airstream will be noted. An awareness of central aperture may also be developed by instructing the client to inhale air and directing his or her attention to the cool sensation from the intake of air. Then instruct the client to exhale the air through the same aperture by which air entered upon inhalation.

3. Instruct the client to put a tongue blade down the midline of the tongue in order to establish a groove for the airstream.

4. Instruct the client to retract the lips sharply and push the tongue forward, attempting to say /s/.
5. Instruct the client to make /t/, holding the release position for a relatively long time, and then retract the lips and drop the jaw slightly. A [ts] should be heard if grooving was maintained properly. Next, extend the duration of the [ts], gradually decreasing the release phase of [t] until /s/ is approximated.

Instructions for Production of the /ɝ/

1. Instruct the client to growl like a tiger (*grrr*), crow like a rooster (*r-rr-rr*) or sound like a race car (*rrrr*).
2. Instruct the client to lower the jaw, say /l/ and push the tongue back until [ɝ] is produced. One can also move from [n] to [nɚ] or [d] to [dɚ].
3. Instruct the client to produce /l/. Then, using a tongue blade, gently push the tip of the tongue back until the depressor can be inserted between the tongue tip and teeth ridge so that an /ɝ/ is produced.
4. Instruct the client to imitate a trilled tongue plus /ɝ/ sound with the tongue tip on the alveolar ridge. Stop the trill but continue producing /ɝ/.
5. Instruct the client to produce /a/ as in the word *father*. As he or she produces the [a], instruct him or her to raise the tongue tip and blade, arching the tongue toward the palate but not touching the palate.
6. Instruct the client to produce /i/ and then lift and retract the tongue tip to produce /ɝ/.
7. Instruct the client to place the tongue lightly between the incisors as in /θ/ and then retract the tip quickly into the /ɝ/. Instruct the client to keep the tip of the tongue near the alveolar ridge to avoid the intrusion of a vowel sound.
8. Instruct the client to say /z/ and to continue to do so while dropping the jaw and saying /ɝ/.
9. Instruct the client to position the tongue for /d/ and then retract it slightly, at the same time dropping the tongue tip and saying /ɝ/. Other clusters such as /tr/, /θr/, and /gr/ may also be used.
10. Spread the sides of the child's mouth with his or her finger, then ask him or her to produce a prolonged /n/ and then curl the tongue backward, continuing to make the sound.
11. Contrast pairs of words beginning with /w/ and /r/. This task may make the distinction between these two sounds more obvious for the client who substitutes /w/ for /r/. Practice word-pairs might include:

wipe–ripe	*wan–ran*	*woo–rue*	*wing–ring*	*way–ray*	*wake–rake*
wag–rag	*wail–rail*	*woe–roe*	*weep–reap*	*wed–red*	

Instructions for Production of /l/

1. Instruct the client to produce /l/ with the mouth open in front of a mirror.
2. Instruct the client to position the tongue for /l/ and then lower it to produce /a/. Alternate these movements. The result should be [la], [la], [la]. This procedure can be varied by using /i/ and /u/ instead of /a/.

3. Instruct the client to imitate the clinician's singing of the nonsense syllables [leɪ], [li], [laɪ].

4. Using a lollipop, peanut butter, or tongue blade, touch the place on the client's alveolar ridge where the tongue tip makes contact to produce a correct /l/. Then tell the client to place the tongue at that point and say /l/.

5. Instruct the client to pretend that the tongue is one part of a bird's beak and the roof of the mouth is the other part of the beak. Tell him or her to put the tongue directly behind the teeth and move it up and down quickly, as a bird's beak might move when it is chirping, and say /a/.

Instructions for Production of /f/ and /v/

1. Instruct the client to touch the lower lip with the upper front teeth and blow. The breath stream may be directed by placing a feather or strip of paper in front of his or her mouth while /f/ or /v/ is being produced.

2. Instruct the client to say [a], place the lower lip under the edge of the upper teeth, and blow the breath stream between the lip and teeth so that frication is audible.

Instructions for Production of /k/ and /g/

1. Press underneath the posterior portion of the child's chin and ask him or her to say [kʌ] in a whisper as the pressure is suddenly released.

2. Hold the tongue tip behind the lower teeth, using a tongue blade if necessary. Instruct the client to hump the back of the tongue and build up oral pressure. The tongue contact should be released quickly, thus releasing the pressure built up behind the constriction.

3. Instruct the client to imitate the clinician as the clinician pretends to shoot a gun, producing a lingua-fricative, as in [ka].

4. Instruct the client to alternate the raising of the back and front of the tongue in a rocking movement from [k] to [t].

Instructions for Production of /t/ and /d/

1. Instruct the client to press the tongue tip firmly against the upper dental ridge in front of a mirror. Then have him or her quickly lower the tongue; air pressure will be released, producing approximations of /t/ or /d/.

2. Instruct the client to make a /p/. Then ask him or her to place the tongue tip between the lips and again to try to say /p/. This gives the tactual sensation of a stop made with the tip of the tongue but is not the correct position for /t/ or /d/. Finally, instruct the client to make a similar sound with the tongue tip in contact with the upper lip only. Repeat with the tongue tip touching the alveolar ridge.

References

Elbert, M., B. Rockman, and D. Saltzman, *Contrasts: The Use of Minimal Pairs in Articulation Training*. Austin, Tex.: Exceptional Resources, 1980.

Fairbanks, G., *Voice and Articulation Drill Book*, New York: Harper & Row, 1960.

Goda, S., *Articulation Therapy and Consonant Drill Book*. New York: Grune and Stratton, 1970.

Griffith, J., and L. E. Miner, *Phonetic Context Drillbook*. Englewood Cliffs, N.J.: Prentice Hall, 1979.

Nemoy, E. M., and S. F. Davis, *The Correction of Defective Consonant Sounds*. Magnolia, Mass.: Expression Company, 1954.

Schoolfield, L. D., *Better Speech and Better Reading*. Magnolia, Mass.: Expression Company, 1951.

Author Index

Subject Index

A

Acoustic phonetics, 8, 45–46
  amplitude, 45–46
  duration, 45–46
  frequency, 45–46
Additions, 177
Affricates, 17–18, 45–46, 285
Affrication, 278
African American Vernacular English (AAVE),
    152–154
  characteristics, 152–153
  phonological development, 153–154
Airflow (aerodynamics), 42–45
Air pressure (intraoral), 42–45
Allophone, 2–3
  complementary distribution, 3
  free variation, 3
Analysis procedures of articulation/phonological
    assessments, 274–280, 281. *See also* Assess-
    ment of articulation/phonology
Ankyloglossia, 189–190
Antecedent events, 300
Apraxia, 203–205
Appalachian English, 154–155
Approximation, 314–315
Arizona Articulation Proficiency Scale, 284, 324
Articulation. *See also* Phonology
  assessment of. *See* Assessment; Articulatory tests
  automatization, 362
  consistency of, 184–185, 252–253

development/acquisition. *See* Phonological acquisi-
    tion/development
error categories, 176–179
maintenance, 361–365
related factors, 172–223
  auditory perception factors, 174–187
  cognitive-linguistic factors, 207–216
    academic performance, 214–216
    intelligence, 208–210
    language development, 210–214
  neuromotor factors, 202–207
  psycho social factors, 216–223
    age, 216–217
    familial tendencies, 219–221
    gender, 217–218
    personality and adjustment, 222–223
    siblings, 221
    socioeconomic status, 218–219
  speech mechanism factors, 187–196
    major structural variations, 190–193
    minor structural variations, 187–190
    motor, 197–198
    oral sensory, 193–196
    tongue thrust, 198–202
  treatment/remediation. *See* Therapy
Articulatory phonetics, 8
Articulatory tests/assessment procedures, 238,
    245–250, 281
Asian languages, 158–161
  acquisition of tone, 159–160